MW01618689

PRAISE FOR

LEADING CAMPUS DRUG & ALCOHOL ABUSE PREVENTION

"Anderson and Hall have 75 years of experience working with drug and alcohol misuse prevention, and it shows in this encyclopedic roadmap for higher education leaders. Given the increased complexities in the lives of students, this book will help leaders 'think and do' better with and for them. If you are committed to actualizing the potential of students, and ensuring their safety and well-being, add this book to your library and give it to others."

—**Patricia A. Perillo,** Vice President for Student Affairs and Affiliate Faculty Member–Student Affairs, University of Maryland

"This book is an extraordinarily comprehensive work addressing campus alcohol and substance abuse prevention undergirded by theory and evidence-based approaches and processes. It is a must-read for all involved in this issue on college and university campuses."

—**John D. Welty,** President Emeritus, California State University, Fresno

"As a senior campus leader whose work focuses on holistic student well-being, I found Anderson and Hall's insights to be an essential resource for seasoned professionals and a perfect primer for those new to the field."

—**Frank E. Ross III,** Vice President for Student Affairs, Butler University

"Drawing on the authors' own experiences and those of other well-known leaders in the field, this engaging book will help orient the next generation of prevention professionals, re-energize the experienced practitioner, and inform campus leadership on the drug and alcohol issues that affect student success."

—**Katrin Wesner-Harts,** Interim Associate Vice Chancellor for Student Affairs, University of North Carolina Wilmington; Immediate Past President, American College Health Association

"This is a must-read book for anyone working with college students! Anderson and Hall wonderfully weave together foundational theories, evidence-based strategies, case studies, and examples in an easy to follow guide, helping any professional cultivate change in college drinking culture."

—**Louise Harder,** Executive Director, Prevention Network

"This addition to the literature accentuates scientific inquiry with everyday occurrences that will assist many in managing this important continuing issue on our campuses."

—**Thomas G. Goodale,** Retired Faculty and Student Affairs Administrator

"*Leading Campus Drug & Alcohol Abuse Prevention* provides a roadmap to drug and alcohol abuse prevention that is both comprehensive and practical. The case studies from practitioners with years of experience are amazing sources of information for both new and experienced practitioners. This book is a valuable contribution to the field of AOD prevention work."

—**M. Scott Tims,** Assistant Vice President, Campus Health, Tulane University

"This book is an incredible resource for higher education professionals that highlights the work being done in the field, which is used to identify the work needed to make a difference. The professionals who contributed to this book offer insight, inspiration, as well as worksheets that engage with readers in a way that prompts them to implement similar programs suited for their campuses."

—**Hawra Ahmad,** Program Coordinator, Michigan Higher Education Network

LEADING CAMPUS DRUG & ALCOHOL ABUSE PREVENTION

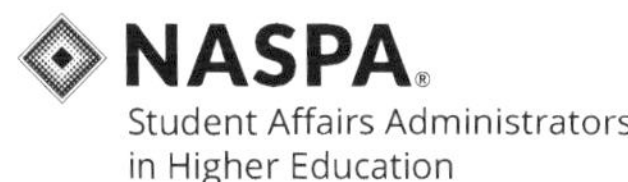

LEADING CAMPUS DRUG & ALCOHOL ABUSE PREVENTION

GROUNDED APPROACHES FOR STUDENT IMPACT

David S. Anderson & Thomas Hall

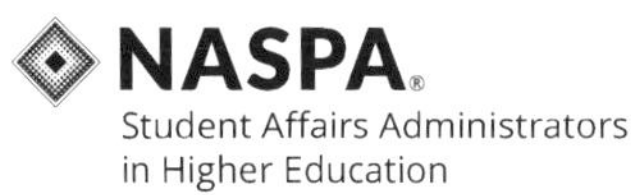

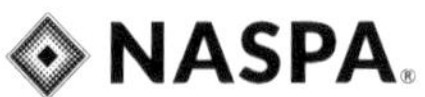
Student Affairs Administrators
in Higher Education

Published by
NASPA–Student Affairs Administrators in Higher Education
111 K Street, NE
10th Floor
Washington, DC 20002
www.naspa.org

Additional copies may be purchased by contacting the NASPA publications department at 202-265-7500 or visiting http://bookstore.naspa.org.

NASPA does not discriminate on the basis of race, color, national origin, religion, sex, age, gender identity, gender expression, affectional or sexual orientation, veteran status, or disability in any of its policies, programs, publications, and services.

Library of Congress Cataloging-in-Publication Data
(Prepared by The Donohue Group, Inc.)

Names: Anderson, David S., 1949- author. | Hall, Thomas (Thomas Virgil), 1961- author. | NASPA-Student Affairs Administrators in Higher Education, issuing body.
Title: Leading campus drug and alcohol abuse prevention : grounded approaches for student impact / David S. Anderson and Thomas Hall.
Description: Washington, DC : NASPA-Student Affairs Administrators in Higher Education, [2021] | Includes bibliographical references and index.
Identifiers: ISBN 9781948213288 (paperback) | ISBN 9781948213295 (ePub)
Subjects: LCSH: College students--Alcohol use--United States--Prevention. | College students--Drug use--United States--Prevention. | Alcoholism--United States--Prevention. | Drug abuse--United States--Prevention.
Classification: LCC HV4999.Y68 A54 2021 (print) | LCC HV4999.Y68 (ebook) | DDC 362.29084/2--dc23

Printed and bound in the United States of America

FIRST EDITION

To those whose shoulders are broad, courage is strong, insight is visionary, passion is deep, and commitment is lasting. Upon you rests the future of students at colleges and universities.

CONTENTS

CONTENT

COLLABORATION

FIGURES AND TABLES

CONTRIBUTIONS

CASE STUDIES

LESSONS FROM THE FIELD

INNOVATORS

WORKSHEETS

Preface

The preparation of this book has been a labor of love. The project grew out of our love for college and university campuses—for the students enrolled, the prevention specialists striving to make a difference, the faculty and staff working at these institutions of higher education, and the surrounding communities. Moreover, the project grew out of our love of higher education—and our belief in it as an important anchor in society for inquiry, sound reason, and the achievement of human potential.

This book is based on our collective experience coming from programmatic, policy, and clinical backgrounds. Between us we have 75 years of experience working with drug and alcohol misuse prevention. We have seen numerous ways in which drugs and alcohol have wreaked havoc on many campuses and the lives of numerous students and their families. One of us helped carry the body of a lifeless undergraduate to an ambulance, whose emergency lights were no longer needed. One of us helped nurture a campus back to health after a midafternoon drunk driving crash killed two key campus administrators. And one of us counseled countless students through their decisions related to substances, with some ultimately seeking treatment, some avoiding relapse, and others negotiating inhospitable campus environments.

Our effort with the hundreds of hours spent conceptualizing and writing this book, and encouraging colleagues from throughout the nation to tell their stories, was a heartfelt one. It was based in the belief that so many of the drug and alcohol problems facing colleges and universities are preventable. Further, it was grounded in the dedication to maximizing the productivity and potential of students during their college years, and in preparation for their lives as healthy and productive individuals, family members, community leaders, and members of society.

To further illustrate the need to address drug and alcohol issues, particularly at the highest levels of institutional leadership, an example is helpful. For one of the authors who was concluding a site visit and consultation for a campus, his professional observation was that about half of the students had a problem with alcohol. To this conclusion, the college president responded, "I don't disagree with that assessment of our students. But so what? We are no worse than anyone else."

We created this book based on our belief that colleges and universities, as microcosms of society, can indeed do better than being "no worse than anyone else"; we believe that higher education institutions can be much more committed, more organized, more grounded, more comprehensive, and more effective with reducing problems associated with drugs and alcohol. We believe that campuses can aggressively promote the health, well-being and potential of their students. Our belief is that higher education leaders must demonstrate clear and visible leadership with drug and alcohol issues.

We are inspired by the good work of so many people. And we are inspired by the heartfelt commitment of so many professionals who truly want to make college and university campuses healthy and safe places to study, to learn, to grow, and to serve the larger society. We believe that the challenges surrounding campus drug and alcohol efforts are achievable; with perseverance and hard work, together, we can make a difference.

David S. Anderson
Thomas Hall

September 2020

Introduction

A half-century ago, although higher education administrators were aware of students' use of drugs and alcohol, and many were concerned, little was done. Some of the rationales for not acting were that substance-using behavior was a rite of passage, that colleges and universities were a microcosm of society, and that students would grow out of it. College campuses typically addressed the misuse and abuse of drugs and alcohol by having a policy, offering a few educational events, and then hoping for the best. At that time, however, the complexities and stressors of student lives were significantly lower than they are today. In addition, the awareness of, and tolerance for, the problems, concerns, injuries, and deaths associated with these substances are now notably heightened. Those involved in leadership roles with drugs and alcohol—whether at the national, state or local level—acknowledge that so many of these problems are preventable.

Leading Campus Drug and Alcohol Abuse Prevention: Grounded Approaches for Student Impact is designed as a roadmap for higher education leaders to orchestrate meaningful results on college and university campuses. Acknowledging that many differences exist among higher education institutions, and that thus a "one size fits all" approach is not sufficient, this book provides the tools to develop, revamp, revitalize, and review campus drug and alcohol prevention strategies. The book is an essential tool for campus personnel at all levels, and offers a practical approach for guiding drug and alcohol abuse prevention initiatives. Featuring insights from numerous practitioners, researchers, and national professionals who have worked on or with college and university campuses, the book provides processes and strategies that will help prevention specialists and leaders organize and implement their campus efforts. Central to this volume is a focus on accountability. Institutions of higher education are encouraged to demonstrate a leadership role in society by showing commitment to the health and well-being of students, staff, faculty, and community members. Based on their historical grounding and pragmatic foundations, colleges and universities are strongly encouraged to have the commitment and courage to develop, support, and sustain quality strategies to reduce drug and alcohol problems.

FOUNDATIONS FOR THIS BOOK

Problems and issues surrounding drugs and alcohol are widespread on college and university campuses, much as they are throughout society; however, the vast majority of these problems are preventable. Higher education institutions, by their very nature, have unique opportunities and obligations to provide leadership. As organizations that promote scientific grounding, critical thinking, and human potential, and that emphasize high standards and excellence, colleges and universities must address substance misuse to be consistent with their foundations. Institutions are particularly well suited to organize and plan strategies and develop resources that achieve positive outcomes with issues like drug and alcohol problems. This is particularly important with drug and alcohol issues, as these challenge and harm the institutional fabric and the lives of students, faculty, and staff.

This perspective about the important leadership role of higher education institutions is a certain foundation for this book. Another major foundation is the perspective about drugs and alcohol, and related issues. The vision of the Substance Abuse and Mental Health Services Administration (SAMHSA) is that "SAMHSA provides leadership . . . toward helping the Nation act on the knowledge that:

- Behavioral health is essential for health;
- Prevention works;
- Treatment is effective; and
- People recover from mental and substance use disorders." (SAMHSA, 2011, p. 4)

Despite hundreds of substance-related college student deaths in the United States each year, and the many costs and harms to individuals and property, campus-based drug and alcohol initiatives are often provided limited attention, low resources, and few personnel. Drug and alcohol issues cause a disproportionately high amount of problems for campuses; however, efforts to address these issues receive a disproportionately low level of priority. The attention and resources provided to drug and alcohol misuse should be commensurate with the extent of the problem itself. This book provides the foundations, strategies, and tools to address the imbalance of drug and alcohol problems and prioritization of these issues.

This book acknowledges that drug and alcohol misuse prevention is a tremendous undertaking. Much has been learned over the past half-century; yet so much more remains to be learned and done. Professionals working on the front lines to address these issues are highly dedicated and skilled. However, their time and resources are limited. This book challenges those with higher level, decision-making authority on campuses to commit to provide resources and direction to facilitate and support strategies designed to reduce drug- and alcohol-related problems.

This book incorporates the views of dozens of professionals with decades of experience working with drug and alcohol misuse issues in varied settings. It is based on their individual and collective extensive experience and research grounding; their insights and recommendations are timely and relatively timeless, and thus appropriate and helpful for campus efforts. While current events with the COVID-19 health pandemic have resulted in extreme disruption in individual lives, campus systems, economies, lifestyles, visions, and so much more, the content and processes articulated by these many contributors and the authors remains highly relevant. Although so much has been transformed for students, faculty, staff, administrators, and campuses as a whole, the larger institution of higher education, and factors associated with college student development, remain the same. Drug and alcohol misuse issues can reasonably be expected to grow, following patterns of other major catastrophes. While methods of interaction and program delivery will be adjusted, the important thrusts embodied in this book remain. As the needs regarding drug and alcohol use deterrence remain high—and perhaps even higher than before due to the COVID-19 pandemic—the opportunities and the responsibilities for higher education are vitally important.

THE BOOK'S ORIENTATION

The content, style, and processes embedded in this book represent a nexus of theory and practice. This text is written as a practical guide; the emphasis is on the processes used, with the acknowledgment that each campus will develop strategies based on its needs, interests and capabilities. While much can be learned from others' experiences, each campus's culture, history, needs, and priorities are different. Regardless of what approaches are identified, the essential foundation is that campus prevention efforts must be grounded in theory and evidence-informed approaches, coupled with innovation designed to work best for the circumstances on the campus.

The book is written in the context of a rapidly changing society. Specifically, while significant technological change has occurred in recent years (e.g., the first iPhone became available only 15 years ago) and cultural upheaval has been extensive (e.g., the COVID-19 pandemic has affected lives and lifestyles), the theory and foundations undergirding meaningful effort do not change. This recurring message on incorporating sound foundations with campus strategic planning permeates this book.

Central to this book is the prevention framework within the Institute of Medicine's continuum of care. As detailed in Chapter 3, this framework focuses on universal, selective, and indicated strategies. These three elements serve as anchors for a reasonable and appropriate comprehensive campus program, and are thus helpful for planning and implementing successful strategies.

This book is written primarily with the campus prevention specialist in mind. Each of the book's four sections provides an introduction for new personnel and as a refresher and reminder for experienced personnel. In addition, this book is intended for those in campus decision-making roles, whether a chief student affairs officer, a president, a provost or chancellor, a residence life director, a chief health officer, or a chair of the faculty or staff senate; for these individuals who are not involved with drug and alcohol issues on a full-time or regular basis, the book provides an overview of the nature, complexity, and processes associated with a comprehensive campus effort. This volume can help leaders throughout the campus prioritize the attention to ameliorating the negative consequences associated with drug and alcohol misuse; as such, the book helps with their leadership to prevent drug and alcohol problems.

Even with the level of commitment held by prevention specialists and campus leaders to address drug and alcohol problems, their efforts are often stymied based on numerous challenges. They face highly constrained budgets, limited personnel, entrenched perspectives, low prioritization, and lack of overall understanding by key administrators of the needs as well as responsibilities to address drug and alcohol issues. The book offers a practical approach to help those who are committed to addressing this issue make progress. It provides processes, tools, strategies, and tips that can be applied to address a variety of concerns. With the processes identified, the book supports campus leaders in engaging and collaborating with others within the context of a shared responsibility. Acknowledging the symbiotic relationship between student well-being and the nature and scope of campus prevention efforts, the priority is given to emphasize the overall campus culture.

ORGANIZATION OF THIS VOLUME

Although this volume includes some checklists and proposed processes, its premise is that grounded, locally appropriate efforts are what will make a difference. Such efforts are also more likely sustainable over time. As such, this book is not so much a "how-to" guide; instead, it is a "how to think" guide. The processes and planning efforts involve collaborative engagement of key constituencies; as such, the entire effort constitutes a significant amount of hard work. With this in mind, the book revolves around this quote from Benjamin Franklin: "Tell me and I forget. Teach me and I may remember. Involve me and I learn" (Good Reads, n.d., para. 4).

To help orient those using the book, the overall organization encompasses four broad sections: Context, Content, Collaboration, and Choices. The Context section offers chapters focusing on societal and campus data, campus culture issues, and theories and frameworks. In the Content section, the chapters focus primarily on the three prevention strategies from the Institute of Medicine: universal, selective, and indicated. Also addressed are policy issues, training, and evaluation. The Collaboration section highlights a nine-step planning model, and its chapters encompass coalition strategies as well as advocacy considerations. The book ends with Choices, with chapters discussing approaches to reporting results from prevention initiatives and long-term perspectives about the changes associated with campus efforts.

In the chapters, three types of contributions bring attention to specific issues and topics: Case Studies, Lessons From the Field, and Innovator perspectives. The case studies and lessons learned provide insights from individuals of varied backgrounds who share experiences helpful for campus leaders. Further, because innovation is vital for making progress, and within the context of evidence-informed strategies, each chapter highlights a professional who made a mark (and continues to do so) by taking risks and demonstrating leadership.

The conclusion section of each chapter provides a brief review of key content and attends to four central points deemed essential for quality campus planning efforts.

- Prevention specialists and campus leaders benefit from emphasizing grounded and theory-based approaches.
- Innovation should be explored as a way of best reaching aims.

- The processes of planning and engagement benefit from being thorough and thoughtful.
- Campus efforts are more likely to succeed if they are prepared with the unique features of the campus in mind; succinctly stated, they should be locally appropriate.

These four foundational elements are integral to achieving the student impact emphasized with the processes articulated throughout this volume.

FINAL THOUGHTS

Through its emphasis on sound processes, this book provides a helpful roadmap for college and university leaders. The roadmap is not an "answer key" per se; rather, it identifies many essential elements for planning and implementing the campus effort. This book is designed for the reader to draw guidance, inspiration, and hope from those dedicated personnel who have shared their insights. The book is not designed to provide detailed content about topics such as how drugs work on the body, the science of substance use disorders, the components of treatment, or the strong impact of cultural influences. Rather, it highlights the hard work required to make a difference.

The book incorporates controversies—as have been central to drugs and alcohol for centuries, many of which are highlighted in Ruth Engs's (1990) book *Controversies in the Addictions Field*. Some of the perspectives of the authors and contributors in this book may differ from commonly held views. These varied points of view are provided to push and propel campus strategies—to cause campus leaders and prevention specialists to stretch their limits—with the ultimate aim of making colleges and universities healthier and safer places.

In his essay *The Fixation of Belief*, Charles Peirce penned this thought in 1877: "The irritation of doubt is the only immediate motive for the struggle to attain belief" (p. 6). Examining belief is counterintuitive because truth informs belief. Change is like an irritant, something that moves us forward, away from an unexamined consensual reality.

Because this book is about thinking and understanding before doing, campus leaders may question the relevance of some observations. These leaders also may reformulate existing beliefs or revalidate them. Further, systems change can raise additional challenges; Gladwell's (2000) *The Tipping Point* illustrates the context for current campus systems and opportunities.

The varied points of view presented throughout this book are consistent with the focus on utilizing locally informed, campus-based efforts. Acknowledging that "one size does not fit all," it is vital that those responsible for planning and leading campus prevention strategies guide thoughtful deliberations about what is best for the campus at a particular point in time. These leaders can help engage others in rigorous discourse regarding topics and issues included in this book, and thus orchestrate locally appropriate and grounded strategies. Overall, this book aims to provide direction and the requisite foundations for making meaningful decisions about health promotion (generally) and drug and alcohol misuse prevention (specifically) processes and strategies grounded in theory and validated in practice.

Central to this book—for the prevention specialists, the campus leaders, the stakeholders, and to all reached by them—is a pointed question: What are you willing to commit yourself to do? This question, whether explicitly asked or implied, helps the prevention specialist and others advance the conversation and the planning. Having clear answers and specified commitments demonstrate leadership and, ultimately, maximize student impact.

REFERENCES

Engs, R. C. (1990). *Controversies in the addictions field.* Kendall Hunt Publishers.

Gladwell, M. (2000). *The tipping point: How little things can make a big difference.* Little, Brown, and Company.

Good Reads. (n.d.). *Benjamin Franklin quotes.* https://www.goodreads.com/author/quotes/289513.Benjamin_Franklin

Peirce, C. S. (1877, November). The fixation of belief. *Popular Science Monthly, 12,* 1–15.

Substance Abuse and Mental Health Services Administration. (2011). *Leading change: A plan for SAMHSA's roles and actions 2011–2014* (Publication No. [SMA] 11-4629). https://www.dshs.wa.gov/sites/default/files/BHSIA/dbh/documents/SAMHSA_Leading_Change_01-FullDocument.pdf

CONTEXT: "The Why"

This first of four sections of this book provides the empirical and conceptual basis for orchestrating a comprehensive campus strategy to address drug and alcohol misuse. Its three chapters serve as the foundation for prevention specialists as they initiate, revise, renew, or expand their efforts. Central to effective strategies is that they be grounded in current and anticipated needs, with particular attention to local issues. Looking beyond prevalence data, campus leaders examine risk and protective factors and the reasons students use drugs or alcohol. Keeping in mind current and desired campus culture, prevention specialists use thoughtful processes to incorporate evidence-informed approaches into their logic model. Key theories and frameworks as well as organization and staffing considerations help with these grounded approaches, and further inform the campus efforts. The important role of leadership, particularly based on the role of institutions of higher education in society, serves to provide the *why* for campus prevention strategies.

CHAPTER 1

The Impact of Substance Abuse on Campus

"When I first arrived on campus as a student who rarely drank prior to coming into college, I experienced culture shock when I realized how prominent drinking can be. I met a new group of friends, but quickly realized alcohol was always a part of the festivities. I really liked these people, but I had also felt external pressure to fit in."

—Senior at a large suburban university

The use of drugs and alcohol by college students is a long-standing problem that continues to challenge higher education leadership seeking remediation and solutions. The use patterns, the consequences, the damage to the academic and learning environment all serve as motivation for action, and a sound understanding of "the nature of the problem" is essential if decision makers are to establish thoughtful and appropriate strategies.

A review of students' use of drugs and alcohol—and associated consequences—highlights "what is" as well as "what has been" and can determine "what could be" and "what should be." Data, both quantitative and qualitative, are essential for making strategic decisions, helping to define the context within which general and specific approaches are suitable for our institutions of higher education.

The essential point is that many of the problems associated with students' drug and alcohol use are, in fact, preventable. With the use of grounded, evidence-informed strategies, the negative consequences facing individuals, communities, worksites, schools, and society at large would likely be reduced significantly. National data must be complemented by local-level data to guide leaders toward action—thus making a meaningful, valuable difference.

Three contributions from professionals who have years of experience with collegiate drug and alcohol issues illustrate practical applications. A case study about faculty engagement with substance misuse and one practitioner's approach for identifying risk, as a Lessons From the Field segment, offer rich insights. At the conclusion of this chapter, Frances Harding, identified as an Innovator, shares her experience with making a difference.

COLLEGE STUDENT DRUG AND ALCOHOL USE AND RELATED ISSUES

The use of drugs and alcohol by college students has been studied by numerous researchers, practitioners, and government agencies over many decades. One of the best sources of data is the Monitoring the Future (MTF) study, hosted by the University of Michigan and funded by the National Institute on Drug Abuse; this decades-old research highlights college students, adults, high school students, and adolescents (Miech et al., 2020; Schulenberg et al., 2020). The 2020 MTF report by Schulenberg et al. cites lifetime, annual, 30-day, and daily use of a wide variety of substances by full-time college students. The annual prevalence of any illicit drug is 46.5%; illicit drug use, when excluding marijuana, was 16.8%; and marijuana use was 43.0%. Annual alcohol use was reported by 77.6% of students, with reports of being drunk at 58.7%. The study cited the annual use of many other substances, including hallucinogens (5.3%), cocaine (5.6%), narcotics other than heroin (1.5%), and amphetamines (8.1%).

Reports of monthly substance use—as opposed to annual or

lifetime—are generally more useful data, as this information reflects current and likely more regular behavior. The MTF study (Schulenberg et al., 2020) found illicit monthly drug use among 29.7% of students; with marijuana removed, illicit use decreased to 7.6%. Marijuana use was at 26.3%, and other drugs showed much lower use: amphetamines (3.4%), cocaine (2.4%), hallucinogens (1.4%), and narcotics other than heroin (0.4%). Alcohol use was 62.2%, while 34.8% of respondents reported having been drunk in the past month. The study also reported daily alcohol or drug use, with 5.9% of students using marijuana daily and 1 in 50 students (2.0%) using alcohol daily. Respondents also reported the consumption of five or more drinks in a row during the past 2 weeks (32.7%).

Other sources provide complementary data. The National College Health Assessment (American College Health Association, 2019) showed 30-day use patterns of alcohol at 58.4%, marijuana at 22.1%, and cocaine at 1.8%. The National Survey on Drug Use and Health (NSDUH; Substance Abuse and Mental Health Services Administration, 2019a), which focused on young adults aged 18 to 25, found past-month alcohol use to be 55.1% and binge alcohol use to be 34.9% (note that the term *binge use* is defined for men as consuming five or more drinks on the same occasion at least once during the previous 30 days; for women, this is four or more drinks). This survey reported the annual use of illicit drugs at 38.7%; marijuana, 34.8%; cocaine, 5.8%; methamphetamines, 0.8%; and hallucinogens, 6.9%. The 2018 NSDUH study indicated that 18- to 25-year-olds use mood-altering substances more frequently than the cohort examined in Schulenberg et al.'s (2020) MTF study, which surveyed college students 1 to 4 years beyond high school.

Parallel to this important finding about the higher rates of substance use is the role that campus prevention strategies play in addressing the problem. Typical campus prevention strategies focus on undergraduate students; however, heightened rates of drug and alcohol use have been found with law students and medical students (Ayala et al., 2017; Louros, 2016; Report of the AALS Special Committee on Problems of Substance Abuse in Law Schools, 1994; Schwartz et al., 1990). This finding has resulted in specific targeted strategies for these audiences (Anderson et al., 1995; Butler Center for Research, 2017; Singleton et al., 2005).

These study results, from different sources, give a general picture of overall substance use; each source of data provides much more detail with analyses by factors such as individual demographics, attitudes and beliefs, and the social context (e.g., peer norms, exposure to drug use, perceived availability). National data, coupled with in-depth reviews of findings, can be used by campus leaders to identify areas of concern and attention; national data can also serve for comparison purposes with locally collected data. Reviews of national data and associated trends allow for more current baseline information that can inform and guide campus needs assessments and planning efforts. Campuses have a particular interest in a review of data for high school youth, as many local students may transition to colleges and universities close to home.

Although these and other national data sources capture new and emerging substances, on-campus prevention specialists benefit from using varied methodologies (see Chapter 9). With evolving laws about medicinal and commercial use of marijuana, the mixing of substances, vaping, and emerging patterns of students' use of substances, maintaining timely knowledge of students' knowledge, perceptions, and patterns of behavior is key for these practitioners. Only with this knowledge can the real impact of substance use on campuses be known.

DRUG AND ALCOHOL USE PATTERNS OVER TIME

A broad perspective shows patterns and changes over time, so knowledge of various substances' emergence, reduction, or continuance can help prevention specialists plan timely and appropriate campus efforts. Monitoring use patterns, consequences, attitudes, knowledge, perceptions, and more assists with identifying what could warrant attention. Understanding overall national trends allows prevention specialists to pinpoint desirable changes and areas of concern. Such national-level data can inform local policies, programs, services, and strategies, as well as local data-collection efforts and queries.

Annual data from the MTF study on college students date to 1980; such breadth provides helpful perspectives. For example, over the past 2 decades, 30-day illicit drug use excluding marijuana has fluctuated between 6.9% and 10.0%; marijuana use has risen almost continuously over this time from 20.0% to its 2018 level of 24.7% (Schulenberg et al., 2020). Monthly alcohol use had a high of 69.0% in 2008 and reduced to 59.6% in 2018; rates of high-risk consumption (defined as five or more drinks in a row) have also fallen, hovering around 40% from 1980 to 2008 before dropping fairly continuously to a current rate of 28.4% (Schulenberg et al., 2020). The fact that this high-risk behavior has been reduced significantly is noteworthy, as the data demonstrates that positive change is feasible; this fact can be used with campus planning efforts, providing rationale for articulating and testing causal linkages as part of the campus logic model.

The MTF study began in 1975 with a focus on high school students. For 12th-grade students, the high point for illicit drug use (including marijuana) was 54.2% (1979) and its low point was 27.1.0% (1992); when marijuana is excluded, the highest rate of annual illicit drug use was 34.0% (1981), and the low was 11.5% (2019; Miech et al., 2020). Annual marijuana use for 12th-grade students was 50.8% in 1979; it dropped to 21.9% in 1992, has been above 30% since 1994, and has hovered around 35% since 2010 (Miech et al., 2020). Thirty-day prevalence among 12th-grade students showed alcohol use at 29.4% (2019), its lowest since 1975, and with a peak of 72.1% (1978; Miech et al., 2020). The trends revealed a 50% range in the 1990s, a 40% range in the early 2000s, and a rate below 40% since 2013. Again, these high school focused data demonstrate the feasibility of change (with alcohol) and continued concerns (with marijuana) for youth who may transition to institutions of higher education.

It is helpful to look at data regarding some of the consequences associated with drug and alcohol use. While these data are not specific to college students, the societal context is important, as colleges and universities are embedded in the larger society. Alcohol-related traffic fatalities have remained relatively constant over the past decade, reported at 10,759 in 2009 and 10,511 in 2018; the fatality rate per

100 million vehicle miles traveled was 0.36 in 2009 and 0.33 in 2018 (National Highway Traffic Safety Administration, 2019).

Another relevant data point is drug overdose deaths. The year 2017 saw 70,237 fatal overdoses, a 9.6% increase from 2016 (Centers for Disease Control and Prevention, 2020). Opioids were the cause in 47,600 of these deaths; among them, 15,000 involved heroin. In 2019, opioid deaths had become the second leading cause of death in the United States, and prescription and opioid drug analogue deaths accounted for more overdoses than those from heroin.

Another consideration for campus prevention specialists deals with specific audiences or subpopulations. As highlighted in Chapter 6, Selective Prevention Strategies, defined groupings of students report higher levels of risky behaviors in terms of substance use. Notably, data show that higher risk use patterns are traditionally found with first-year students; those affiliated with a fraternity or sorority; and student-athletes. Regarding this third category, for example, the National Collegiate Athletic Association (NCAA) has surveyed student-athletes at member institutions for decades. Its data show that 77.1% of student-athletes used alcohol within the last year, binge alcohol use was 42%, and marijuana use was a 24.7% (NCAA, 2017). Compared with students in general, student-athletes use alcohol at a comparable level; however, binge use is higher, and marijuana use is much lower. NCAA also reports data by sport; with binge drinking, highest rates were in lacrosse (with 69% for men and 57% for women), hockey (64% for men and 56% for women), and swimming (55% for men and 49% for women). Division III saw higher alcohol use overall.

The important takeaway for prevention specialists is twofold. First, reviewing national- or state-level data can provide a broad perspective of substance use issues for students, subpopulations, or specific audiences. This review can spark more interest and encourage data mining. Second, prevention specialists must understand what is needed or appropriate locally. Local information that parallels national- or state-level data can be gathered, and insights of a qualitative and interpretive nature can be ascertained. Data of long-term trends as well as current information are most helpful for use with local planning efforts.

Worksheet 1.1: Campus Issues of Concern guides campus planners in identifying items of relevance.

OTHER CONSEQUENCES OF SUBSTANCE USE

Of equal relevance are the data about the range of consequences associated with drug and alcohol use, most of which are evident and raise considerable concerns. The most serious consequence of alcohol abuse is death, and an estimated 1,500 college students each year die from alcohol-related causes, including motor vehicle crashes (National Institute on Alcohol Abuse and Alcoholism, 2020). Assault by a student who has been drinking is estimated at 696,000 students annually; sexual assault or date rape is estimated for 97,000 students each year (National Institute on Alcohol Abuse and Alcoholism, 2020).

Drinking and driving over the last 30 days is reported by 19.0% of students; drinking and driving after having five or more drinks is reported by 1.3% of students (American College Health Association, 2019). Students' self-reported alcohol-related behavior in the previous 12 months include the following: doing something later regretted (31.5%), unprotected sex (21.9%), physical injury (12.1%), and forgot where they were or what they did (26.5%). Of these and the other six items identified (i.e., got in trouble with police, had sex with someone without their consent, someone had sex with them without consent, physically injured self, physically injured another person, seriously considered suicide), nearly half (49.5%) of students reported experiencing at least one alcohol-related consequence.

College and university administrators cite alcohol's involvement with various student behaviors: property damage (43%), campus policy violation (52%), residence hall damage (49%), and violent behavior (47%; Anderson & Santos, 2018). Administrators also cite alcohol's involvement with acquaintance rape (68%), unsafe sexual practices (58%), physical injury (38%), emotional difficulty (31%), risk of suicide (29%), and health center contacts (18%; Anderson & Santos, 2018). Finally, alcohol use has academic-related consequences: missed classes (31%), diminished performance on tests or projects (27%), lack of academic success (24%), and student attrition (19%; Anderson & Santos, 2018). Although alcohol-related problems have reduced over the past 2 decades, alcohol alone contributes significantly to many campus difficulties and issues.

Worksheet 1.2: Campus Incidents provides a starting point for organizing data collection and monitoring efforts. Although these national and local data are substantive and significant, other, not quantified factors must also be considered as consequences.

- Take into account the emotional stress faced by students, faculty, and staff when a student dies, whether due to an automobile crash, a drug overdose, or alcohol poisoning.
- Think about the trauma faced by a student, his or her roommate, friends, teammates, or others when an incident of sexual assault or physical injury occurs.
- Reflect on the general disruption to the campus environment when there is noise and physical damage associated with parties or drunken behavior.
- Consider the cost factors associated with students departing campus, whether because of the sanctions related to drug or alcohol use, poor academic performance due to the impact of drugs or alcohol, or depletion of financial resources because of drug/alcohol use.

Each—and more—must be considered among the consequences of drug and alcohol misuse on campus. In Case Study 1.1, Ellen Bass discusses the importance of engaged, concerned faculty members.

CASE STUDY 1.1

An Engineering Faculty's Journey Into Undergraduate Alcohol Abuse Prevention

Ellen J. Bass, PhD
Interim Senior Associate Dean for Research, College of Computing and Informatics
Professor and Chair, Department of Health Systems and Sciences Research
Professor, Department of Information Science
Affiliate Professor, School of Biomedical Engineering, Science and Health Systems
Drexel University

I was waiting for an undergraduate who had missed several meetings with his senior design team, but he stood me up as well. How could such an excellent student suddenly behave like this? Later, I found out that people close to him had recently died from two separate incidents related to alcohol. Concerned about this student, I reached out to the Office of the Dean of Students; the advice to contact the university's alcohol and substance abuse prevention team changed my entire perspective on my role as a faculty member. I requested permission for that student to change his senior design topic to one focused on health promotion, and together we were able to introduce some of his findings into a course I was teaching.

Following this experience, I embarked on a journey to integrate health promotion into my academic life. In collaboration with the alcohol and substance abuse prevention office,

I advised senior design teams to develop and evaluate social norms marketing campaigns to reduce hazardous drinking and to analyze the resulting data (see, e.g., Montealegre et al., 2011; White et al., 2008). The students were critical to the success of the efforts—not only did they bring passion to the work, but also they were experts in student culture. With faculty in my home department and with support from the prevention office, I introduced health promotion curriculum into engineering courses (see Bass, et al., 2019). These efforts excited the students about the topic of healthy behavior and led to conversations with peers outside of the classroom. They also led to me becoming a co-advisor for a PhD student in the School of Education on the topic of curriculum infusion and to being invited as a keynote speaker at the National Conference on the Social Norms Approach.

I encourage faculty to work with the prevention office and with students, staff, and other faculty to address the difficult issues surrounding alcohol abuse and related negative consequences. No one should wait for excellent students to come to office hours—or worse, for students for whom it may be too late to help.

RELATED FACTORS AND AFFILIATES OF SUBSTANCE USE

Other issues are relevant when examining the impact of drugs and alcohol on college students, as they can influence students' decisions about whether to use of substances. One issue is the perceptions of others' use, as dramatic differences exist between perceptions and reality. According to an American College Health Association (2019) study, for alcohol, 2.6% of college students reported never using alcohol, yet students believed that 4.9% of their peers are lifetime non-users. Similarly, 58.4% reported using alcohol during the past 30 days;

the perception is that 92.9% of their peers have used alcohol during this time period. With marijuana, over one half (57.6%) of college students reported having never used it; the perception is that 7.9% of their peers have never used marijuana. Marijuana use over the last 30 days was reported by 22.1% of students; the perception is that 87.1% of their peers had used it during this time period (American College Health Association, 2019). These dramatic differences can inform social norms marketing efforts, which can shape the desired campus culture. More detail about social norms efforts is found in Chapter 6, with a resource bibliography in Appendix B.

Another issue is how people assess harm, as personal substance use is inversely related to perceived harm. College students' beliefs about the harmfulness of various substances show between 21% and 31% of young adults within varying age groups (18, 19–22, 23–26, and 27–30) reported significant risk with regular marijuana use; this is half the rate (between 57% and 66%) reported 2 decades ago (Scheulenberg et al., 2020). The implications for marijuana, and for other substances, are clear: "The study has shown that perceived risk often is a leading indicator of change, and also that cohort effects help to predict forthcoming changes at later ages" (Scheulenberg et al., 2020, p. 5).

Prevention specialists must understand the risk and protective factors associated with substance misuse if they are to address substance misuse and substance use disorders (SUDs). According to the Substance Abuse and Mental Health Services Administration (2019b), risk factors "increase the likelihood of beginning substance use, of regular and harmful use, and other behavioral health problems associated with use" (p. 5). Protective factors "directly decrease the likelihood of substance use and behavioral health problems or reduce the impact of risk factors on behavioral health problems" (p. 5).

The social-ecological model (Centers for Disease Control and Prevention, 2020) helps explain risk and protective factors, specifying the multiple elements that contribute to the development (or nondevelopment) of substance misuse. The four main elements of this model are Individual, Relationship, Community, and Societal (see Figure 1.1); the compilation of these elements takes into account genetics, family background, schools, interpersonal relationships, worksites, communities, and overall society. An individual's risk for substance misuse increases with more risk factors, so the goal is to reduce the presence and effect of risk factors and to increase resistance or resiliency through enhancing protective factors.

Figure 1.1
Substance Misuse Prevention for Young Adults

SOCIETAL
CULTURE — HISTORICAL TRAUMA — NORMS AND ACCESS — SOCIOECONOMIC STATUS — MEDIA — LAWS AND POLICIES
COMMUNITY
FAITH-BASED INSTITUTIONS — SCHOOLS — WORKPLACES — NEIGHBORHOODS
RELATIONSHIP
PEERS — PARENTS — TEACHERS
INDIVIDUAL

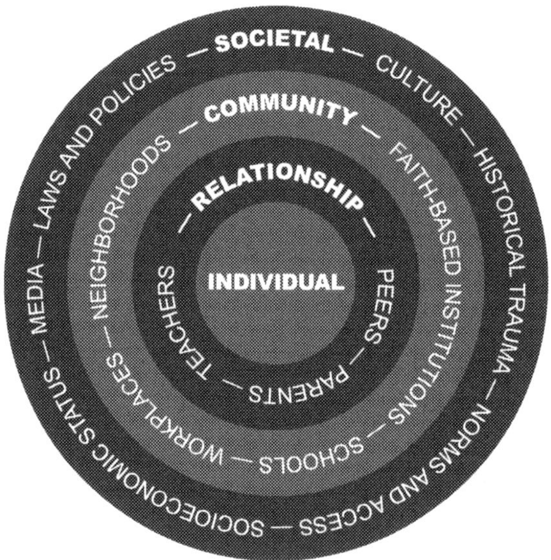

Note. Reprinted from *Substance Misuse Prevention for Young Adults* (p. 6), by the Substance Abuse and Mental Health Services Administration, 2019b (https://store.samhsa.gov/product/Substance-Misuse-Prevention-for-Young-Adults/PEP19-PL-Guide-1). In the public domain.

Designing appropriate strategies means considering those risk factors that students face. For example, students from rural backgrounds may have a greater risk of abusing alcohol and methamphetamines (Lambert et al., 2008). Also, males as well as students not in a committed relationship have a heightened risk for substance misuse (Stone et al., 2012). Schulenberg et al. (2020) reported that attendance at a college or university is a risk factor for binge drinking: "Both relative and absolute increases in most indices of alcohol use among college students in the first few years following high school are quite striking and point to full-time college attendance as a risk factor for binge drinking" (p. 354). No single calculus can be used to predict accurately the causal factors associated with an individual's high risk or problematic use or potential for a SUD, so prevention specialists are wise to pay attention to these myriad considerations.

Understanding the reasons students choose to use substances helps to promote appropriate strategies. A core question for students who misuse substances focuses on what the perceived benefit of substance use is. Understanding this question aids in determining and addressing "root causes." A useful framework for organizing these reasons encompasses physical, cognitive, social, and emotional factors. For example, stress is associated with interpersonal relationships; prevention specialists may address both the stress aspect and the relationship quality. Similarly, with academic performance issues, prevention specialists can emphasize time management, study skills, and writing, as these strategies can improve academics and perhaps deter substance use.

Consider also the presence of substance-related problems and SUDs (see Chapter 7). Some students arrive on campus with a diagnosis of a SUD; some are in recovery. Others have drinking or drug use patterns that move them along the continuum of a SUD toward a clinical diagnosis. And other students may engage in drinking or drug use patterns that cause problems or may result in injury or death. What is important is acknowledging the range of behaviors among students—from nonuse to low-level use or experimentation, to moderate use, to occasional problematic use, to regular problematic use, to a diagnosis of a SUD. Prevention specialists should focus on reducing problems overall and helping individuals lower their interpersonal risks.

Embedded with this understanding is a logic model about the causation of substance misuse and abuse. Specifically, what is the relative role of students' attitudes about substance use, longer term harm, or consequences? What do students know about the short-term and long-term effects of substance use? Are students aware of available campus resources, and what are student attitudes about accessing services for prevention, intervention, treatment, or recovery? The social-ecological model informs understanding of these and other precursors to substance abuse. Worksheet 1.3: Applications of the Social-Ecological

Model illustrates issues within its framework, and organizes strategies associated with risk and protective factors.

ORCHESTRATED EFFORTS TO ADDRESS DRUG AND ALCOHOL ISSUES

Over recent decades, numerous efforts have been made at the national level to address drug and alcohol issues, and some may have resulted in reductions with drug and alcohol use among the general population, college students, and high school and younger youth. Many of these efforts were initiated decades ago and remain; others have had their moment but are no longer available. The agencies and organizations that follow represent the most commonly cited efforts with the most significant reach; others have had efforts, large and small, to specifically address substance abuse issues in higher education. Primary among the federal agencies addressing collegiate drug and alcohol issues, historically, are the National Institute on Alcohol Abuse and Alcoholism (with its Whole College Catalog About Drinking in 1976, and more recently CollegeAIM) and the U.S. Department of Education (with its Fund for the Improvement of Postsecondary Education; Network of Colleges and Universities Committed to the Elimination of Drug and Alcohol Abuse [1987–2015]; Office of Safe and Drug-Free Schools; and the Higher Education Center for Alcohol, Other Drug, and Violence Prevention). Collegiate efforts were also based in the U.S. Department of Transportation's National Highway Traffic Safety Administration and the Center for Substance Abuse Prevention (CSAP).

Federal legislation relevant to these efforts includes the Drug-Free Schools and Communities Act (1986) and the Drug-Free Workplace Act (1988). Other federal agencies involved with collegiate efforts include the Office of National Drug Control Policy, the National Institute on Drug Abuse, and the Substance Abuse and Mental Health Services Administration. More recently, the Drug Enforcement Administration initiated its campus drug prevention initiative.

Various higher education associations, such as the American

Council on Education, the North American Interfraternity Council, the American College Health Association, and the National Collegiate Athletic Association, have developed standards, authored reports, and sponsored various initiatives to help their members address alcohol and other drug issues. Beyond these, many states have orchestrated efforts, often based in the state departments of education, health, transportation, or liquor control.

Other initiatives have been instrumental with the collegiate prevention effort. The American College Health Association developed standards on alcohol issues, the Foundation for Addressing Alcohol Responsibility (formerly The Century Council) developed collegiate resources with its Promising Practices: Campus Alcohol Strategies efforts, NASPA–Student Affairs Administrators in Higher Education developed a knowledge community on alcohol and other drug issues, and ACPA–College Student Educators International had a commission on drugs and alcohol. Currently, the Coalition of Higher Education Associations for Substance Abuse Prevention (formerly the Inter-Association Task Force on Alcohol and Other Substance Abuse Issues, and founded in 1983) promotes collaboration among numerous higher education associations. Finally, the Higher Education Center for Alcohol and Drug Misuse Prevention and Recovery offers resources and training.

Overall, attention to collegiate drug and alcohol issues has been widespread at the national level for decades. With different federal agencies and organizations providing leadership and resources, different areas of emphasis have been addressed. These national efforts are complemented by state and regional initiatives, often coordinated by various state agencies such as departments of education, health, public safety, and alcohol beverage control.

Efforts to address drug and alcohol misuse and abuse among college students are not new; they range from early national publications, such as the *Whole College Catalog About Drinking* more than 40 years ago, to the CSAP-published *College Series* (including a white paper and resources for faculty and program administrators), to the Higher Education Center's multiple publications, resources, training, and support services. There has also been legislation, with EDGAR Part 86 Drug-Free Schools and Campus Regulations. Simply put, numerous efforts have been undertaken to address the various problems such as injuries, deaths, property damage, and other harmful consequences associated with drug or alcohol misuse. The resources here and beyond exist for campus leaders to incorporate into their locally appropriate initiatives. Utilization of these resources varies from institution to institution and state to state.

WHY COLLEGE LEADERS SHOULD BE CONCERNED

The importance of addressing drug and alcohol issues among the nation's colleges and universities is straightforward. Institutions of higher education are organizations of knowledge, research, social justice, culture, inquiry, leadership, and more for their communities and society. They are founded for the positive development of students, with the goal of preparing them for their lives as thoughtful, qualified, ethical, healthy, and productive adults who can have positive impacts on their families, communities, worksites, and society at large.

As such, these institutions have an obligation to achieve this goal. Many accrediting organizations, state agencies, and national governing bodies prescribe standards and guidelines. Further, parents, legislators, educators, and community members expect that those in leadership positions at colleges and universities will do everything they can to maximize positive outcomes for students; they expect vision, courage, and action to facilitate student success. As Brubacher and Rudy (1968) pointed out decades ago, two types of universities were developed: One was "representing public action by the democratic community in the realm of higher learning" and the other constituted "great endowed institutions, centers of advanced learning and research" (p. 144). More recently, Stearns (2016) stated that "the big balancing act now is between preservation and innovation, both essential but both by themselves inadequate in dealing with what universities need to do in the near future" (p. 3). On each campus, all leaders—from the governing boards to the chief executive, from the chief academic officer to the chief student affairs officer—have responsibilities to maximize the desired outcomes. This means providing direction, support, focus, and prioritization of efforts that help achieve these results; it also means addressing challenges and obstacles that deter the forward movement and promoting a campus culture that maximizes both living and learning environments.

Not only must institution leaders seek to reduce problems, but they must also promote the potential of students, faculty, and staff. Some of the practical outcomes of a well-grounded, thoughtful, and planned effort for addressing drug and alcohol issues are reduced student death and injury, reduced sexual assault, lowered violence, lower property damage, and lower costs. Associated with these outcomes are increased safety, enhanced academic performance, and improved learning opportunities. If drug and alcohol problems were reduced dramatically, the likely result encompasses greater quality and quantity of thought leaders, more knowledge communities, and enhanced preparation of individuals who enter the workforce, families, communities, government, and civic engagement. Worksheet 1.4: Reasons to Be Concerned Planning Sheet aids prevention specialists in gaining understanding and consensus about campus issues. Further, perspectives such as those provided by Robert Chapman in Lessons From the Field 1.1 can help to reduce these problems.

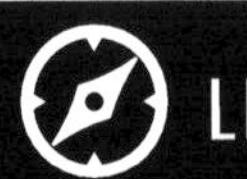

LESSONS FROM THE FIELD 1.1

Identifying Risk: Right Church, Wrong Pew

Robert J. Chapman, PhD
Alcohol and Other Drug Program Coordinator (former)
La Salle University

Sometimes even the practice and principles of Motivational Interviewing are insufficient to elicit change talk in an interviewee—even one who is a model student.

John was a graduating senior who consistently made the dean's list. He would be starting a full-time position upon graduation and making a substantive salary. He had no previous campus violations, no alcohol-related traffic offenses, and no aggressive behavior, financial difficulties, or "blackouts." Despite this dearth of traditional issues associated with high-risk drinking, John reported drinking ten 12-oz bottles of beer three nights a week—clearly high-risk drinking.

Despite my concerns, John did not see his drinking as risky. My inner voice said: *Give him a calculator and ask him these questions.*

I gave John my calculator and asked him to calculate the following: 10 x 3 x 15 x 2 x 140. He arrived at a figure of 126,000. Asked if he knew what that number represented, he said no. I informed him that that was the number of calories he consumed his senior year following his reported pattern of drinking: 10 beers 3 times a week for 15 weeks for 2 semesters, times 140 calories per 12-oz bottle of his favorite brand.

John looked at me, then at the calculator, then back at me: "I drink a lot of beer, don't I?" He then agreed to discuss "dialing it back a bit" because he was concerned—not about the risk but about the calories.

> John's engagement in "change talk" speaks to the fact that innovation may result from little more than a flash of insight—the realization that you were in the right church for your niece's wedding but seated in the wrong pew.

BRINGING IT LOCAL

National-level data about drugs and alcohol can be overwhelming; however, they can also be instrumental for understanding a wide variety of factors and issues. That said, six cautions arise.

- It is important *not to be overwhelmed* by the data. Much is known, and the campus practitioner will be well served to be intentional with what can be used.
- The data cited are those with the greatest depth and breadth. *Much more research exists*, whether at the state or national level.
- Campus personnel should *expand their focus* beyond current students. While students are the primary focus of most campus efforts regarding drugs and alcohol, it is essential to "look beyond the borders" and ascertain what is relevant.
- The data cited has limited attention to many of the *underlying factors or root causes* of substance use and misuse.
- Much of the data cited is quantitative. A more complete understanding is gained from *gathering qualitative information.*
- It is vital to *make things local*. The core issue is ascertaining what is needed and appropriate for institutions in relation to its community and state at this given point in time. Community and institution-specific information are essential in understanding local needs and available resources.

The important theme of "bringing it local" permeates this volume. The rationale for this focus is that campus issues are addressed most effectively when the areas of concern for that campus are specifically identified and documented; further, when campus personnel design the strategies, local ownership and likelihood for support and sustainability are enhanced. Collective wisdom, shared resources, and mutual support benefit tremendously from these local efforts, as documented by Frances Harding in Innovator 1.1.

INNOVATOR 1.1

Building the First Statewide Alcohol and Substance Abuse Prevention Model for New York

Frances M. Harding
Director (retired)
Substance Abuse and Mental Health Administration's Center for Substance Abuse Prevention

Prevention programming has certainly changed over the 39 years I have been working in the prevention field. My interest in finding strategies to reduce alcohol misuse began when I worked for a couple of colleges and learned firsthand the devastating effects of alcohol and drug misuse among students. When I started working for New York State in 1982, I was hired to write a manual on preventing alcohol and drug misuse on college campuses. I had no idea this assignment would expand into the development of statewide guidelines for prevention programs in settings beyond colleges.

Several years later, when I was New York's lead for alcohol and substance misuse prevention, I developed a strategic plan for the state to address the high rates of underage drinking and the alarming number of high school and college students dying in alcohol-related traffic crashes.

This strategic plan required each of the state's 62 counties to receive regular site visits from my agency's prevention staff. The visits' purpose was to assess and update the counties' existing prevention plans for their schools and communities by training them to use their data to select evidence-based programs.

The state's communities, including colleges and universities, needed significant support to prevent the tremendous loss of young people to impaired driving crashes, alcohol poisoning, and hazing—just to name a few consequences. With assistancee from a federal grant, the state selected the Communities That Care (2020) program, primarily because of Hawkins and Catalano's (1992) development of the risk and protective factors model, which looked closely at the various factors that contributed to, and helped to protect against, alcohol and drug misuse.

Getting this prevention science and messaging out to the prevention professionals who needed to learn it was somewhat difficult. Prevention professionals were interested in maintaining the status quo and continuing to do what they had always done—which resulted in a lack of positive outcomes. I was advocating for them to learn about innovative research that not only was effective but also could be adapted to meet the needs of the state's diverse communities. This was particularly challenging as my responsibilities included working with the largest U.S. city as well as some of the most rural counties. It was the most difficult and yet exciting work I ever did.

In the late 1990s, New York took two innovative steps forward in helping both the state and the country. First, the agency I led (New York State's Office of Alcoholism and Substance Abuse Services) brought representatives from the 10 different college coalitions into a statewide steering committee to advise the agency. Second, the agency convened both the community- and campus-based coalitions to work on common issues. They were instrumental in statewide efforts to prevent alcohol and drug use among college students, including administering a survey to measure alcohol and drug use, updating the programming manual, and hosting a conference. I believe this is why New York was viewed as a national prevention leader on these issues. To this day, some of these coalitions remain—more than 2 decades after they launched. New York has truly embraced and grown in the coalition structure, which continues to address current and emerging issues related to alcohol and drug misuse. I was fortunate to have played such a prominent role in starting this innovative strategy in New York.

CONCLUSION

Having sound foundations to address campus drug and alcohol issues is vital for attaining desired results. Particularly helpful are many resources available at the national level, including ongoing research and other documentation. Campus leaders and prevention specialists benefit from grounding their efforts with local data collection and needs assessments, with attention given to metrics such as drug and alcohol use, patterns over time, consequences of substance use, and related factors. Current and ongoing data collection aids in establishing campus strategies to maximize outcomes that are current and meaningful for the campus. Through engagement in thoughtful planning and with active participation from the community of scholars and learners, specific evidence-informed and innovative strategies can be defined, planned, and implemented.

REFERENCES

American College Health Association. (2019). *National college health assessment.* https://www.acha.org/documents/ncha/NCHA-II_SPRING_2019_US_REFERENCE_GROUP_EXECUTIVE_SUMMARY.pdf

Anderson, D. S., Hanna, J., & Maddalena, G. (1995). *Smart start resource manual: A substance abuse prevention program for law schools.* George Mason University; Phi Alpha Delta Public Service Center.

Anderson, D. S., & Santos, G. M. (2018). *College alcohol survey: The national longitudinal survey on alcohol, tobacco, other drug and violence issues at institutions of higher education.* George Mason University.

Ayala, E. E., Roseman, D., Winseman, J. S., & Mason, H. R. C. (2017). Prevalence, perceptions, and consequences of substance use in medical students. *Medical Education Online, 22*(1), Article 1392824.

Bass, E. J., Foster, H. A., Lee, D. W., Bruce, S., & Bailey, R. R. (2019). Curriculum infusion through case studies: Engaging undergraduate students in course subject material and influencing behavior change. In W. Karwowski, T. Ahram, & S. Nazir (Eds.), *Advances in human factors in training, education, and learning sciences: Proceedings of the AHFE 2019 International Conference on Human Factors in Training, Education, and Learning Sciences, July 24–28, 2019, Washington D.C., USA* (pp. 203–214). Springer.

Brubacher, J. S., & Rudy, W. (1968). *Higher education in transition: A history of American colleges and universities, 1636–1968.* Harper & Row.

Butler Center for Research. (2017). *Substance use disorders: Research update.* Hazelden Betty Ford Foundation. https://www.hazeldenbettyford.org/education/bcr/addiction-research/substance-abuse-legal-professionals-ru-317

Centers for Disease Control and Prevention. (2020). *The Social-Ecological Model: A framework for prevention.* https://www.cdc.gov/violenceprevention/publichealthissue/social-ecologicalmodel.html

Communities That Care. (2020). http://www.communitiesthatcare.net

Hawkins, J. D., & Catalano, R. F. (1992). Risk and protective factors for alcohol and other drug problems in adolescence and early adulthood: Implications for substance abuse prevention. *Psychological Bulletin, 112*(1), 64–105.

Lambert, D., Gale, J. A., & Hartley, D. (2008). Substance abuse by youth and young adults in rural America. *The Journal of Rural Health, 24*(3), 221–228. https://doi.org/10.1111/j.1748-0361.2008.00162

Louros, J. (2016). *Elephant in the room: Mental health and substance abuse in law school.* ABA for Law Students. https://abaforlawstudents.com/2016/07/18/mental-health-and-substance-abuse-in-law-school

Miech, R. A., Johnston, L. D., O'Malley, P. M., Bachman, J. G., Schulenberg, J. E., & Patrick, M. E. (2020). *Monitoring the future national survey results on drug use, 1975–2019: Volume I, secondary school students.* Institute for Social Research, The University of Michigan.

Montealegre, L-E., Bass, E. J., Bruce, S. E., & Foster, H. A. (2011, April 29). Cavman, Wonder Woman, or too drunk to tell: An evaluation of the effectiveness of a Halloween social norms marketing campaign. In K. A. Neely (Ed.), *2011 IEEE Systems and Information Engineering Design Symposium* (pp. 65–70). IEEE. https://ieeexplore.ieee.org/document/5876846

National Collegiate Athletic Association. (2017). *Student-athlete substance use survey.* http://www.ncaa.org/about/resources/research/ncaa-student-athlete-substance-use-study

National Highway Traffic Safety Administration. (2019). *Alcohol-impaired driving.* https://crashstats.nhtsa.dot.gov/Api/Public/ViewPublication/812864

National Institute on Alcohol Abuse and Alcoholism. (2020). *Consequences.* https://www.collegedrinkingprevention.gov/Statistics/consequences.aspx

Report of the AALS Special Committee on Problems of Substance Abuse in the Law Schools. (1994). *Journal of Legal Education, 44*(1), 35–80. http://www.jstor.org/stable/42893309

Schulenberg, J. E., Johnston, L. D., O'Malley, P. M., Bachman, J. G., Miech, R. A., & Patrick, M. E. (2020). *Monitoring the future national survey results on drug use, 1975–2019: Volume II, college students and adults ages 19–60.* Institute for Social Research, The University of Michigan.

Schwartz, R. H., Lewis, D. C., Hoffman, N. G., & Kyriazi, N. (1990). Cocaine and marijuana use by medical students before and during medical school. *Archives of Internal Medicine, 150*(4), 883–886. https://doi.org/10.1001/archinte.1990.00390160125024

Singleton, O. L., Baker, A. C., & Escobar, E. (2005). *Substance abuse in law schools: A tool kit for law school administrators.* American Bar Association.

Stearns, P. N. (2016). *Guiding the American university: Contemporary challenges and choices.* Routledge.

Stone, A. L., Becker, L. G., Huber, A. M., & Catalano, R. F. (2012). Review of risk and protective factors of substance use and problem use in emerging adulthood. *Addictive Behaviors, 37*(7), 747–775. https://doi.org/10.1016/j.addbeh.2012.02.014

Substance Abuse and Mental Health Services Administration. (2019a). *Key substance use and mental health indicators in the United States: Results from the 2018 National Survey on Drug Use and Health* (HHS Publication No. PEP19-5068, NSDUH Series H-54). https://www.samhsa.gov/data/sites/default/files/cbhsq-reports/NSDUHNationalFindingsReport2018/NSDUHNationalFindingsReport2018.pdf

Substance Abuse and Mental Health Services Administration. (2019b). *Substance misuse prevention for young adults* (Publication No. PEP19-PL-Guide-1). https://store.samhsa.gov/product/Substance-Misuse-Prevention-for-Young-Adults/PEP19-PL-Guide-1

White, M. H., Odioso, M. S., Weaver, M., Purvis, M. C., Bass, E. J., & Bruce, S. E. (2008). Horses? There are horses at Foxfield? An analysis of college student hazardous drinking and related decision making behaviors. In G. E. Louis & K. G. Crowther (Ed.), 2008 *IEEE Systems and Information Engineering Design Symposium* (pp. 283–288). IEEE. https://ieeexplore.ieee.org/document/4559726

CHAPTER 2

Changing the Campus Culture

Norms and Assumptions

"I remember sitting on the campus lawn for 2 hours before my college orientation started because I arrived 2 hours early. I was nervous, I knew no one and knew no place. But the first coffee shop I went to became my favorite, and continues to be a safe place in the big city. There is power in space and making places your own, and a part of you can make new environments less alien."

—Junior at a large public urban university in the Pacific Northwest

So much of what comprises a college or university revolves around its culture. Typically incorporated into the mission statements of institutions of higher education are cultural aims such as educating the entire human being, promoting academic discourse, emphasizing preparation for life, stressing quality efforts, highlighting grounded and critical thinking, aspiring to a liberal arts education, and preparing for a productive life. Through experiences within and outside of the classroom, colleges and universities prepare students for a life of inquiry and compassionate human relationships. The culture of the campus affects these ideals and aspirations; some parts of the culture help these aims, and some parts hinder them.

Many campus problems are associated with drugs and alcohol, which detract from the stated institutional aims. Much of the human and property damage related to substance misuse continues unabated, whether through campus leadership's inattention, minimization, low prioritization, unawareness, old paradigms, or other factors. Essential to a campus achieving its aims, and for students to attain theirs, is identifying how drug and alcohol prevention can contribute to positive outcomes. This proactive approach aids colleges and universities in reducing many of the negative and harmful aspects of campus culture.

This chapter tackles the need for change—moving far beyond the "wink-wink, nod-nod," "we're no worse than anyone else," "when I was in college . . . ," and "hoping for the best" approaches. The emphasis of this chapter is to provide campus prevention specialists with the requisite grounding so they can provide leadership for localized strategic planning and shaping of the campus culture.

Illustrating various ways that institution leaders and prevention specialists can address the campus culture are this chapter's five contributions from professionals who have varying responsibilities and histories. Three Lessons From the Field segments discuss the important role of "prevention influencers," the importance of relationships in the context of hospitality, and faculty members' roles within an online environment. Case Study 2.1 tells of an administrator standing up for what was deemed best. The Innovator for this chapter, Dolores Cimini, highlights ways of moving forward strategically.

CULTURE AND NORMS

When thinking about campus culture, two considerations are appropriate. One part is the general culture, with factors such as human respect, behavioral norms, decision-making styles, traditions, and general human interactions. The other part revolves around drugs and alcohol; this has to do with the "party culture," the "drinking culture," the rites of passage in campus life, the norms and behaviors surrounding socializing, how drugs and alcohol are related to group membership, and how drug and alcohol policies are viewed and enforced. These two broad perspectives of culture ground and shape the specific campus strategies and focused initiatives associated with a comprehensive drug and alcohol prevention effort.

Overall culture consists of the general beliefs, values, norms, or traits shared by a group of people. It incorporates areas of alignment and assimilation and includes purpose, collaboration, order, and sharing. Culture can encompass "world culture," the "U.S. culture," and "Southern culture." It can apply to generations (Baby Boomers, Generation X, Generation Y), race and ethnicity, religion, and sexual orientation. Culture can also come into play with organizations and affiliation groups. Anthropologists have noted how to define a culture's boundaries, how various cultures overlap, and how individuals can "belong" in multiple cultures simultaneously.

The culture surrounding drugs and alcohol is complex and long-standing. How alcohol use has been addressed throughout U.S. history shows shifting views; consider Prohibition, its repeal, the role of social host liability, and the idea of alcohol as "the devil's brew" and "demon rum." Heroin, at its start, was a legal "heroic" drug, and use of marijuana was once seen as "Green Death" and "Reefer Madness." The culture surrounding these and other substances continues to evolve. Many adults see marijuana use as "no big deal," similar to how underage alcohol consumption is sometimes viewed as a "rite of passage."

Currently, alcohol consumption, and likely the use of other substances also, is seen as having a direct relationship to external factors such as pricing, availability, advertising, and potential consequences; however, other contextual factors influence individuals' choices to consume. Meanings attributed to drinking and drug use are important, and they stem from the cultural context within which individuals find themselves. Further, influencers' attitudes and expectations have a great deal of sway.

The campus itself has several subcultures, many of which parallel those of society in general and some are unique to the college setting. Some prominent campus affiliation groups are fraternities and sororities (individually and collectively), student-athletes (overall and by the team), residential students, student-veterans, international students, adult learners, LGBTQIA+ students, and groups based on race/ethnicity. Others may include student government, various student organizations, recreation and intramural groups, honors societies, service organizations, and individuals in recovery. These distinct and overlapping groups have cultural nuances and norms associated with membership and affiliation.

A norm is the dominant view or standard of operation. All too often, the term *norm* becomes conflated with *normal*, and thus as acceptable behavior or status; similarly, the term *abnormal*, while technically meaning not the norm or average, is often interpreted as deviant or undesirable. Thus, behavior outside the standard (such as abstaining from alcohol use while underage) may be, technically, abnormal. Similarly, if the norm is one of cheating academically, or violating campus rules, that is not to suggest that these are acceptable or desired behaviors. A norm of driving 10 miles over the speed limit does not make it legal or safe. Thus, much of campus prevention efforts involve examining current norms and determining what is desirable moving forward. Another way to think of norms is within the sociological notion of deviance. Deviant behavior is not by definition good or bad; deviance is a willful departure from a group norm.

Also important is identifying injunctive norms and descriptive norms. Injunctive norms are those that are desired and include perceptions of what others would approve or not approve. Descriptive norms report what is occurring and are based on observations of behavior. Social norms' marketing approaches take account of both types and are based on correcting misperceptions of others' actual behavior as well as others' approval or desirability. Because discrepancies abound (typically with regard to students believing higher levels of peer drug or alcohol use, or peers' acceptance of substance use, than is actually true), marketing campaigns address these misperceptions, including desired actions, to promote healthier behaviors.

Overall, the challenge of changing the campus culture must incorporate an understanding of the broader societal culture as well as those unique to the campus and any subgroups. Prevention specialists can help with the ongoing process of moving the campus environment away from those undesired elements. This process continues with the turnover of the student body, changes in key campus leaders, and the evolution of the external culture. This process is further aided by "prevention influencers" on campus, as Carlton Hall demonstrates in Lessons From the Field 2.1.

LESSONS FROM THE FIELD 2.1

Now Is the Time for Campus-Based Prevention Influencers

Carlton Hall, MHS
President and CEO
Carlton Hall Consulting

Prevention science points to the efficacy of community involvement, advocacy, and policy change in mitigating harmful behaviors; however, for many college campuses, a critical deficit has been found in employing effective engagement and policy advocacy to address substance misuse (Jernigan et al., 2019). Cultivating campus-based prevention influencers offers one strategy to address this engagement gap on campuses and to encourage a focus on important policy, programmatic, and strategic remedies.

As a *prevention influencer* in your campus community, you need to be seen as credible and fully informed about the issues you are addressing. In short, *if you want people to follow you, you must give them confidence that you know where you are going.*

You must focus on skills that will enhance your abilities to engage and influence campus policy makers, students, gatekeepers, and others:

Describe the specific drug- or alcohol-related issues or problem that you want to address. It is not enough to say: "I want to prevent or stop drug use!" Although this is noble, you must be much more specific about what aspect of the problem you want to tackle.

So, you will need to **research** the issue, including documenting the problem with data and finding out who is impacted negatively or even positively by it. Ideally, this means local data, but state or national data may be included, too.

Identify the specific **strategies** you are promoting to address the issue. It is not enough just to say, "We have a problem!" You must also have proposed strategies to address it.

Every day brings needs and with them opportunities to influence and change policies and services that impact the entire campus community. As a prevention influencer, you can become a true leader in ways that promote the prevention of substance misuse by community members today and in their future.

CHALLENGES TO SOCIAL ORDER

Shaping the campus culture overall, and specifically drug and alcohol programs, requires attention to various challenges. Attending to them throughout the planning process allows prevention specialists to anticipate their influence—and promotes the achievement of desired outcomes.

First, *any challenge to the social order* can be seen as disruptive. Within a culture or subculture, shared values and interests help the group to coalesce and to attract new members. Many of the structures and operational standards have been established over time, with members taking pride and ownership of them. Disruptions are often resisted—even when the current social order is contrary to policy or has negative consequences. Consider a social organization with a heavy partying lifestyle; although this is the "order" of that group, the behavior and attitudes can be damaging to individuals' health and safety and potentially detrimental to the organization and institution. Further, some or many organization members may dislike or disapprove of that lifestyle. Also consider, for the organization or the campus, a social order that encompasses interests financial in nature (e.g., sales of alcohol), reputational (e.g., a "party school"), or historical (e.g., traditions). Efforts to effect desired change must necessarily consider the social order.

Many challenges with *drug and alcohol issues* deserve specific consideration: individual issues, such as student mental health concerns; limited coping skills; beliefs; attitudes; feelings; and perceived lack of healthy opportunities. There are institutional challenges such as denial, lack of interest, competing priorities, risk avoidance, different viewpoints, limited data, and poor role modeling. Professional challenges include limited staffing, lack of dedicated time, compassion fatigue and burnout, lack of resources, and competing job responsibilities. Community challenges also abound, such as limited resources, alcohol or cannabis access, local priorities, limited enforcement, and decisions or policies made by local governing officials that affect campus life. Strategies for understanding and addressing community concerns are found in Chapter 10. Worksheet 1.1: Campus Issues of Concern helps with identifying items of relevance for campus planners.

The 21st-century college experience brings with it unique elements for consideration. The increasing use of technology for academic courses, with distance education, online resources, and virtual classrooms, reduces the opportunity for face-to-face interaction and human engagement. This online environment creates unique challenges for faculty members, particularly with regard to addressing student needs with drugs and alcohol. Diane Rullo illustrates this problem in Lessons From the Field 2.2.

Further compounding technological issues is the fact that social media permeates society and affects norms on so many levels. With information validity often left unchecked, as well as the presence of "Internet courage" where individuals say something on social media or with a text that they would not say in person, the established social order and interaction styles can be easily disrupted. A further factor is the role of micro-influencers on norms and the dissemination of information. The idea that traditional news outlets cannot be trusted leads to individuals seeking support from online followers rather than established sources. This is further compounded by the fact that many campus leaders are Baby Boomers, born between 1946 and 1964; they tend to base their decisions on their generational values, which are often much different from those held by the vast majority of undergraduates. The shifts in this century's political climate affect campus culture, as increasing partisan behavior dominates political discourse and decision making at the local, state, and national levels. Related is the role of activism on campus (so prevalent during the formative years of those from the Baby Boomer generation); the nature of activism, what is acceptable, free speech, and the balance between individual rights and collective responsibilities all contribute to culture.

Whether confronting the overall nature of changing the social order, issues unique to drugs and alcohol, or factors prominent in the 21st century, prevention specialists must delineate which is the influential driver if they are to orchestrate planned change.

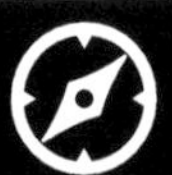

LESSONS FROM THE FIELD 2.2

The Online Environment and Student Assistance

Diane Rullo, PhD

School of Social Work and Human Services

Walden University

More than a century old (Verduin & Clark, 1991), distance learning has become a staple in education (Allen & Seaman, 2013), with technology and the Internet (Lee, 2017) allowing millions to access online education. Increasingly, courses have gone totally online or followed a hybrid approach. Faculty and administrators recognize that students may experience many challenges, including addiction and mental health issues, which can affect the quality of their academic learning experience (Walden University, 2020). A major challenge with the online learning environment is that faculty have very limited opportunities to identify these issues.

Online education programs offer formats that are synchronous and asynchronous (Perrotta, 2020). Through the use of video conferencing software, synchronous programs give faculty a slightly better opportunity to recognize students' behavior. In asynchronous programs, however, faculty rarely have any face-to-face contact with students. Some disciplines (psychology, counseling, social work, and nursing) have additional educational components that may include a residency or clinic where the faculty engage students for in-person training and evaluation. This gives instructors a better chance of picking up on mental health and addiction issues.

Generally, the online environment hinders the identification of student problems. Although faculty members in the social sciences are more apt to have the expertise to identify an addiction or mental health issue, the online setting poses a barrier. In fact, a survey found more than 70% of faculty in all disciplines did not feel qualified to recognize signs of psychological distress (Kugler, 2017). Even though student assistance programs are offered in online environments, these programs rarely receive referrals from online faculty for addiction and mental health (Rochelle Gilbert, personal communication, April 3, 2020).

Looking forward, school administrators in conjunction with mental health specialists would benefit from a three-pronged approach. First, identify strategies that increase personalized student engagement in the online academic setting. Second, train faculty members in problem identification (signs, symptoms, and other clues) and referral. Third, redefine faculty members' roles to include these important identification and referral roles, to help troubled students and promote academic success. Although such changes may not be particularly comfortable for many faculty members, especially those outside the social sciences, these adjustments are necessary to enhance student engagement and welfare.

THE FOUNDATIONS OF CHANGING CAMPUS CULTURE

Preparation for changing the campus culture considers the external culture, the campus as a whole, subgroups on campus, and the surrounding community. Through all of these considerations, the role of relationships and the context of responsible hospitality is vital; Jim Peters emphasizes this point in Lessons From the Field 2.3. Further, while Chapter 10 articulates a step-by-step model for ongoing planning and review efforts, including a leadership group and guiding principles, this current chapter provides background information and insights regarding how drug and alcohol issues contribute to and detract from the campus environment as a whole.

Essential to the change effort is, first, understanding *what the campus culture is* and, second, specifying *what is desired*. The planning steps help achieve the desired state of affairs by reducing gaps between these two elements. Ideally, and ultimately, the current and desired states of affairs will overlap, thus resulting in campus leaders identifying ways to maintain, strengthen, enhance, and expand what is desired.

Consider aspirations to be a research university, classified as R1 by the Carnegie Commission on Higher Education. The campus culture may have high graduation rates, limited student debt, and high levels of employment after graduation. The nature of the campus environment, the quality of services and resources available, and many additional features of studying and living in that campus setting contribute to a campus culture supportive of the desired outcomes. In terms of drug and alcohol issues, there may be few acute intoxication emergency transports to hospitals, limited overdoses, no deaths, few injuries, minimal property damage, high bystander engagement, and overall positive attitudes about drugs and alcohol. Campus leaders will identify what contributes to these (and other) positive outcomes and continue to enhance them; they will also modify them as needed according to changing attributes, needs, and interests.

Typically, however, a gap (sometimes large) exists between the current and desired campus culture. Academically speaking, it may include low standards and high tolerance for academic misconduct; faculty may not be actively engaged in scholarship or research, and students may not be challenged with critical thinking. Campus recreational, cultural, and social opportunities may be limited or unappealing, and norms for responsible decision making about drugs and alcohol may be few. Negative consequences associated with drugs and alcohol may be rampant, and the rowdiness of the parties may be a measure of social engagement. "Party school" ratings are typically viewed differently by different groups, as some may see this as an indicator of a vibrant social life, and others may believe that designation detracts from the academic mission or reputation of the school. The distinction between current and desired campus cultures points the way for critical efforts.

The first foundational step is to *document the current campus culture*. Prevention specialists should consider elements such as the quality of the learning environment, opportunities for promoting critical thinking among students, respectful human interaction, attention to diversity and cultural differences, opportunities for creative exploration, opportunities for exposure to the arts, variation in recreational activities, spiritual engagement, understanding of varied lifestyles, aspiration for healthy living, and joy of life. The specific nature of what should be examined with the current campus culture—with an eye toward what might be desired—will be based on the interests and values of the campus leadership. Worksheet 2.1: Campus Self-Assessment provides a starting point for this documentation and encompasses many major areas regarding the campus culture and current prevention efforts.

The drug and alcohol aspect of the campus culture may include a focus on individual factors as well as systemic elements. The individual-based elements include the extent to which students' knowledge is accurate and current, their personal decision-making skills, their sense of self-responsibility, the extent to which they are accountable for their actions, their understanding of and attitudes about substance use disorders, the quality of their communication and conflict management skills, and their respect for the dangers associated with substance misuse. From a systemic perspective, consideration should be made to organizational elements, such as comprehensive policies; equitable enforcement of policies; thorough procedures, quality measures for group-event planning; consequences for groups and individuals commensurate with the nature of the violations; high-quality training for staff, faculty and paraprofessionals; and thorough documentation. Further, campus culture considerations include the nature and scope of harmful consequences associated with drugs or alcohol, such as deaths, personal injuries, emergency transports and hospital admissions, property damage, interpersonal violence, and other violation of specified community standards.

This documentation of "what is" helps not only with understanding the current state of affairs but also with *specifying the desired state of affairs*. For example, having multiple alcohol-related medical transports can lead to the aim of reducing occurrences of acute intoxication. The desired campus culture, often identified as the vision, can also be envisioned based on what is sought by campus leaders, whether from learning about what other campuses are doing or attending to the campus mission statement, or it may reflect the values of those currently in leadership positions within the organization. Worksheet 2.2: Campus Vision Development is useful for group discussion and guiding participants toward this desired state of affairs. Also, Worksheet 2.3: Obstacles and Challenges for Achieving Visions guides campus prevention specialists in considering what might be limiting the attainment of their visions.

Two questions are at the heart of any efforts to change the campus culture so that it is within the realm of what the campus leaders envision, are proud of, and want to promote. First, in terms of the campus culture, both current and desired, *where do drug and alcohol issues fit?* Second, *how much of a priority is it to address drug and alcohol issues?* If drug and alcohol issues are, in fact, minimal, there may not be much of a problem to address. If drug and alcohol issues are noteworthy, the question is then what campus leaders think of them. If these issues are seen as "no big deal," "not worse than anyone else," "tolerable," and "part of the college experience," then the challenge becomes a different one. The emphasis for prevention specialists then becomes documentation, convincing, and advocacy that stresses how quality prevention efforts can result in more desirable and shared outcomes. It is through sound individual and organizational leadership that shifts in perspective and action can be achieved.

LESSONS FROM THE FIELD 2.3

Life Is About Relationships

Jim Peters, MEd
Founder and President
Responsible Hospitality Institute

Sociability is key to how we form and develop relationships. College is where students learn how to socialize, create meaningful relationships, and engage with the community. For many, alcohol consumption is closely linked to the college social experience; however, how college students socialize with alcohol can create unique risks.

Whether in the home or in a venue (e.g., café, bar, pub, restaurant, nightclub), *hospitality* is creating spaces for people to socialize. *Responsible hospitality* is ensuring safety, security, and community engagement in venues where people share food and drink, enjoy live music, and dance. When students prepare to go out and when they converge at social venues, four critical intervention points enhance sociability and reduce risk.

- **Off-campus housing** blurs the line between campus and community. Although students are educated about being good neighbors, residents still bear the brunt of negative impacts: house parties, noise, litter, bio-waste, vandalism, parking, and traffic. Face-to-face interaction among students and permanent residents can build positive relationships and open communication and reduce risks.
- **Pre-load** (pre-drink, pre-game) behavior occurs at house parties and tailgate parties, and in cars, parks, and fields. However, intoxication can be detrimental to relationships and may increase liability to the venues patronized. Promising approaches include shifting the focus from drinking to socializing—and training venue staff to identify signs of intoxication and deny entrance.
- **Party buses** grew in popularity in part due to increased awareness of impaired driving; however, this option brings risks, including underage drinking, pre-loading, injury, or death. With news stories about party bus accidents nationwide, policies for licensing, restrictions on alcohol service, chaperones, and vehicle standards keep riders safe from harm.

- **Sexual assault** and sexual violence often include alcohol as a factor. Nightlife venues can incorporate prevention by training staff, empowering bystanders to intervene with predators, and helping to change social norms.

A community alliance and strategic engagement among campus personnel (e.g., student leaders, administrators, security) and town/city police, compliance agencies, residents, and nightlife venues can facilitate harm reduction strategies.

THE ROLE OF LEADERSHIP

Leadership is central to changing the campus culture. Leadership can come from various sources, such as the institution's president or provost, chief student affairs officer, chair of the faculty senate, student government association, athletics department, or other influential individuals or groups. The prevention specialist will benefit from working with any of these individuals or groups, as well as other intact groups and organizations. Leadership is essential to make progress and not remain stagnant; leaders have a vision, confront and reduce problems, garner support, engage various constituencies, communicate boldly and frequently, and thus enhance the likelihood of achieving the desired outcomes.

A key leadership issue regarding alcohol and other drugs (AOD) concerns *the campus organization structure*. AOD efforts are usually housed within campus health services and sometimes within counseling services; they are generally housed within a student affairs division. They are often blended with, or subsumed within, a campuswide initiative on wellness or health promotion. This hierarchy makes sense conceptually, as AOD prevention factors into enhanced health; however, from a practical perspective, prevention efforts often become "buried," whether within health services or under a wellness "umbrella." The lack of congruence between prevention aims and organizational structure is what limits program effectiveness. How health threats are prioritized is vital: Is the prevention of substance use–related problems prioritized, or is the reaction to problems prioritized?

Leadership that genuinely cares about addressing the dominant problem should prioritize the most appropriate administrative placement for the campus prevention effort. Consider the extent to which alcohol—alone—was reported to be involved in many campus problems, such as campus behaviors, personal behaviors, and academic issues (Anderson & Santos, 2018):

- Alcohol's Involvement with Campus Behaviors: Property damage (43%); Policy violation (52%); Violent behavior (47%)
- Alcohol's Involvement with Personal Behaviors: Risk of suicide (29%); Emotional difficulty (31%); Physical injury (38%); Unsafe sexual practices (58%); Acquaintance rape (68%)
- Alcohol's Involvement with Academic Issues: Student attrition (19%); Lack of academic success (35%); Diminished performance on tests or projects (27%); Missed classes (31%)

With alcohol misuse alone being responsible for approximately one third of a campus's overall problems, campus leadership should make this issue a high priority to address. High-level attention and visibility must be provided to an issue causing a significant portion of problems. Without this kind of leadership, limited change will likely result. Offering priority attention through the organizational structure and placement within the administrative hierarchy will demonstrate both commitment and visibility for these efforts—and be read as a good-faith effort to change campus culture.

Leadership takes many forms, including instrumental leadership and expressive leadership; each is relevant for individuals and groups. *Instrumental leadership* focuses on tasks, and *expressive leadership* emphasizes process; both shape and reshape the campus culture.

Instrumental leadership, central for goal attainment, focuses on task completion, management, productivity, and results. These individuals, structures, groups, and priorities are focused primarily on the job, with emphasis on direction and planning. Often found is attention to the "status quo" and keeping things running smoothly, prioritizing campus traditions, attending to policies and procedures, and limiting risk taking. Although the achievement of goals and objectives is important, instrumental leaders must take care not to overlook personal engagement and shared ownership.

Expressive leadership emphasizes the people, the process, group cohesion, and quality relationships. With group work, the emphasis is on the agency or group as a whole, and the maintenance of staff and personnel cohesion. Participatory decision making and the well-being of the participants are of central importance. Expressive leaders may be seen as challenging the status quo or traditions. These individuals and groups may test the limits, identify new norms, and redefine the organization's boundaries.

Both types of leadership can shape the campus culture, and each style is essential: Instrumental leadership makes progress with outcomes, and expressive leadership ensures collective engagement throughout the process. Finding ways to engage both types of leadership is central for sustainable change. Anthony Jenkins, in Case Study 2.1, discusses the importance of leadership in change.

CASE STUDY 2.1

Leadership and the Art of Change

Anthony L. Jenkins, PhD
President
Coppin State University

There is no debate that alcohol, drugs, and substance use disorders have a huge impact on public health in the United States, and institutions of higher education are not immune.

According to the Centers for Disease Control and Prevention (2019, 2020), overdose deaths involving prescription opioids reached almost 450,000 between 1999 and 2018. In Florida, opioid-related deaths increased 35% in 2016 alone (Florida Medical Examiners Commission, 2017). In an effort to combat the opioid epidemic, the University of Central Florida (UCF) was among the first universities in the nation to require campus police to carry Narcan.

It is important to note that any effort to address such societal issues on a university campus must include campuswide buy-in at the highest level. Therefore, the president must provide support and clearly communicate that bolstering students who face alcohol- and drug-related challenges is a priority.

At the outset, we grounded our overall efforts at UCF in best practices and supported our students with the appropriate campuswide wrap-around services. We sought to avoid a "one-size-fits-all" approach. We felt it crucial to know the needs of our students and the culture of our campus—as well as what the campus infrastructure could support.

When I helped lead the implementation of the use of Narcan at UCF, my team sought to first understand the implications of our actions. Our goal was to save lives and transform campus into a community that was more caring, forgiving, and supportive. We believed that providing campus police with Narcan was an essential part of our campuswide effort. There were those who opposed our efforts—who suggested that we were fostering a culture of drug use without accountability, and that our plan to implement Narcan sent a message of enabling, not deterring. I disagreed.

For our implementation, we trained our first responders on how to use Narcan, we educated our campus community about the rationale and logistics of our policy, and then we amended our Student Life Conduct Policies to include a medical amnesty clause. Though never intended as a "cure-all," this policy is one part—albeit initially a controversial one—of the full range of services and strategies.

INCULCATING CAMPUS NORMS

The ultimate aim is having a healthy, desirable campus—one that inspires pride in its students, staff, faculty, leaders, and alumni. The overall campus culture and the drug and alcohol culture are part of this aim; each one can enhance or detract from the other. The objective of reducing the gap between the current campus culture and the desired campus culture is both valid and vital. It is useful because it is needs based and goal directed; it is essential because it supports the public mission of the institution of higher education of quality educational experiences.

Leadership moving toward a positive and appropriate change of campus norms must first provide *attention*. Campus leaders must prioritize movement toward a positive, desired campus culture. Though movement will likely be slow, progress can be achieved. Without awareness, no positive action is likely and institutional drift may lead to movement in the less desirable, more problematic direction.

Leaders should emphasize goals that are *deliberate, intentional, and manageable*. The specified outcomes should be clear and attainable and encompassed within a logic model. Various pieces, from policies and programs to training and assessment, should have a reason for inclusion. The role of instrumental leaders is most appropriate here.

It is important to nurture *optimism and hopefulness*. While skepticism ("that's unrealistic") and naysayers ("that's not who we want to be") will exist, a positive, can-do spirit is essential. Change is difficult for institutions generally, and for drug and alcohol issues specifically, for many reasons. Expressive leaders can be most helpful here, as collective support sustains commitment and energy.

Bold leadership is vital for promoting culture change; this includes being outspoken and compelling. Spokespersons can be confident with sound grounding and inclusive planning for the campus efforts. Using the leader's "bully pulpit," vision, passion, strategies, and anticipated results can be shared. Leaders can articulate what they want from individuals and groups and specify how others can demonstrate their support. The nature of this bold leadership is stated succinctly with the title (and within the contents) of the publication *Be Vocal, Be Visible, Be Visionary* (Higher Education Center for Alcohol and Other Drug Abuse and Violence Prevention, 1997).

With regard to leadership, prevention specialists must provide attention to the *Instrumental Trinity*. Generally speaking, this includes the president/provost, the chief student affairs officer, and the student government association. The specific titles vary; nonetheless, it is crucial to have a blend of the top academic or institutional leader, the student affairs professionals, and the students. These key campus constituents must all be supportive of and engaged in the campus prevention effort.

Complementing this trio is the *Expressive Trinity*, which includes student, faculty, and staff disruptors; key stakeholder informants; and social media influencers. Student, faculty, and staff roles may include those individuals who seek a campus culture that aligns with the campus academic and reputational standards. Stakeholder groups may consist of athletics departments, fraternity and sorority members, alumni, community leaders, staff members, and parents. Social media influencers can generate interest in and support for both broad and specific initiatives. Further, although a "trinity" is cited here, prevention specialists should be sure to engage multiple voices and offices representing various constituencies.

Changing campus culture is a *shared responsibility*. Campus prevention strategies should not be "relegated" to one office or individual and not compartmentalized into one division. The primary leadership for guiding the campus efforts may be focused, but the campus effort should, ideally, work like a three-legged stool—all three legs are critical.

This is true for the Instrumental Trinity as well as for the Expressive Trinity. It is upon the legs of those two stools that the orchestration of the campus effort can occur.

Also essential is the *visibility* of the campus prevention effort. Because drug and alcohol problems are prominent and visible and also counterproductive to the attainment of overall campus aims and individuals' goals, the campus prevention effort should not be hidden or buried within a department. Campus leaders should be very intentional about its placement, as that placement communicates the priority, particularly during a time of focused attention to culture change. If the institution has a vice president for wellness issues, then this office may be an appropriate setting. Absent that, consider collaborative reporting relationships, such as to the chief student affairs officer as well as to the president, chancellor, or provost. This is akin to the role of an ombudsperson, with direct reporting to the top campus administrator.

Finally, *accountability* is critical for culture change. Action plans typically incorporate clearly defined roles and responsibilities, as well as activities, timelines, and evaluative criteria and metrics. The attention to sound, efficient decision-making and implementation systems incorporates individual and group responsibilities and follow-up efforts. Accountability can also incorporate the extent to which the measurable objectives were attained, what contributed to or hindered their attainment, the impact of communication efforts, the consistency of implementing policies and procedures, the receptivity of different audiences to various strategies, and the engagement of key participants and stakeholders.

Collectively, these nine factors change the campus culture; this is an action-oriented approach focused on change. To instill new norms, prevention specialists must consider new strategies, grounded in science and sound practice. The nine steps identified in the planning model of Chapter 10 will guide campus leaders through a useful, rigorous process for organizing or reorganizing the campus prevention effort. Dolores Cimini, in Innovator 2.1, gives a long-term perspective. Her tips about innovation provide practical approaches that can be adapted and expanded upon by prevention specialists and other campus leaders as they work collectively to create the desired campus culture.

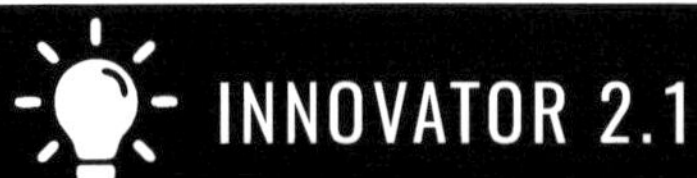

Driving Innovation in Prevention Work

M. Dolores Cimini, PhD
Psychologist and Director
University at Albany

When I began my career as a prevention professional 3 decades ago, I made many of my choices based on an instinct that what I was implementing would reduce AOD misuse among students. After all, who could resist the power of a fraternity member or student-athlete who spoke about taking a friend's life while driving under the influence of alcohol? Who would not reduce their substance use immediately upon witnessing a crashed car in the middle of our residence quadrangle, walking into a trailer containing an exhibit of the personal effects of a college student who died from a heroin overdose, or spending an hour sitting in a mock jail cell to experience some of what it's like after a drug arrest?

Although my instincts were well intentioned—and such initiatives do have a place within a comprehensive, multicomponent effort based on a public health approach—effectiveness is not defined by the above strategies. We, as preventionists, have a responsibility to our campuses and communities to think carefully about our choice of strategies and programs, to integrate evidence-based or evidence-informed practices in the campus strategy, and to embrace innovation.

We must remember that innovation in prevention begins with good ideas that are developed using what we have learned from prevention science; they are delivered using clearly defined protocols, implemented with fidelity, and evaluated regarding how well they work. Following are tips for selecting, implementing, and evaluating prevention strategies.

Seek innovation. The prevention field has identified both efficacious and promising strategies that result in significant reductions in AOD misuse and related consequences. Be an eager and engaged consumer of research, and do not hesitate to consult researchers and practitioners in the prevention field who have developed, implemented, and tested innovative strategies about evidence of efficacy.

Tailor what is innovative to meet your campus needs. When implementing innovative strategies on college campuses, prevention specialists must remember that "one size does not fit all." Adaptations or modifications may be needed, based on student demographics, availability of resources, and other factors. When making such adaptations to programs and strategies, prevention specialists must develop and document the protocols employed, implement them with fidelity, and not stray very far from the original intervention study protocols from which effectiveness was demonstrated.

Recruit partners in innovation. In evaluating the fit of evidence-based programs (EBPs) and strategies for their campuses, many preventionists have found it helpful to partner with faculty members who have experience in research methodology. These colleagues can assist in designing evaluation protocols to determine whether the implemented EBPs are working. Faculty colleagues in this role often benefit from partnerships with prevention practitioners by being able to collect data for publications necessary to advance their own careers.

> Driving innovation in AOD prevention is not easy, nor is the journey straightforward. With a spirit of inquiry and a bit of persistence, we can take significant steps forward in identifying what works in addressing AOD misuse—and translate these strategies into practices that change the lives of students and promote a healthy campus community.

CONCLUSION

Central to campus AOD prevention efforts is attention to the campus culture as a whole—what each institution of higher education stands for. Through valid assessment methods, campus leaders can ascertain how their campus and its culture are viewed by various constituencies—and what is important moving forward. Attending to the culture at the institutional as well as subgroup levels supports grounded and locally appropriate campus prevention efforts. Learning how challenges to social order are perceived undergirds thoughtful processes for campus efforts. Understanding instrumental and expressive leadership roles permits engaged planning efforts. Taking into account nine factors for action ultimately changes the campus culture in desired directions.

REFERENCES

Allen, I. E., & Seaman, J. (2013). *Changing course: Ten years of tracking online education in the United States.* https://files.eric.ed.gov/fulltext/ED541571.pdf

Anderson, D. S., & Santos, G. M. (2018). *College alcohol survey: The national longitudinal survey on alcohol, tobacco, other drug and violence issues at institutions of higher education*. George Mason University.

Centers for Disease Control and Prevention. (2019). *Annual surveillance report of drug-related risks and outcomes: United States, 2019.* https://www.cdc.gov/drugoverdose/pdf/pubs/2019-cdc-drug-surveillance-report.pdf

Centers for Disease Control and Prevention. (2020). *Opioid data analysis and resources.* https://www.cdc.gov/drugoverdose/data/analysis.html

Florida Medical Examiners Commission. (2017). *2016* annual report. http://www.fdle.state.fl.us/MEC/Publications-and-Forms/Documents/Annual-Workload-Reports/2016-Annual-Workload-Report.aspx

Higher Education Center for Alcohol and Other Drug Abuse and Violence Prevention. (1997). *Be vocal, be visible, be visionary.* https://safesupportivelearning.ed.gov/sites/default/files/sssta/20130315_plgvisionary.pdf

Jernigan, D., Shields, K., Mitchell, M., & Arria, A. (2019). Assessing campus alcohol policies: Measuring accessibility, clarity, and effectiveness. *Alcoholism: Clinical and Experimental Research, 43*(5), 1007–1015.

Kugler, K. (2017). Optimization of online substance use interventions targeting college students. *Annals of Behavioral Medicine, 51*(Suppl. 1), p. S2350.

Lee, K. (2017). Rethinking the accessibility of online higher education: A historical review. *Internet and Higher Education, 33,* 15–23. http://dx.doi.org/10.1016/j.iheduc.2017.01.001

Perrotta, K. (2020). Getting HIP: A study on the implementation of asynchronous discussion boards as a high-impact practice in online undergraduate survey history courses. *The Journal of Social Studies Research, 44,* 209–217. https://doi.org/10.1016/j.jssr.2020.02.001

Verduin, J. R., & Clark, T. A. (1991). *Distance education: The foundations of effective practices*. Jossey-Bass.

Walden University. (2020). *MyWalden University portal.* https://my.waldenu.edu/portal/c/19655.htm

CHAPTER 3

Organization and Frameworks

"As a kid growing up with older family members with past alcohol issues, I knew that my experiences in college would be similar to those I grew up around. I did not want to fall into the same position they had been in, and they had advised me to do so. Being responsible for yourself is a big step that mostly every student will face throughout their journey, and learning how to consume is one of those big steps."

—Sophomore at a public Midwest college

Substantive grounding and an appropriate organizational structure are essential for an effective prevention effort. These foundational elements will permeate all aspects of the prevention initiatives, from the rationale, theory, and planning processes to final review. Although decisions and plans are local and prepared based on relevant circumstances, common and clear conceptual foundations allow for maximized success.

Constructing a house, a road, or an office building all require general and more detailed plans in the form of blueprints, and campus prevention planning should take a similar approach. It is essential to establish the aims, identify parameters, specify strategies and timelines, and incorporate needed resources and personnel. No one expects a plan of "ready, fire, aim" to succeed; therefore, the desired course of action should be more intentional and have a grounded process with sound thinking and shared goals.

Essential as a starting point is ensuring the campus prevention effort is grounded with a sound theoretical basis and having a clearly defined conceptual framework. These elements are complemented by the organizational structure, crucial for garnering support from various aspects of the institution. This vital preparation work helps with strategic aims and institutionalization of quality services.

This conceptual and theoretical grounding is brought to life by four contributions from professionals working on these issues for decades. The *CAS Professional Standards for Higher Education* overview offers a case study about an important framework. Two Lessons From the Field segments provide insights—one about the role of faculty members and the other about having a positive focus. Richard Lucey, highlighted in this chapter as an Innovator, discusses three constructs surrounding innovation for campus prevention specialists.

THE ROLE OF THEORY

A theoretical foundation is central to campus drug and alcohol prevention efforts. Currently, many campus efforts do not have an articulated theory undergirding their actions; this may be due to lack of comfort with theories by those leading the effort, boredom by participants when discussing theory, limited time for development or preparation, or perceived irrelevance by key players. Although no single best approach exists to address drug and alcohol issues, a sound theory is essential for shaping or redirecting the campus efforts. In short, theory helps guide practice.

As prevention specialists organize and prioritize strategies, they must first address the foundations of the effort. As, ostensibly, societal and cultural leaders in critical thinking and sound decision making, professionals in higher education institutions must prepare substantiated initiatives with ethical and theoretical foundations; to do otherwise is unwise, unsound, and, in fact, hypocritical.

Planning efforts are guided by logic models, which are implicitly based in theory. Prevention specialists must articulate why they believe that implementing a particular strategy will result in a specific outcome. No single approach is specified as the "best" one, as there are specialties in college student development, young adult theory, and adolescent development. Beyond population-focused theories, others exist in organization, management structures, planned change, and interpersonal relationships. Further, psychological, sociological, and anthropological theories may be useful; examples include behavioral- and nonbehavioral-based approaches. Specific methods include the social-ecological model, the health belief model, the transtheoretical model, social norms theory, social capital theory, transformational leadership, student engagement theory, or the social change model for leadership development. The entire approach of positive youth behavior is worthy of consideration. Regardless of the theory selected to undergird a prevention effort for drug and/or alcohol use, linkages and assumptions embedded in the logic model are vital. Further, blending theories is appropriate. For example, a strategy may specifically use the transtheoretical model (and focus on the contemplation stage) and integrate it with the health belief model (and emphasize perceived benefits and self-efficacy).

As part of the theoretical grounding, consider the role of evidence-based practices. Campus prevention specialists and their allies seek to implement strategies that work, and several specialists, as well as funders, specify that evidence-based practices must be used; however, many prevention specialists adopt an evidence-based approach without first assessing its fit or suitability for the unique, current, local needs. Adaptation, innovation, and theoretical foundations are all important factors for effective campus efforts.

Helpful for blending the theoretical underpinnings, the logic model, and evidence-based practices is the construct of "best fit." Prevention specialists benefit from seeking the most appropriate approaches for their local needs and issues. As the Substance Abuse and Mental Health Services Administration (SAMHSA; 2018) explained: "The best candidates for inclusion in a community's comprehensive prevention plan are programs and practices with a strong conceptual fit, practical fit, and evidence of effectiveness" (p. 5). Similarly, the National Academies of Sciences, Engineering, and Medicine (2019) cited the importance of local customization of efforts. With this in mind, and with rapidly changing needs and audiences, SAMHSA (2018) acknowledged the role of innovation: "Innovation, like any other prevention-related decision and effort, should be based in evidence. While a new program or practice cannot be deemed evidence-based until after it has been evaluated for effectiveness, it can and should be evidence-informed" (p. 13). Thus, as new issues with opioids, stimulants, high-risk drinking, marijuana, or other substances emerge, new or adapted efforts to address them are appropriate.

Further, considering that many specialists are working with Generation Z students, strategies that capture their learning styles and influence factors should be implemented. Thus, while evidence-based practices can help inform local decision making, they should not constrain or limit campus efforts. Instead, theory-based approaches are essential to guide the planning and the strategies.

PREVENTION THEORIES

The key feature of campus efforts that address drug and alcohol issues is prevention. Essentially, prevention encompasses strategies that reduce the incidence of engagement with drugs and alcohol. Clarity regarding "what" is being prevented is essential; this may be usage, harm, illegality, negative consequences, or increased problems. SAMHSA (2019) made clear that prevention practice is "a type of approach, technique, or strategy . . . intended to prevent initiation or escalation of substance use" (p. 5).

Prevention is embedded within the *continuum of care*, which attends to the general nature of services provided. With *prevention*, the focus is to address behavior before any use occurs. It seeks to delay the initiation of substance use and to prevent harms associated with it. *Intervention* is often needed to halt or reduce problematic use, such as harmful behavior of an acute nature (e.g., someone attempting to drive a vehicle while impaired by drugs or alcohol) or of a more progressive, longer term nature (e.g., referral for counseling and potentially for treatment services). *Treatment* may follow and includes individual and group counseling, self-help, mutual aid, medication, life skills development, and education. *After-care and recovery* follows, with a focus on reducing the likelihood of relapse after treatment for a substance use disorder, and continues in various forms for the rest of one's life. It includes self-help groups such as Alcoholics Anonymous and Narcotics Anonymous.

Complementing this understanding of prevention is the distinction between *prevention* and *promotion.* Prevention seeks to keep down the negative; it emphasizes what one does not want to see (i.e., use, injury, death, harm, negative consequences). It is complemented by what one wants to promote; this is what one does want to see (i.e., healthy decisions, self-esteem, positive attitude, confidence, quality interpersonal relationships). With prevention, these two elements go hand in hand, as the latter helps with resiliency skills and protective factors. Jeff Linkenbach's Lessons From the Field 3.1 contains strategies for emphasizing promotion with a positive approach.

Considerations regarding the supply and demand framework, often used in economics, is helpful for demonstrating the interplay between availability and desire for a substance. As availability is increased and drugs/alcohol are easier to obtain (i.e., supply), usage (i.e., demand) often goes up at the same time. Thus, to reduce usage, approaches to reduce supply often include environmental strategies, such as limiting access, reducing hours of availability, limiting advertising, specifying conditions for use (e.g., setting, age, identification), increasing costs, and managing distribution. To reduce demand, attention focuses primarily on the individual; these include factors such as increasing knowledge, promoting resiliency skills, limiting enticements, reducing interest, encouraging values-oriented reflection, and promoting attractive and available alternatives (e.g., activities, events, beverages, food). Attention to both the supply and demand side of the equation is important.

Several other theories and constructs can support prevention efforts, and three are highlighted here. In terms of strategies, the health belief model (Becker & Rosenstock, 1984; Hochbaum, 1958) is most useful. To obtain receptivity (and ultimately action) by targeted audiences, prevention specialists benefit from considering this model's six elements. *Perceived susceptibility* addresses the extent to which one believes they may be affected by a situation or condition. *Perceived severity* focuses on how extreme or damaging the consequences would be if affected. *Perceived benefits* illustrates the potential constructive outcomes that can be achieved by taking action. *Perceived barriers* focuses on what might be in the way of taking action, including costs of a financial, intellectual, physical, emotional, or social nature. *Cues to action* is what helps suggest and encourage taking action, and *self-efficacy* focuses on one's confidence for moving forward. With Worksheet 3.1: Action Framework Based on the Health Belief Model, those organizing the campus effort, including its communication components, will find a tool for determining specific areas of focus for campus strategies.

Complementing the health belief model is the stages of change or transtheoretical model (Prochaska & DiClemente, 1983), an approach that considers individuals' or groups' patterns of use and attends to an individual's readiness for change when determining strategies. The first stage, *precontemplation,* acknowledges no intention of making change, including lack of awareness, limited applicability, or denial of need. *Contemplation* follows with consideration of the desirability and feasibility of change, due to awareness, greater motivation, or desire to depart the current state of affairs. *Preparation* involves making plans for movement and change; this stage includes goals and action plans. *Action* follows with the actual shift in behavior; this includes the need for feedback, reassurance, and review of challenges. *Maintenance* is the continuation, ideally forever, of the changed behavior, so support and validation of the change are important. For some, however, *relapse* occurs, and a return to earlier stages of the model are required. Worksheet 3.2: Stages of Change Worksheet provides a summary overview of this model's components, and helps campus planners organize their change strategies.

The commonly cited framework of universal, selective, and indicated approaches constitutes the "prevention" part of the overall model prepared by the Institute of Medicine (IOM; Springer & Phillips, 2007); it is this framework that serves as the primary focus for this book and around which prevention planners can organize thoughts and efforts. Although some elements of the IOM's continuum of care

are incorporated in this volume, its primary focus is on the prevention aspect of this "protractor," illustrated in Figure 3.1.

Figure 3.1
The IOM "Protractor"

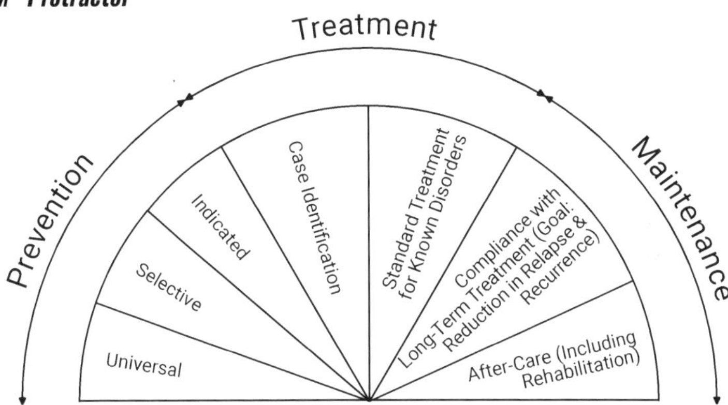

Note. Reprinted from *The Institute of Medicine Framework and its Implication for the Advancement of Prevention Policy, Programs and Practice* (p. 3), by J. R. Springer and J. Phillips, 2007, U.S. Department of Health and Human Services (http://ca-sdfsc.org/docs/resources/SDFSC_IOM_Policy.pdf). In the public domain.

Within the prevention segment are three components. *Universal* approaches address the entire audience, including students, faculty, and staff. Also within this type of approach may be a campus policy, an informational campaign, training activities, educational efforts, or other services. *Selective* approaches may consist of many of the same content elements. Still, the focus is a subset such as first-year students, fraternity and sorority members, student-athletes, student government leaders, residence hall staff, students preparing to graduate, or other focused groups. It may also encompass faculty, or alumni, or owners of shops, restaurants, and bars near campus.

The groups may be identified because of actual or potential risk factors or for enhanced engagement opportunities. The *indicated* grouping is more specific and is typically based on an incident or problem (e.g., alcohol poisoning, drug overdose, hospital admission, impaired driving arrest). This stage will involve assessment and, potentially, some treatment services. Overall, the framework helps campus organizers allocate limited resources and personnel time and maximize the likelihood of success for individuals and groups. Campus planners can use Worksheet 3.3: Prevention Task Force Planning Guide to determine ways of best applying the IOM framework for campus efforts.

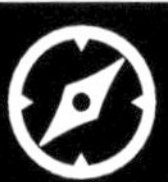

LESSONS FROM THE FIELD 3.1

Seven Steps for Positive Cultural Transformation

Jeff Linkenbach, EdD
Director
The Montana Institute

The Montana seven-step model has been fostering positive campus and community cultures for 3 decades (Linkenbach, 2003). The seven steps first emerged through a focus on "re-norming" fraternity and sorority alcohol and drug use (Linkenbach, 1991); they were later revised to become the foundation for social norms marketing and then the positive community norms approach to prevention (Linkenbach, 2019). These basic steps have been applied to a wide array of topics, including substance abuse, domestic and campus violence, traffic safety, and more (Linkenbach et al., 2012).

1. **Plan and advocate.** Form a coalition and include a broad array of campus and community stakeholders. The coalition then develops a common core identity by developing seven core principles based on the science of the positive framework (Linkenbach, 2007). These principles then guide both internal and external planning and advocacy.

2. **Assess cultures**. As vibrant environments rich with diverse cultures and communities, campuses identify and define numerous cultural norms to reveal baseline measures and opportunities.
3. **Establish a common frame and prioritize opportunities**. Recurring themes establish a common frame for fostering transformation. This common frame may reveal perceptions and misperceptions; further, fostering stakeholder engagement will reveal critical gaps in attitudes and behaviors, helpful for prioritizing opportunities.
4. **Develop a portfolio of strategies.** A portfolio of strategies can be developed appropriate for different campus–community cultures. Each strategy should be based on the best available science regarding cultural sensitivity, effectiveness, and outcomes.
5. **Pilot test and refine.** Strategies and messages must be respectful of different cultures; pilot testing, rapid-return research, and demonstration projects are vital and optimize outcomes.
6. **Implement portfolio strategies.** Strategies are implemented broadly across the campus and community systems, with ongoing monitoring and feedback. Maintaining close contact with stakeholders in the coalition is critical for success.
7. **Evaluate effectiveness and needs.** The process of cultural transformation is never complete; with every cycle, new opportunities to improve campus health and safety will be revealed and inform future efforts. Returning to planning and advocacy (Step 1) offers new insights and wisdom from engaging in the seven-step cycle.

THE ROLE OF PLANNING FRAMEWORKS

Just as having theoretical foundations are important, a planning framework is critical to organize, guide, and focus the campus efforts. This structure allows prevention specialists to operate in an organized way—essential for maximizing efficiencies and increasing the likelihood of reaching desired outcomes. Consistent within the construct of "planned change," a framework avoids involvement in unorganized, disparate, unplanned, and unfocused change efforts.

Having such a framework not only organizes and establishes the prevention efforts with sound theoretical and conceptual grounding, but also allows specialists to review assets, resources, and challenges. With an organized process, stakeholders, intermediaries, academic departments, and personnel can be engaged in meaningful ways; these individuals and groups can also gain a broader understanding of substance use prevention issues and generate potential win–win scenarios for programming, research, and services. Built-in review processes for outcomes and processes as well as lessons learned and refinement of assumptions, strategies, measures, and more can be incorporated into future efforts.

Currently, personnel preparing campus efforts have limited specified resources. Campus administrators report moderate use of existing resources and guidelines (Anderson & Santos, 2018), including the National Institute on Alcohol Abuse and Alcoholism's (NIAAA's) *College AIM–College Alcohol Intervention Matrix*, the *CAS Professional Standards for Higher Education*, and other indices of best practices. Further details about the CAS standards are highlighted in Case Study 3.1 by Jennifer Wells and Laura Dean.

Prevention specialists' planning efforts are best served by several fundamental approaches and resources. Blending them, with attention to local needs and styles, will help specialists orchestrate their campus strategies. Campus leaders will benefit from reviewing these resources and others to determine where they best fit and deliver the most impact. Incorporating them within the step-by-step approach in Chapter 10 will further enhance campus outcomes.

When organizing the campus effort, prevention specialists benefit from drawing upon the theories discussed here as well as additional, complementary frameworks. For example, with the construct of indicated prevention (Chapter 7) is the screening brief intervention and referral to treatment model as well as BASICS; the *IMPACT Evaluation Resource* could aid with evaluation efforts (Chapter 9).

One key framework, the social-ecological model (Centers for Disease Control and Prevention, 2020) focuses on both the individual and the population, addressing dynamic interactions and interrelations among various elements affecting individuals' behaviors. Its premise is that because behavior has many influencers, interventions must also be planned at several levels. The first level is the *individual*, concentrating primarily on knowledge, attitudes, and skills. It incorporates one's genetic background and physical composition and strength (which can be altered harmfully, and made more vulnerable, by factors such as poor diet, limited exercise, stress and lack of sleep). *Interpersonal* factors encompass family, peers, mentors, and other relationships. Third, *institutional* factors address school and workplace; for college students, this area includes their previous as well as current settings. Fourth, *community* consists of the social and physical environment as well as activities and local norms. Finally, *policy* includes the larger structure of economics, health, education, and societal mores; this includes laws, rules, regulations, and procedures.

A well-established approach, SAMHSA's (2017) strategic prevention framework (SPF) has been used for decades by communities and organizations. Its five steps begin with *assessment*, which identifies needs, issues, and opportunities and emphasizes gathering locally appropriate information of both a quantitative and qualitative nature. *Capacity*, SPF's second step, looks at the local resources and assets, as well as the organization's readiness to change (per the stages of change model); these resources include personnel, structures, policies, and support systems. Third, *planning* identifies approaches and strategies incorporated within the context of a localized logic model; planning ensures efforts are targeted for cost effectiveness and impact. *Implementation* includes the actual delivery of the planned approaches, including steps and resource allocation. Finally, *evaluation* reviews outcomes and processes, including what results were achieved, what strategies were used and how they were received, and ways in which all efforts, including documentation and measures, can be improved. These steps center on *cultural competence* (attending to different needs of various groups) as well as *sustainability* (or institutionalization over the long term). Worksheet 3.4: Strategic Prevention Framework provides an outline of this tool's keep components and helps with planning appropriate campus initiatives.

Prepared by the Drug Enforcement Administration (2020), the *Strategic Planning Guide* applies the SPF for colleges and universities. Its detailed applications and resources are organized around five steps. The first step is to *assess*, stressing primary and secondary effects of substance misuse and reviewing risk and protective factors. Second, *build capacity* gives attention to individuals and groups, including stakeholders and allies. *Plan,* the third step, prioritizes efforts and thoughtful planning of appropriate evidence-based efforts. Fourth, *implement,* enacts the effort with attention to consistency and the continued engagement of stakeholders. *Evaluate,* the final step, deals with process and outcome evaluation and use of results.

CollegeAIM, prepared by the NIAAA (2019), dovetails with the social-ecological model. *CollegeAIM* has collated published research on strategies addressing college students' misuse of alcohol and is organized broadly into two constructs: *individual* and *environmental*. Prevention specialists can review potential strategies based on costs (lower, mid-range, and higher), effectiveness (higher, moderate, lower, not effective, and too few studies to rate), public health reach (broad or focused), barriers (higher, moderate, lower), primary modality (in-person individual, in-person group, online, or office), and research amount (based on the number of studies). Worksheet 3.5: *CollegeAIM* Strategy Planning Worksheet provides a tool that applies this resource.

These frameworks and constructs are all worthy of consideration by prevention specialists as they develop locally appropriate logic models for their campus efforts. These various theoretical and planning frameworks can guide the discussion when specialists prepare to organize their campus effort via the step-by-step model (Chapter 10). Such an ordered process will structure and guide the process and inform decisions along the way. Although such preparation requires a significant investment of time and effort, it is essential for impact in the short and long term.

CASE STUDY 3.1

Using Professional Standards to Guide Practice and Assessment

Jennifer B. Wells, PhD
Assistant Professor
Kennesaw State University

Laura A. Dean, PhD
Professor
University of Georgia

One of the challenges in working to create grounded and effective programs and services for students is figuring out what should be included, how things should be structured, and what considerations are most important in each area. The term *best practice* is often invoked—but with little evidence about what constitutes "best." The Council for the Advancement of Standards in Higher Education (CAS) was created to define standards of practice that can be used to guide the development, administration, and evaluation of programs, services, and graduate programs in student affairs.

Built on a philosophy of self-assessment, the *CAS Professional Standards for Higher Education* (CAS, 2019) and associated materials have been created and updated for 47 functional areas, each with broad input, vetted by experts, and designed to be applied in light of the specific, local context in which they are used. This interdepartmental, interprogram collaboration characterizes both the creation of the standards and the recommended approach for those working on campus.

The Alcohol and Other Drug Programs (AODP) standards and guidelines were originally developed in 1990 with the assistance of many collegiate organizations. AODP has since been revised and updated several times (1997, 2003, and 2013) with the continued assistance of expert and practitioner feedback. The focus of AODP is on diversifying and enhancing campus prevention efforts, including both programming and interventions. The standards offer guidance about a range of areas, including the program's mission, goals, specific services, structure, intended outcomes, access, equity, leadership and staffing, collaborations, ethical and legal issues, policies, finance, technology, and facilities.

As an example, one standard statement is: "AODP must develop, provide, and advocate strategies that model practical applications of prevention theories and research results and that are evidence-based or evidence informed such as environmental approaches, risk reduction approaches, brief interventions, and student support programs" (CAS, 2019, p. 42). The specific strategies are left up to the judgment of the campus practitioners, with the clear expectation that they will be solidly grounded. Thus, the CAS standards can be used to provide guidance in both creating and assessing strong, grounded, and effective programs. "Sound standards guide leadership, and in turn, leadership guides organizations and communities. That is why the effective and meaningful frameworks offered through CAS are so important to prevention efforts" (CAS, 2019, p. 41).

ORGANIZATION AND STAFFING

One of the primary considerations for prevention specialists is how to provide leadership for and organize the overall campus initiative. As decisions are made about what strategies are appropriate for inclusion in the campus's efforts, issues of staffing and resources are integral. Using the processes outlined with the step-by-step planning framework in Chapter 10, specialists can determine the necessary and desired functions of the campus-based initiative to address drug and alcohol issues. Although the phrase "form follows function" typically applies to architecture, it is also valid here; the specific responsibilities, skills, and attributes (i.e., the form) will be based on the strategies and services (i.e., the function) needed to address—most effectively and most appropriately—the needs of the campus.

Central to this issue of organizing the campus effort is coordination. Depending on the size of the institution and the resources allocated for prevention efforts, coordination may be handled by an individual and/or office. Currently, the vast majority (87%) of 4-year institutions have a designated alcohol/substance abuse educator or specialist (Anderson & Santos, 2018).

With the "form follows function" construct, decisions among top administrators will be based on how much of a problem drugs and alcohol are, how seriously they want to address it, and what they envision for the desired campus culture generally and vis-à-vis substance issues. For historical context, in 1998 the Inter-Association Task Force on Alcohol and Substance Abuse Issues, the predecessor of the Coalition of Higher Education Associations for Substance Abuse Prevention (n.d.), held a national policy conference. A proposal made there, which was narrowly defeated in a vote by those in attendance, called for one full-time professional for every 4,000 students. With campuses of 20,000 students, for example, this proposal would result in five professional staff members, an allocation that makes sense based on the varied responsibilities and attributes needed to manage effectively comprehensive campus efforts.

The challenges with organizing and leading the campus drug and alcohol prevention effort is further compounded by the range of diverse roles and responsibilities held by campus coordinators. Currently, these coordinators' time allocations for different functions shows the following: education (33%), counseling (15%), administrative (14%), assessment (12%), training (10%), task force (8%), research (6%), and other (2%; Anderson & Santos, 2018). Similarly, other time is spent on various topics: alcohol (36%), violence (30%), wellness (17%), drugs (11%), and tobacco (6%; Anderson & Santos, 2018). These numbers illustrate the reality that personnel leading campus programs on drug/alcohol issues need to manage myriad responsibilities with varying skill sets. Clearly, an opportunity exists for prevention specialists, in consultation with campus leaders, to clarify the extent to which various elements should and should not be part of the campus strategy.

One significant consideration with having a coordinating point person or office is that this person or office should not be seen as "the doer of all efforts." All too often, this coordinator or office does it all; in some senses, this role becomes a dumping ground. Although inevitably that individual/office will possess a preponderance of specialized skills, the main role must be that of coordination. It is appropriate to have a central organizing individual or unit, and that leadership encompasses the coordination of a broad range of personnel, offices, resources, and strategies.

A related issue is where to house the campus drug and alcohol prevention effort. Because drugs and alcohol are involved with so many problems facing students, it is incumbent upon the institution's leadership to position the prevention effort within the organizational hierarchy in an accountable and influential way. Essentially, to avoid being "buried" or relegated to a token placement, the prevention effort should have its organizational reporting at a very high level. This leadership should be visible, as its success is vitally important to the future and the success of both students and the institution. It is reasonable to have this effort as a direct report to the chief student affairs officer (CSAO); if the campus has a high-level wellness executive parallel to the CSAO, then perhaps have the position report there or jointly to the CSAO. Often, however, prevention leadership is housed within the health center, counseling center, or residence life office—and then it may be further located within a wellness office or initiative. Though such placement is conceptually sound, the de facto consequence is that drug/alcohol issues become buried. With regard to the concept of form follows function, campus decision makers must decide how *best* to achieve the aims of visibility and impact (function) with the organizational placement decisions (form).

It is likewise important to have a steering committee that serves as the core leadership group. With representation from key campus offices and stakeholders, students, and potentially the surrounding community, this group will give direction, advice, and support for the campus effort. Details on various configurations and considerations are provided in Chapter 10.

A peer-based component (whether as peer educators, peer advisors, peer helpers, or peer advocates) is a critical organizational element. This approach not only can be cost-effective but also can serve a valuable role in its impact on students. Students respond well to the messages, insights, and voices of other students, particularly those peers who are well trained and passionate about their work. This role goes beyond merely having students "at the table" when decisions are made (as highlighted in Chapter 4); the impact on the peer educators themselves, in terms of their education and self-esteem, is an equally important consideration and has been well established with the helper therapy principle (Reissman, 1965).

Beyond issues associated with organizational placement and staffing, funding for campus drug and alcohol prevention work, excluding personnel, currently totals $4.10 per student annually (Anderson & Santos, 2018). At the Inter-Association Task Force Policy Conference in 1998 noted earlier, the recommended funding was $2 per student per semester for programming, and $0.50 per student per year for evaluation, totaling $4.50 per student annually; this would be $7.06 per student in today's money.

Ultimately, coordination, collaboration, and resources help the campus effort succeed and thrive. The nature of this effort is necessarily based on the unique characteristics, history, and culture of each institution, so different approaches will be used in different schools.

GARNERING SUPPORT

Central to the success of the campus drug/alcohol prevention effort is high-level institutional support. Not only do substance abuse issues cause a disproportionate amount of campus problems, they also are atop reported areas of concern for campus presidents and chancellors. Thus, substantive support for prevention efforts is warranted. This support can involve minimal effort on leadership's part; what is essential is that attention is paid to providing visible support and to minimizing perceived or unintentional resistance.

The following strategies will help garner campus leaders' support:

1. **Link the effort to the institution's mission statement.** Show how these efforts are consistent with and supportive of the campus's overall aims. When mission statements or core components get revised, seek engagement from various sources to elevate the inclusion of substance abuse prevention.
2. **Gather information that documents current needs as well as results achieved.** Include both quantitative data and qualitative insights, such as compelling stories and scenarios designed to illustrate the importance of the campus effort.
3. **Solicit support from various parts of the campus and community.** Demonstrate the value of both cross-campus collaboration and the effort overall.
4. **Have others serve as advocates.** Faculty members, key administrators, student leaders, and community leaders are key influencers.
5. **Seek opportunities to brief the president/chancellor as well as the institution's governing body.** Address the nature of the issue, the institution's efforts, remaining needs, and vision. Include briefing documents and testimonials.
6. **Provide regular updates to various constituencies.** Cite the variety of issues and opportunities surrounding drug and alcohol abuse.

7. **Reinforce the broader societal context regarding campus needs and issues.** Consider the institution's leadership role in the community and society.
8. **Appeal to logos, pathos, and ethos.** Highlight the logical, data-driven strategy, the heart-strings of decision making, and the incorporation of the "right" approaches.

Again, no single best approach exists for garnering support from the institution's leadership personnel. Gathering support from multiple places can demonstrate to campus leadership the effort's importance and relevance. In Lessons From the Field 3.2, Tavis Glassman provides additional insight about engaging faculty members with campus prevention efforts.

LESSONS FROM THE FIELD 3.2

Role of Faculty With Prevention on Campus

Tavis Glassman, PhD
Professor
School of Population Health
University of Toledo

The role of faculty involvement in college health represents a tremendous opportunity to expand prevention efforts. All too often, health promotion initiatives on campus are underfunded and understaffed. Even among the best-funded programs, the health issues are so complex and vast that additional support and expertise is invariably needed. Further, with the fiscal challenges looming in higher education, many programs—prevention and otherwise—will suffer from budget cuts affecting staff members and what little discretionary or operating money they might have.

Rebound effects will then likely occur, since health issues will not be addressed in a prevention or health promotion manner, thus increasing the nature, severity, and costs of problems.

Thus, the need to collaborate and share resources is evident. Prevention and health promotion leaders benefit from working with faculty in several ways. One example is for prevention specialists to create internships for students who want experience working in college health. Another example is engaging faculty as specialists with theoretical grounding, strategic planning, marketing and messaging, and evaluation or program design. Third, many opportunities exist for research for the faculty and their students.

More extensive collaboration can be obtained with a graduate assistant (GA) from an academic program working with health promotion staff; the health promotion department could pay the GA stipend, while the academic program or college provides a tuition waiver. This mutual investment can be a game-changer for all. With joint supervision of the GA, the professor leads the intervention/research activity(s)—that is, research methods and data analysis—and the prevention professionals manage the day-to-day activities and administrative duties. The student could assist the professor with a health-related class, thus imparting to the student content knowledge. The graduate assistant would augment preexisting prevention efforts, and faculty with expertise could aid health promotion specialist(s) to ensure evidence-based, theory-driven interventions are conducted to maximize return on investment.

INSTITUTIONALIZATION

Campus drug and alcohol abuse prevention efforts must have ongoing initiatives. This need has existed for a long time and is embedded deep within the campus culture. Although substance abuse issues can never be solved, per se, they can be managed much better. Solutions lie in the process and boast both shared responsibility and a long-term comprehensive plan. Effectively addressing drug and alcohol abuse issues can be integral to the life and health of the institution and its students.

Prevention specialists' efforts for institutionalization dovetail with gaining support from the campus's top administrators. With strategic planning efforts that are well-organized and inclusive, and with thorough documentation and review processes in place, prevention specialists are much more likely to achieve greater permanence with the overall initiative. Having a blend of short-term results and longer-term impact, and sharing these results, helps with the desired campus culture change.

Basing campus efforts in theory and employing quality planning processes aid with institutionalization. The planning, based on a logic model, includes anticipated connections between aims and strategies and outcomes. The collaborative nature of the campus efforts, with the steering committee and advisory bodies, and as a type of ganglion effort with outreach, networks, and relationships, can be useful for long-term integration.

Throughout the efforts of planning and implementing the campus strategies, prevention specialists must continually maintain vigilance with documentation and reporting of results. Collecting data, performing needs assessments, and monitoring feedback will help specialists ensure that efforts are relevant and on track. These review processes monitor the evolution of student needs, changing norms, and learning and socialization styles; they also attend to changes with substances and substance use patterns. Leaders should remember the lag between innovation and practice. In science, the dissemination of innovation can stretch for a decade or longer. For example, many of the strategies currently labeled as evidence based were studied 10 or more years ago. Traditional evidence-informed strategies do not control for emerging technologies. Campus prevention strategies require continual review and revision to remain relevant.

This focus on institutionalization creates a greater permanence for campus prevention efforts. The "target" is broad and keeps evolving; substantive attention, in an institutionalized way, helps with maintaining effectiveness and significance. With the turnover of staff, faculty, and student leaders, and with changing student needs and issues, campus prevention goals are more likely to be achieved with organized, consistent, and institutionalized initiatives.

Of course, institutionalization does not mean stagnation; rather, it focuses on permanence and importance. Part of that process is about staying relevant—and doing that requires innovation. Richard Lucey, who brings decades of experience working on drug and alcohol issues in the collegiate environment at both the state and federal levels, dives into this point in Innovator 3.1.

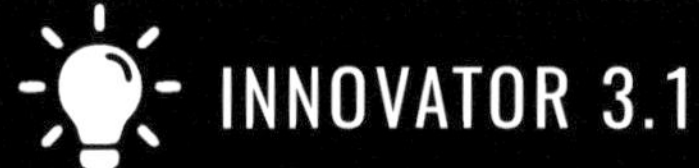

Innovation in Preventing Drug Misuse Among College Students

Richard Lucey Jr., MA
Senior Prevention Program Manager
Drug Enforcement Administration

One of the key things I have learned during my nearly 3 decades of experience working in the field of preventing drug misuse is that results don't happen overnight. In fact, it is critically important to acknowledge there are no shortcuts in prevention. Unfortunately, one of the struggles we face in prevention is impatience. There is pressure from many fronts to produce results quickly. So, staff might rush to replicate programs and policies being used at other campuses—even when not enough information is available to know if those programs/policies are a good match for their campus or if these efforts can produce favorable outcomes locally.

Another key thing I have learned is that although implementation and evaluation of evidence-based strategies and programs are very important, so is development of innovative and promising approaches to prevent drug misuse. The challenge here is that the concept of innovation is subjective; it can have varied interpretations. In this segment, I offer three takeaways about innovation.

INNOVATION BASED ON RESEARCH

Early in my career, the science of prevention was forever changed by the introduction of two significant research areas. The first were studies done by Hawkins and Catalano (1992) about risk and protective factors, and the second are the three classifications of prevention identified by the Institute of Medicine (1994).

As the agency I worked for began to apply these research findings broadly to prevention efforts statewide, I was asked to identify how this research specifically applied to institutions of higher education. This groundbreaking research was not only new but also poised to influence the prevention field for decades to come. To this day, colleges and universities that are invested in comprehensive and effective prevention will identify and address not only specific factors that put their students at risk for drug misuse but also factors that will protect students from the costs and consequences of drug misuse.

INNOVATION AS AN OPPORTUNITY

When I started my federal career, I worked on a grant program to identify model prevention programs at colleges and universities. A review criterion was evidence of an innovative program integrated into the campus's overall comprehensive prevention effort.

Disagreement among peer reviewers about "innovation" resulted in a consistent benchmark that became a standard for future use. Essentially, the discrepancy was between the view of innovation as a groundbreaking approach versus an approach new for the campus that had not been considered or implemented previously.

INNOVATION AS A STRATEGY

Currently, I continue to identify ways to enhance the Drug Enforcement Administration's (DEA's) outreach to colleges and universities and produce resources to support their efforts to prevent drug misuse. The DEA's (2020) decision to publish *Prevention With Purpose: A Strategic Planning Guide to Preventing Drug Misuse Among College Students* was based on filling a gap. Although the strategic prevention framework, which serves as the foundation throughout the guide, has been around for about 25 years, the specific linkage to preventing drug misuse among college students did not previously exist. This innovative publication provides a roadmap to help colleges and universities be intentional and purposeful, and to develop a strategic approach to comprehensively prevent drug misuse among their students.

In closing, whether using innovation based on research, as an opportunity, or as a strategy, always ensure your efforts are strategic and aligned with prevention science to achieve positive outcomes.

Note. The contents of this book represent the scholarship and professional opinions of the editors and chapter authors. Neither the Drug Enforcement Administration nor any other federal or state agency cited in this book states nor implies any endorsement, association, or recommendation with regard to the authors and their affiliations, or the book's publisher, or its products or services.

CONCLUSION

It is essential that a quality campus prevention effort be grounded in a logic model, and even more useful are evidence-informed foundations that are coupled with theoretical underpinnings. The IOM model and its three prevention strategies are critical, as this framework guides planning, resources, and campus strategy. Innovation's role complements localized planning and should be based in theory as well as evidence. Clear thinking about organization and staffing—including placement and resources—is a crucial component of any planning effort. Theory helps guide practice, just as form follows function.

REFERENCES

Anderson, D. S., & Santos, G. M. (2018). *College alcohol survey: The national longitudinal survey on alcohol, tobacco, other drug and violence issues at institutions of higher education.* George Mason University.

Becker, M., & Rosenstock, I. M. (1984). Compliance with medical advice. In A. Steptoe & A. Mathews (Eds.), *Health care and human behavior* (pp. 135–152). Academic Press.

Centers for Disease Control and Prevention. (2020). *The social-ecological model: A framework for prevention.* https://www.cdc.gov/violenceprevention/publichealthissue/social-ecologicalmodel.html

Coalition of Higher Education Associations for Substance Abuse Prevention. (n.d.). *History*. http://coheasap.myacpa.org/about/history

Council for the Advancement of Standards in Higher Education. (2019). *CAS professional standards for higher education* (10th ed.).

Drug Enforcement Administration. (2020). *Prevention with purpose: A strategic planning guide to preventing drug misuse among college students*. http://www.campusdrugprevention.gov/preventionguide

Hawkins, J. D., & Catalano, R. F. (1992). Risk and protective factors for alcohol and other drug problems in adolescence and early adulthood: Implications for substance abuse prevention. *Psychological Bulletin, 112*(1), 64–105.

Hochbaum, G. (1958). Public participation in medical screening programs (DHEW Publication No. 572). Public Health Service, U.S. Government Printing Office.

Institute of Medicine. (1994). *Reducing risks for mental disorders: Frontiers for preventive intervention research.* National Academies Press. https://pubmed.ncbi.nlm.nih.gov/25144015

Linkenbach, J. (1991). *Our chapter, our choice facilitator's guide—Workshop manual: Redefining alcohol and drug norms through Greek empowerment.* National Interfraternity Conference.

Linkenbach, J. (2003). The Montana model: Development and overview of a seven-step process for implementing macro-level social norms campaigns. In H. W. Perkins (Ed.), *The social norms approach to preventing school and college age substance abuse: A handbook for educators, counselors, and clinicians* (pp. 182–205). Jossey-Bass.

Linkenbach, J. (2007). *The seven core principles of the science of the positive workbook.* The Montana Institute. http://www.montanainstitute.com/publications

Linkenbach, J. (2019). The seven-step Montana model of positive community norms communications. In D. S. Anderson & R. E. Miller (Eds.), *Health and safety communication: A practical guide forward* (pp. 87–88). Routledge.

Linkenbach, J., Ward, N. J., & Otto, J. (2012). *An action framework for transforming traffic safety culture.* Montana State University, Center for Health and Safety Culture, Western Transportation Institute. http://www.westerntransportationinstitute.org/documents/centers/culture/An_Action_Framework_for_Transforming_Traffic_Safety_Culture.pdf

National Academies of Sciences, Engineering, and Medicine. (2019). *Promoting positive adolescent health behaviors and outcomes: Thriving in the 21st century*. National Academies Press. https://doi.org/10.17226/25552

National Institute on Alcohol Abuse and Alcoholism. (2019). *Planning alcohol interventions using NIAAA's CollegeAIM alcohol intervention matrix* (Publication No. 19-AA-8017). U.S. Department of Health and Human Services, National Institutes of Health. https://www.collegedrinkingprevention.gov/CollegeAIM/Resources/NIAAA_College_Matrix_Booklet.pdf

Prochaska, J., & DiClemente, C. (1983). Stages and processes of self-change in smoking: Toward an integrative model of change. *Journal of Consulting and Clinical Psychology, 5*, 390–395.

Reissman, F. (1965). The "helper" therapy principle. *Social Work, 10*(2), 27–32.

Springer, J. R., & Phillips, J. (2007). *The Institute of Medicine framework and its implication for the advancement of prevention policy, programs and practice* (SMA-4205). U.S. Department of Health and Human Services. http://ca-sdfsc.org/docs/resources/SDFSC_IOM_Policy.pdf

Substance Abuse and Mental Health Services Administration. (2017). *Focus on prevention* (Publication No. [SMA] 10–4120). https://store.samhsa.gov/product/Focus-on-Prevention/sma10-4120?referer=from_search_result

Substance Abuse and Mental Health Services Administration. (2018). *Selecting best-fit programs and practices: Guidance for substance misuse prevention practitioners.* https://www.samhsa.gov/sites/default/files/ebp_prevention_guidance_document_241.pdf

Substance Abuse and Mental Health Services Administration. (2019). *Substance misuse prevention for young adults* (Publication No. PEP19-PL-Guide-1). https://store.samhsa.gov/product/Substance-Misuse-Prevention-for-Young-Adults/PEP19-PL-Guide-1

CONTENT: "The What"

This six-chapter section focuses on the *what* of campus prevention strategies. Central to the entire comprehensive campus approach is the Institute of Medicine's prevention framework, which incorporates universal, selective, and indicated prevention strategies. Universal prevention approaches address public safety risks using proactive measures, and incorporate primarily information dissemination and environmental strategies. Selective prevention approaches target groups with a defined membership that have a documented higher risk for problems associated with drugs and alcohol; selective approaches also target individuals with characteristics known to increase their risk for problems. Selective approaches focus on both reducing the risk for these problems, as well as promote engagement with resiliency-oriented approaches. Indicated prevention strategies focus on individuals with harmful involvement with drugs and/or alcohol, including the individual's progression toward a substance use disorder; indicated prevention also addresses issues surrounding ongoing recovery from a substance use disorder. Helping anchor these three components of the Institute of Medicine's framework are three additional elements: policies, training, and evaluation. Central to campus drug and alcohol misuse prevention efforts are comprehensive policies and procedures. Training of staff, students, and student leaders helps these key constituencies understand the rationale for their understanding, support, and engagement. Finally, evaluation aids with documenting proximate and longer-term outcomes as well as the strategies and processes used. Collectively, these chapters undergird an accountability focused campus effort designed to be evidence based and use theoretical, historical, and forward-thinking approaches.

CHAPTER 4

Policy and Procedural Interventions

"As a senior in high school, I could not wait to attend college and live independently for the first time in my life. Along with my newly gained independence, however, came a lot of different decisions, most of which regarded the balance between achieving academic success and having a social life. I looked to older girls in my sorority to help me stay on track while also having fun."

—Junior at a large Southern university

In society, policies and procedures exist to support the functions of bureaucracies; colleges create policies and procedures to protect the health and welfare of the campus community. The development and implementation of policies about drugs and alcohol may differ on campuses from that of the community at large, in part because college is viewed as a time when individuals are navigating a newfound freedom of adulthood. But this idea is dated. Generation Z students are more open to structure than their millennial peers and Baby Boomer parents or grandparents. Policy development and implementation is an essential prevention strategy. Campus leaders can leverage policy to support campus health and welfare. Student input on the creation and modification of policy offers the opportunity to foster community and mutual trust.

Policy, broadly defined, serves as the foundation for overall campus planning efforts. Policy includes, but is not limited to, rules and regulations as well as standards and guidelines. Specifically, policy also includes the values, beliefs, and priorities of institution leaders, often emanating from the campus mission statement. As such, policy encompasses the entire thrust of the campus prevention effort. Rules and regulations, while essential, must be complemented by much more, such as programs and training, campaigns and advocacy, evaluation and support services, and curriculum and engagement. Thus, when using or hearing the term *policy,* it is helpful to specify if it refers to simply "the rules" or if it incorporates the overall campus effort and its philosophical underpinnings.

Many practical issues surround the implementation of policies and procedures. Some insight about these issues can be found in Case Study 4.1, about amnesty policies, and Lessons From the Field 4.1, about alcohol consumption and college sports events. Professor Peter Lake, an Innovator, shares observations about legal considerations and perspectives, including his "*pro*vention" approach.

WHAT IS MEANT BY POLICY

The campus policy is the foundation of any approach by campus to address drug and alcohol issues. Broadly speaking, policy encompasses the overall philosophy and beliefs about how these substance issues are going to be treated; in a narrower sense, policy addresses the rules and regulations about these substances. The rules, then, become an outgrowth of the philosophy; the specific policies and procedures are the visible articulation of the campus's stance regarding the prevention effort as a whole.

When formulating or revising the campus policy, some initial questions can inform and guide campus leaders:

- How does the campus mission statement, and institutional and departmental goals, guide the policy?
- Do distinct policies exist for students, faculty, staff, and visitors?
- How are accountability and self-responsibility specified?
- Are the themes of compassion and understanding addressed?
- How are individual and group rights balanced with responsibilities?

- How is concern for the overall community communicated and accomplished?
- Do standards incorporate individuals' prior substance use history (i.e., experimentation, prior offense, in recovery)?
- What are the responsibilities of the institution and individuals to deter and respond to problematic or illegal behavior?
- What interventions and messages are appropriate regarding illegal behavior?
- How is caregiving implemented within the context of strict enforcement?
- Where do punishment and positive reinforcement fit in?
- In what ways are protective factors and risk factors addressed?

Although these questions do not address all the broad, conceptual policy issues, they do illustrate much of the complexity surrounding such issues and are meant to stimulate thought among campus leaders. Overall, it is essential that prevention leaders address these and related issues as part of the strategic planning efforts, which include the development of guiding principles (see Chapter 10).

Beyond the broad policy discussions, vitally important is creating and specifying appropriate and clear rules and regulations; in addition, attention to the details regarding the procedures associated with their implementation is critical. Also included within policy development is enforcement, so that consistency exists between behavioral expectations, follow-through and oversight, and consequences of noncompliance. For example, a comprehensive approach in traffic safety is referred to as the 3 *E*s: engineering, education, enforcement. Policy undergirds all of them; a desire for speed control and responsible driving informs infrastructure (speed bumps, narrow roadways, lineage), public information (awareness campaigns and motivational efforts), and behavioral monitoring with consequences (tickets and fines).

In brief, policy articulates the values and principles to which the institution ascribes. Having sound policies and procedures is an opportunity to be expressive as well as grounded.

THE ROLE OF POLICY ON CAMPUS

Policy development and implementation have a critical place on the college campus. Not only do they establish order, but they also provide standards for behavior and strategies for handling conduct outside those standards. Policies offer the opportunity for prevention specialists to convey their vision for the campus, interpersonal relationships, and human behavior.

Overall policy plays both reactive and proactive roles on campus. The reactive role is one where problems associated with drugs and alcohol on the campus (or other campuses) are addressed by developing appropriate policies. The proactive role is done by anticipating situations and problems that may arise; with this, standards and frameworks are established to prevent or minimize the occurrence or impact of problems. Some of what will be promulgated will be philosophical or conceptual; other aspects will include specific rules and regulations. Policies and procedures may be designed to set a tone and be entirely proactive in nature; they may also stem from an incident (and, thus, be intended to prevent a future recurrence) or from unsatisfactory results of existing, well-intentioned policies (e.g., with loopholes, avoidance practices, exceptions). Whatever is the rationale for developing a policy, messaging must be clear to ensure understanding and, ideally acceptance, from those constituencies that may be affected. For example, some policies may only affect student-athletes, some may focus on student organizations (such as fraternities or sororities) that sponsor parties, and others may be applicable to paraprofessional staff members.

The general aim of having a policy for drugs and alcohol is to eliminate, ideally, or otherwise reduce death and injury associated with the use of these substances. Most of the drug- and alcohol-related deaths, injuries, and other consequences among college students each year are preventable. Drug and alcohol policies may be based on location (e.g., athletic venue), type of event, circumstances for events (food, alcohol-free beverage, training of server, hours), or audience. Specific rules will be based on the campus's areas of concern, designed to reduce the risk of injury, harm, property damage, other negative consequence, or legal liability.

To be effective, local ownership of policies and procedures is essential—both for design and implementation considerations. The phrases "you own what you help create" and "having skin in the game" apply here. Greater ownership—and thus adherence to the policy—results where there is an investment. Campus history and culture, the nature of the surrounding community, and institutional mission vary; so too will specific standards.

Although locally developed, campus policies should also be prepared within the construct of local, state, and federal standards. Legal guidance from appropriate authorities will help prevention specialists to pinpoint local needs. As this is done, it is important to remember that overlapping jurisdictions exist, as state law, local ordinances, and campus policies all apply to an individual's behavior. Campus personnel may find it useful to articulate key behavioral standards specified in local, state, or national laws or ordinances, whether or not they are specifically included in the campus policies. Colleges and universities often state in their written policies that individuals are accountable for all jurisdictional standards; thus it is critical that students know this. It is also critical that the campus policies align with the external jurisdictional laws and ordinances.

That said, it is critical that policies not be too cumbersome. If a policy strives to anticipate all possible scenarios, then, undoubtedly, some situations will not line up precisely with them (the loopholes and exceptions noted). Thus, some broad considerations—such as welfare, safety, health, or other espoused factors—may guide institution policies. Policy aims to influence and shape the campus culture, so it must evolve in tandem with campus needs.

CONTENTS OF POLICY

One useful starting point for prevention specialists is to account for the various rights and responsibilities of students. Existing ordinances and laws are comprehensive and provide a foundation; prevention specialists should identify those of the greatest relevance and importance for the campus. Examples may include laws about public intoxication as well as the use or possession of alcohol while under the legal age of purchase. Similarly, local ordinances may address the use of marijuana, the use of illegal drugs, or the use of prescription drugs for purposes other than those for which they were intended.

Beyond jurisdictional laws, campus policies should be developed according to local needs and issues. Some areas for consideration include (yet are not limited to) those outlined in Table 4.1.

Table 4.1

Areas to Consider When Developing Campus Drug and Alcohol Policies

Area	Questions
Alcohol Availability	• Is alcohol permitted on campus? • Under what conditions can alcohol be served? • What restrictions exist on the type of alcohol (beer, wine, distilled spirits)? • What restrictions exist on the containers (e.g., kegs, size of cups)? • Are settings specified for alcohol use (e.g., private room)? • Are open containers in public permitted? • Is food required to be provided when alcohol is served? If so, what kind and how much? • Are alcohol-free beverages required? • Are servers required? Do they need to be trained? Do they need to be over 21? • What are the hours of service?
Alcohol and Sports	• Is alcohol permitted in sports venues? Which venues? • Are alcohol sales permitted? Is personal consumption ("bring your own") permitted?
Behaviors of Concern	• What are the behavioral expectations related to public intoxication? • What are the standards regarding others' engagement or bystander intervention (e.g., Good Samaritan policies)? • What are the conditions surrounding medical amnesty? Do they vary based on whether alcohol or an illicit drug was involved? • What occurs with impaired driving incidents? Is this consequence based on the location (e.g., on or off campus)? • What reporting relationships or requirements exist with hospital admissions due to a drug overdose or alcohol poisoning? • What reporting requirements exist with health center personnel when drug or alcohol misuse has been reported or suspected? • What are the consequences of impaired driving or other incidents that occur away from campus (e.g., spring break, summer, study abroad)?

Consequences for Violations	• What are the consequences (e.g., punitive, fine, educational, service, counseling, probation) for individual violations? • What are the consequences (e.g., punitive, fine, educational, service, restricted activities, probation) for group violations? • In what ways are the individual and group consequences different for repeat violations?
Enforcement	• How will each of these policies be enforced in a consistent, equitable way? • What will the consequences be for noncompliance or repeat offenses?
Events	• What standards exist for events when alcohol is served? • What registration is required? • How is access controlled? • What training or preparation is required for event hosts? • What standards need to be in place to maintain and monitor control? • When are law enforcement/security personnel required to be onsite?
Marketing and Advertising	• Can advertising occur? • What are the standards on advertising drink specials? • Is advertising by outside vendors permitted?
Underage Drinking	• What procedures and safeguards are established to minimize access by those under 21? • What types of IDs are used to confirm someone's legal drinking age?

The content and details of campus policies and procedures necessarily dovetail with the laws in the state where the institution is located. Different states have different policies on factors such as social host liability and dram shop liability (where, essentially, the business or a host who serves alcohol to a drinker may be subsequently liable for injuries caused by that intoxicated drinker). The various details of these policies, as well as medical amnesty, Good Samaritan laws, and other guidelines, will be led by state laws as well as other sources of best practices. Some insights about amnesty policies are provided in Case Study 4.1, where Ryan Snow shares his experiences and suggestions; they apply to many different policies and procedures. Also helpful is Worksheet 4.1: Drug and Alcohol Policies and Procedures Checklist, which highlights these and other issues that may be of interest to prevention specialists and campus leaders in designing and reviewing policies and procedures.

An essential resource for best practices for policies and procedures is *CAS Professional Standards for Higher Education,* which has been developed and updated by several organizations. One of the 47 key areas within the standards focuses on Alcohol, Tobacco, and Other Drug Programs (Council for the Advancement of Standards in Higher Education, 2019). Another is the National Institute on Alcohol Abuse and Alcoholism (NIAAA; 2020a) College Alcohol Policies Directory, which includes links to individual college policies. Also, NIAAA's (2020b) Alcohol Policy Information System has insights that can inform campus prevention specialists about a wide variety of alcohol-related topics on a state-by-state basis.

Beyond the overall campus policy itself, prevention specialists must consider guidelines of specific affiliation groups. With fraternities, for example, alcohol and drug guidelines are defined by the North American Interfraternity Conference (2019); for sororities, the National Panhellenic Conference has developed standards. These organizations' national headquarters also have standards set for local chapters. With student-athletes, standards are established by the National Collegiate Athletic Association (2020a; 2020b) for the health and well-being of its members. Other affiliation groups may have their own policies and guidelines.

Staff and other professional groups may also have standards of conduct, including ethical guidelines that address professional behavior with drugs or alcohol. These standards may also encompass staff members' handling of student situations regarding substances. For example, counselors, doctors, nurses, and police officers have professional organizations that offer guidance and standards.

A final consideration with the content of policies themselves surrounds campus employees. What are the standards to which they are held, and do they differ from those for students? One general overreaching standard comes from the Drug-Free Workplace Act of 1988, which requires institutions receiving federal assistance to provide a drug-free workplace by "publishing a statement notifying employees that the unlawful manufacture, distribution, dispensation, possession, or use of a controlled substance is prohibited in the person's workplace and specifying the actions that will be taken against employees for violations of such prohibition" (p. 175).

CASE STUDY 4.1

Understanding and Enhancing Amnesty Policies on Campus

Ryan Snow, MEd
Instructor
Preventionleaders.com

Dealing with the issue of drug- and alcohol-related medical emergencies on a college campus is a top priority—for campus policy makers, students, staff, emergency personnel, parents, and so many others. These incidents can be scary and cause major trauma for college students in particular. It is the first time many of them have had to deal with a situation without their parents' support. Cultivating a positive response to these intense and potentially life-threatening incidents is important to the students' overall health.

Amnesty policies should cover the incident from start to finish. Typically, amnesty policies are designed to protect students' health and safety. Although campuses differ in the specific contents of their amnesty policies and procedures, these guidelines generally emphasize an individual getting help in an emergency drug or alcohol situation—without facing disciplinary consequences (there may be another follow-up, however). Consistency between all policies and procedures, and all responders involved in the incident, is vitally important. Students must be educated about the policy prior to any need to use it; if they don't understand it, are confused, or don't trust it, they will probably not use it, which can result in devasting consequences.

Students need first to understand that there is a policy in

place, and that when they call, police will often arrive on scene with medical staff. Students should be confident that they will not be disciplined for illegally consuming substances if they are calling to get help for themselves or someone in medical need.

After the incident, it is equally important that some follow-up occurs with the student who received assistance; this may involve counseling and/or education. With a drug or alcohol medical emergency, the motivations, emotions, behavior, and changes in lifestyle may be addressed.

If a medical amnesty policy is to be successful, it needs to be well considered and embraced by all members of the college community. From the education and staff training, to the debriefing after an incident, and to the follow-up with the student, all parts are important and critical for students' overall health and safety (Haas et al., 2018).

HOW TO DEVELOP POLICY

Developing or revising the campus drug and alcohol policy is an opportunity for the campus community to come together to guide and shape the campus culture. Policy creation allows campus leaders to engage others in determining the best ways to address drug and alcohol issues. Because the process and the specific contents continue to evolve based on changing needs, this opportunity presents itself regularly, whether internally or externally initiated (i.e., from changes in legislation, the Biennial Review, or changes in needs). With the involvement of key personnel and organizations in policy development, promulgation, and review, and with varying and sometimes competing interests, a more inclusive, enforceable, and appropriate set of standards will likely result. Further, specific situations and/or settings will arise where focused policies and procedures are appropriate; with Lessons From the Field 4.1, Tavis Glassman and Tom Castor examine the issue of event-specific drinking, focusing on college athletics events.

Four initial steps serve as foundations for developing or revising a campus policy:

1. Identify the key issues, situations, and behaviors that need to be addressed. Where have problems occurred in the past, and where are problems anticipated?
2. Learn what standards already exist; examples include those developed by various professional associations (e.g., health, counseling, law enforcement, student affairs), state organizations or agencies (e.g., education, health, liquor control), federal agencies (e.g., Substance Abuse and Mental Health Services Administration, Drug Enforcement Administration, U.S. Department of Education, National Highway Traffic Safety Administration), national organizations (e.g., NASPA–Student Affairs Administrators in Higher Education, American College Health Association, ACPA–College Student Educators International, Association of College and University Housing Officers–International), and national leadership groups (e.g., Coalition of Higher Education Associations for Substance Abuse Prevention).
3. Look at policies for specific affiliation groups. For example, the NCAA (2020a; 2020b) has standards for its member campuses, which can have broad applicability to all campuses. Also, national fraternity and sorority organizations, whether for individual chapters or overall, have guidelines on substance misuse and related issues.
4. Look at what other institutions of higher education have developed. Pay particular attention to those with similar demographics (e.g., size, public/private status, setting, religious affiliation, region of the country).

The process then turns to crafting the contents of the policy. Initially, campus leaders must determine their process and timelines. Essential for buy-in and sound implementation is a transparent and engaged process. The process for developing the policy may be part of the campus's drug and alcohol prevention leadership group (see Chapter 10) or as a stand-alone policy committee. However it is organized, the group should have broad representation from key campus constituencies, including stakeholders and decision makers; this group should actively engage students, including the governing body for undergraduate as well as graduate students. Also central are enforcement personnel, such as security and law enforcement, residence life staff, health and counseling center personnel, judicial affairs staff, and other student affairs professionals.

When crafting the policies and procedures, prevention specialists must use specific language that is clear and unambiguous. It is helpful to include the rationale for the specific policies identified; such inclusion educates both the audience and those interpreting and enforcing the standards. A discussion of potential consequences is likewise useful. The question comes down to whether much of this detail should be included with the published policies or placed in a related resource.

Throughout the process of drafting policy content, both the campus's legal counsel and key approval agents must review proposed policies or changes—they will have perspectives regarding potential ramifications. Because their endorsements are important for ultimate approval, their initial input will assist prevention specialists to remedy areas of concern. Politically helpful in the process is having reviews with various groups on campus, particularly those that might be affected by policy changes.

LESSONS FROM THE FIELD 4.1

Event-Specific Alcohol Consumption Associated With College Sports

Tavis Glassman, PhD
Professor School of Population Health
University of Toledo

Tom Castor, PhD
Assistant Professor, Department of Public Health and Healthcare Leadership
Radford University

An emerging area of research is event-specific drinking, which includes special times or occasions when people drink substantially more alcohol than they normally would—such as on 21st birthdays, New Year's Eve, St. Patrick's Day, spring break, Halloween, and weddings (Miller et al., 2013; Neighbors et al., 2006; Oster-Aaland & Neighbors, 2007). Of particular concern for officials in higher education is the event-specific alcohol consumption associated with college sports, commonly referred to as "game-day." The convergence of thousands of guests on campus and frequent excessive drinking creates public health challenges before, during, and after the game—as well as serious liability concerns.

A variety of interventions can be implemented to create a safer environment during college sporting events. Examples may include total bans, limitations on alcohol sales, and restricting when, where, and how much alcohol can be consumed; the location may include within the stadium as well as tailgate areas (National Highway Traffic Safety Administration, 2020).

Texting alert systems used to report unruly fan behavior; no reentry stadium policies; alcohol-free tailgate areas; safe-ride transportation; restriction or prohibition of alcohol marketing; and consistent enforcement of existing policies are event specific prevention (ESP) strategies (i.e., *prevention typology*) that can minimize harm and promote health on game day (Neighbors et al., 2007). In addition, social norms marketing and health communication interventions could be used to educate students and others about issues specific to game-day safety (Castor et al., 2020).

Due to the high visibility of game-day events and associated policy and prevention efforts, support from university presidents is essential. A variety of resources exist to help university officials and prevention specialists implement evidence-based interventions and tailor them to college sporting events. For example, the seminal publication *Be Vocal, Be Visible, and Be Visionary* (Higher Education Center for Alcohol and Other Drug Abuse and Violence Prevention, 1997a) includes a series of suggestions about how senior administrators can lead prevention efforts.

In summary, presidents and other university representatives need to be proactive regarding prevention issues associated with college sporting events, because they are ultimately responsible for the safety and welfare of those fans in attendance. Not enforcing existing laws and policies regarding alcohol use (e.g., open containers) is confusing to fans and sends mixed messages to students about when it is okay to ignore or break the rules. Implementing risk-reduction strategies—such as allowing alcohol to be consumed at certain times and in designated areas—may result in a safer environment, rather than overlooking these standards. Accordingly, school officials should examine their current alcohol policy, specific to game day, to create a safer environment where students and others can socialize and enjoy the game.

POLICY IMPLEMENTATION

The dissemination process for the policy must ensure that all relevant parties are notified of the new or revised content. Essential with this dissemination is highlighting noteworthy changes that have occurred, including the rationale for the changes; this type of explanation is critical to a sound implementation of the current policy. The dissemination must include the policy itself as well as any requisite accompanying procedures. Multiple channels are appropriate for this process, including regular updates to the student handbook, websites, emails, and social media. Print copies of the updated policy should be maintained, including both complete editions and summary versions. Shorter versions may incorporate an overall summary, highlights of changes, and topic-specific resources (e.g., event planning, medical amnesty and Good Samaritan standards, impaired driving).

The relevant audiences (e.g., students, student groups) must be notified, but so should individuals with enforcement responsibilities. Police and security obviously need the latest policies; however, others such as residence hall staff also require the information if they are to help with policy implementation. Other parties such as advisors of student organizations, health and counseling staff, judicial personnel, coaches and trainers, and faculty members benefit from receiving updated policy and implementation guidelines.

Training may also be needed, particularly with new or potentially controversial elements. This instruction prepares personnel to address their responsibilities and successfully implement the policy. Depending on the roles, focused or generalized training will be appropriate. Residence hall staff, whether professional or paraprofessional, need different levels of training to prepare them to handle situations effectively. Similarly, specialized personnel, such as advisors, health or counseling professionals, or athletics personnel, need audience- and profession-specific training. Campus leaders must specify what is appropriate for faculty members, as their role in campus organization and student support is an evolving area.

Associated with training is the need to do periodic updates throughout the year—whether they relate to specific policy updates or revisions, or to communication efforts. Needs or concerns may emerge based on specific policy elements, their interpretation, the presence of a gap, or areas of high incidence, so timely attention is critical. Prevention specialists should communicate broadly all updates and reminders and especially whenever there is a policy modification.

In review, the entire policy implementation process warrants incorporation of a systems approach, whereby all aspects of the college's system support the policy. The systems approach calls for all parts of the system to be in sync—that includes the wording of the policy, the actual implementation (often documented in procedures and protocols), the communication about the policies and potential consequences, the enforcement by various constituencies, and the interpretation and judgment made by adjudication personnel and judicial bodies. The policy, as it is developed, revised, implemented, and communicated to various constituencies, should maintain a balance between the intent, its reasonableness, its dedication to fairness, and its clarity. Actively engaging various constituencies in the entire set of processes associated with policy development, training, and review aids with buy-in.

POLICY IMPACT REVIEW

Policies and procedures should be reviewed regularly to ensure their continued relevance and appropriateness. Each part should be monitored to be sure it is addressing the needs for which it was developed. The critical question is whether the policy, as implemented, is meeting its objectives; that is, does the implemented policy achieve what it set out to accomplish. Questions about whether the policies are current, needed, consistent, comprehensive, and appropriate are relevant. Central are whether the policies, as implemented, are setting the necessary guidelines and standards for the campus. Just as traffic safety includes guidelines (e.g., speed limits) based on well-being, revisions are based on changes due to the setting (e.g., curves, school zone), situation (e.g., construction zone), and conditions (e.g., rain, fog, darkness). Similarly, campus policies may need occasional adjustment to best meet current needs.

Policy review can address multiple issues:

- Does the policy meet its overall aims?
- Is it aligned with the institutional mission?
- Is it equitable and consistent, and is it perceived as such?
- Do audiences know it exists? Do they know its rationale?
- Is the policy viewed as reasonable and appropriate?
- Does it address current needs?
- Does it anticipate emerging issues?
- Is its implementation and enforcement thorough?
- Do staff members have appropriate training for implementation and follow-through?

Beyond these considerations, federal law also requires that institutions of higher education review their prevention efforts at least every 2 years. Known as the Drug-Free Schools and Communities Act, these standards specify and codify campus efforts to review their actions. Beyond this legal requirement, a review of campus efforts is seen as appropriate, meaningful, and helpful, as well as honoring ethical obligations to the institution itself and its multiple constituencies (Higher Education Center for Alcohol and Other Drug Abuse and Violence Prevention, 1997b). The legal obligation has three parts. One part is that institutions of higher education that receive federal funds must have a program for students and employees that addresses illegal use of drugs or alcohol. Second, institutions must review their drug and alcohol prevention programs every 2 years; this is referred to as a *biennial review*. The third part mandates that information be distributed to students and employees annually. More detail about this biennial review process is emphasized in Chapter 13, which is designed to look at overall program effectiveness.

For the purpose of this chapter, brief attention is paid to how prevention specialists can review the policy's impact; more details about evaluation are provided in Chapter 9.

- **Campuswide survey:** It can address topics such as knowledge, attitudes, perceptions, behavioral intention, and consequences, all associated with drugs or alcohol. It may even promote policy awareness by asking a question such as, "To what extent does the campus enforce its policy of . . . ," thus serving an educational as well as an evaluative function.
- **Focus groups:** Groups of students or others can be asked targeted questions about the policy and its implementation; this feedback sheds light on their understanding and reactions.
- **Interviews with stakeholders:** These efforts help campus leaders understand how various personnel, such as law enforcement, athletics, Greek-letter organization leaders, student affairs staff, and faculty, view the policy receptivity and effectiveness.
- **Public discussions:** Offered in an open town-hall format, these meetings can inform prevention specialists about how to improve the design and implementation of the policy.
- **Targeted group discussions:** These meetings may be appropriate for intact affiliation groups, such as student-athlete teams, Greek-letter organizations, student government, and first-year students.
- **Review of reports:** Data that have been collected for years can provide useful insights about the nature and scope of issues for which policies may be needed or for which revisions may be warranted. Examples include incident reports, maintenance logs, hospital reports, health and counseling center reports, police and security records, reports of special events or approved parties, and other queries existing or proposed. Some data may not provide information specific to the needs, so adjustments with data reporting protocols and forms may be called for. In addition, new data collection needs may be identified for future informational purposes.
- **Observation:** By using the classic approach of "management by walking around," campus leaders may get a sense of the extent to which written reports and documentation match what is experienced on campus. This effort may also include systematic observation or monitoring of settings or behaviors of interest.

With any of these approaches, additional insight can be gleaned by analyzing and reviewing the findings based on different groups or audiences. Such an analysis can assess the extent to which there is a consistent view across various campus groups, such as faculty compared with students, or first-year students compared with graduating students, or across demographics such as gender, age, residence status, or student organization affiliation. Also, comparing results from different sources (e.g., survey vs. discussions vs. observation) can provide a richer understanding of areas for improvement. One resource that may assist with this type of review is Worksheet 4.2: Organizational Self-Assessment, which addresses the perspectives of multiple constituencies on these and other issues.

Professor Peter Lake, in Innovator 4.1, highlights important points about the intersection of the law with the work of prevention specialists and campus leaders. With decades of work in this area, he focuses on specific case law and the concept of "*pro*vention."

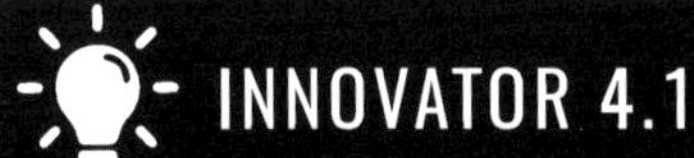

From Deflection to "*Pro*vention": The Law as an Ally in Alcohol and Other Drug Prevention

Peter Lake, JD
Professor
Stetson University College of Law

It is tempting to see the law as creating obstacles to science-based prevention work on campus. Not long ago, college lawyers "counseled"—even *directed*—prevention efforts to stand down for fear of creating potential liability. It was especially difficult to find college lawyers who *championed* prevention work. Colleges often neglected sound public health thinking by deflecting responsibility to others on and off campus (fraternities, for example) and victim-blamed students harmed in the context of alcohol or drug use. A lack of focus on public health modeling was a hallmark of an era I first described as the "Bystander Era," which took root in the 1970s (Bickel & Lake, 1999). Campus leadership, concerned about "assuming duties," regarded prevention as legally risky—even longitudinal data collection might be used against a college, potentially establishing legal "foreseeability" of risks.

As the public health challenges of alcohol and other drugs (AODs) on campus became more publicly visible at the millennium, it was an *educational* approach to prevention that many college attorneys were most comfortable with—often with a focus on individual student responsibility—and to some extent social norming efforts. Despite promising scientific advancements surrounding environmental management strategies, education and information-based strategies appeared legally safer. Even today, many campuses devote relatively little to prevention efforts and devote more of their dedicated resources to education-based AOD prevention strategies than to other matters—a vestige of Bystander Era thinking.

It is hard to claim that college law has made a sudden, complete leap to public health thinking, but there is plenty of evidence that it is moving in the right direction—toward what I like to call "*pro*vention." AOD prevention leaders can help their campuses by understanding these recent developments in the law and continuing to champion science-based approaches to AOD prevention:

1. The law now conceives of students as business customers in legally "special relationships" with their college (*Dzung Duy Nguyen v. Massachusetts Institute of Technology*, 2018). This means colleges have responsibilities—legal duty—to students regarding their safety and well-being.

2. The law has recognized the connection between sexual violence and AOD risks. Federal regulations now require science-based, public health–modeled approaches to prevention on campus for sexual violence (see The Clery Act, 2018). Moreover, the U.S. Department of Education has steadily ramped up enforcement efforts under the Drug-Free Schools and Communities Act (1989). Anemic federal intervention in the early years of the Bystander Era has given way to requirements for active and legally monitored prevention—"*pro*vention."
3. College leaders increasingly understand the need for prevention efforts to reduce the costs and potential brand degradation of relying almost exclusively on intervention and remediation efforts. There are significant correlations between prevention efforts and retention/attrition and attainment rates. Bystanderism is not good business; prevention is good business (EverFi, 2020).
4. Advances in disability law have challenged long-standing legal attitudes that "voluntary" alcohol or unlawful drug use is a moral weakness that justifies blaming a victim who has used alcohol or drugs. Advances in the law related to sexual violence have also reduced similar victim-blaming arguments. The law has also not been lured widely to accept categorical deflection arguments such as AOD problems originate before college or that closing fraternities will solve AOD issues on campus.
5. Some courts have shown significant understanding of how the law can facilitate good public health work, by creating legal standards that support, and are consistent with, research in the field. Public health science is becoming a larger feature of college law.

Over the span of a 30-year career in higher education law, I have seen slow but demonstrable progress toward legal norms that support science-based AOD prevention methods. Ultimately, major changes may come about as a result of consumer pressure for safer, more responsible campuses; these changes, in turn, may drive legal reform (the COVID-19 pandemic may become a catalyst as well). AOD professionals should appreciate that drivers for legal change may come from a variety of directions; it is notable that enforcement of sex discrimination laws has been such a driver.

CONCLUSION

Policy and accompanying procedures are designed to set standards and guidelines for the campus; these are tools that shape student behavior and, thus, the campus culture. Helping ground policy development and review processes are several national resources and standards; further, various specialty groups (e.g., student-athletes, Greek-letter organizations) have their own national guidelines. Local-level data collection can inform prevention specialists and campus leaders as they formulate and revise policies to be appropriately responsive and prevention focused. Prevention specialists should embrace innovative thinking as well as other schools' best practices to create strategies for policy development, relevant procedures, dissemination, and monitoring.

REFERENCES

Bickel, R. D., & Lake, P. F. (1999). *The rights and responsibilities of the modern university: Who assumes the risks of college life?* Carolina Academic Press.

Castor, T. (2020). *Presidents' perceptions of alcohol policies for college sporting events* (Publication No. 28332428) [Doctoral dissertation, University of Toledo, Ohio]. ProQuest Dissertations and Theses Global.

The Clery Act, 20 U.S.C. § 1092(f) (2018), *amended by* Violence Against Women Reauthorization Act of 2013, Pub. L. No. 113-4, 127 Stat. 54 (codified at 42 U.S.C. § 13701 [2013]).

Council for the Advancement of Standards in Higher Education. (2019). *CAS professional standards for higher education* (10th ed.).

Drug-Free Schools and Communities Act Amendments of 1989, Pub. L. No. 101-226, 103 Stat. 1928 (1989). https://bluetigerportal.lincolnu.edu/c/document_library/get_file?p_l_id=142227&folderId=1695938&name=DLFE-18424.pdf

Drug-Free Workplace Act of 1988, 41 U.S.C. § 701 *et seq.* (1988). https://www.samhsa.gov/sites/default/files/programs_campaigns/division_workplace_programs/drug-free-workplace-act-1988.pdf

Dzung Duy Nguyen v. Massachusetts Institute of Technology, (2018). 96 N.E.3d 128 (Mass. Supreme Judicial Court, 2018); *Regents of University of California v. Superior Court*, 413 P.3d. 656 (Cal. Supreme Court, 2018).

EverFi. (2020). *The ROI of prevention: Setting the tone for the future of your institution.* https://everfi.com/white-papers/higher-education/roi-prevention-education-for-higher-education

Haas, A. L., Wickham, R. E., McKenna, K., Morimoto, E., & Brown, L. M. (2018). Evaluating the effectiveness of a medical amnesty policy change on college students' alcohol consumption, physiological consequences, and helping behaviors. *Journal of Studies on Alcohol and Drugs, 79*(4), 523–531.

Higher Education Center for Alcohol and Other Drug Abuse and Violence Prevention. (1997a). *Be vocal, be visible, and be visionary: Recommendation for college and university presidents on alcohol and other drug prevention.* https://safesupportivelearning.ed.gov/sites/default/files/sssta/20130315_plgvisionary.pdf

Higher Education Center for Alcohol and Other Drug Abuse and Violence Prevention. (1997b). *Complying with the drug-free schools and campuses regulations.* https://safesupportivelearning.ed.gov/sites/default/files/hec/product/dfscr.pdf

Miller, P., McDonald, L., McKenzie, S., O'Brien, K., & Staiger, P. (2013). When the cats are away: The impact of sporting events on assault- and alcohol-related emergency department attendances. *Drug & Alcohol Review, 32*(1), 31–38. https://doi.org/10.1111/j.1465-3362.2012.00481.x

National Collegiate Athletic Association. (2020a). *NCAA drug testing program.* https://www.ncaa.org/sport-science-institute/ncaa-drug-testing-program

National Collegiate Athletic Association. (2020b). *Well-being.* http://www.ncaa.org/health-and-safety

National Highway Traffic Safety Administration. (2020). *TEAM coalition.* https://teamcoalition.org/about/about-team-history

National Institute on Alcohol Abuse and Alcoholism. (2020a). *College alcohol policies.* https://www.collegedrinkingprevention.gov/specialfeatures/alcoholpolicies.aspx

National Institute on Alcohol Abuse and Alcoholism. (2020b). *Alcohol policy information system.* https://alcoholpolicy.niaaa.nih.gov

Neighbors, C., Oster-Aaland, L., Bergstrom, R. L., & Lewis, M. A. (2006). Event- and context-specific normative misperceptions and high-risk drinking: 21st birthday celebrations and football tailgating. *Journal of Studies on Alcohol, 67*(2), 282–289.

Neighbors, C., Walters, S. T., Lee, C. M., Vader, A. M., Vehige, T., Szigethy, T., & DeJong, W. (2007). Event-specific prevention: Addressing college student drinking during known windows of risk. *Addictive Behaviors, 32*(11), 2667–2680. https://doi.org/10.1016/j.addbeh.2007.05.010

North American Interfraternity Conference. (2019). *NIC alcohol & drug guidelines.* https://nicfraternity.org/nic-alcohol-drug-guidelines

Oster-Aaland, L. K., & Neighbors, C. (2007). The impact of a tailgating policy on students' drinking behavior and perceptions. *Journal of American College Health, 56*(3), 281–284.

CHAPTER 5

Universal Prevention Strategies

"When I was the president of my fraternity, a brother was using substances and ended up becoming a danger to himself and the fraternity. I was at a loss for what to do, so I reached out to one of the members of a peer alcohol education group I had just joined. The advisor provided me with the resources our chapter needed to effectively mitigate the situation and get the brother back on track."

—Recent graduate of a Southeastern research university

Universal prevention strategies are the first of the three approaches identified in the Institute of Medicine's (IOM's) prevention classification of its protractor (Springer, & Phillips, 2007). The IOM protractor identifies strategies for health prevention, treatment, and maintenance. The prevention segment is divided into three sections—universal, selective, and indicated. Universal strategies represent the most commonly used interventions to address health or well-being at a population level. Seen mostly as benign "posters and coasters," these strategies are often implemented without an expectation of return on investment. They incorporate popularized approaches with positive imagery, catchy slogans, and engaging strategies; as such, they are both widespread among prevention specialists and valued by the general public. Universal prevention efforts are often viewed as an institutional "loss leader" to demonstrate a good faith showing responding to a community health threat. Based on their breadth and visibility, they appear to be the foundation of many campus prevention efforts; however, they may not be viewed as favorably as the IOM's other two prevention strategies (i.e., selective or indicated).

Nevertheless, universal prevention strategies are more than a pretty poster, a catchy slogan, or hashtags on swag. Universal prevention is based on science and has the potential to influence campus health. Universal prevention also addresses the environment and the culture; it includes policies and broad-based efforts focused on a more diverse population.

Universal prevention initiatives incorporate both universal direct and universal indirect approaches. Central are the roles of information dissemination, environmental approaches, and community-building efforts. Information dissemination approaches focus on identifying health threats and protective strategies. Environmental approaches seek to assess, constrain, or correct factors in the environment that cause harm. Community-building efforts seek to garner support from local stakeholders to create momentum for change through advocacy. Due to their prominent roles within the comprehensive campus effort, two of this construct's main strategies—policies and coalitions—are developed much more extensively in Chapters 4 and 11.

This chapter offers a range of practical campus applications, with five professional contributions included. Two case studies illustrate student engagement in campus initiatives; one study focuses on behavioral pledges and the other on community messaging. Lessons From the Field complement these case studies; one lesson emphasizes health communication strategies and the other peer education. At the end of the chapter, Michael McNeil gives a review of universal prevention strategies.

DEFINITION OF UNIVERSAL POPULATIONS

Within the context of substance misuse prevention, universal prevention's net is broader than stopping misuse or reducing the progression of a substance use disorder. Prevention specialists promote healthy people and healthy communities that embrace positive engagement throughout educational, employment, and public life settings. Further, universal prevention targets general populations not explicitly identified based on specific risk factors.

Generally, universal prevention strategies seek to address a *public safety risk*. As stated in Chapter 1, direct impacts include but are not limited to death, personal injury, harm to others, property damage, sexual assault, and impaired driving. Other impacts are based on drug and alcohol influences on high-risk behaviors and situations such as hazing and sexual promiscuity. Common student behaviors, experimentation, feelings of invincibility, underdeveloped social skills, limited coping skills, loneliness, anxiety, and lack of stress-management skills exacerbate these impacts.

Universal prevention strategies can encompass *proactive, positive, and health promotion* approaches. Higher education institutions' core mission is academic performance; universal prevention strategies that address drug and alcohol issues can be instrumental for enhancing student academic performance, attendance, preparation, class participation, and overall achievement. Colleges and universities also stress the development of the "whole person" with "a liberal arts education," and universal prevention's focus on *human potential* is appropriate for promoting a campus culture emphasizing high-quality life. Overall, universal prevention approaches address the positive and enhance protective and resiliency factors; selective and indicated prevention strategies complement these efforts.

Universal prevention interventions that target populations are touted for their cost effectiveness, compared with interventions targeting individuals. Individual interventions that address specific health threats often require cost-prohibitive infrastructure, when compared with the support necessary to implement a universal direct or indirect prevention intervention. Universal prevention designs merely call for knowledge, skill, and persuasion.

To achieve desired results, two types of universal prevention are typically implemented: direct and indirect.

- *Universal direct strategies* emphasize the demand side of the supply/demand framework, seeking to reduce individuals' desires and motivations for using substances. These efforts attend to individual and community well-being; are process oriented; and engage community stakeholders.
- *Universal indirect strategies* are more task oriented, focusing on initiating or modifying laws and policies. These indirect strategies support instrumental population-based programs and environmental strategies and tend to engage members through policy and advocacy interventions.

Also, universal direct intervention strategies target members of a group based on *demographic* characteristics rather than *risk* characteristics, such as those found with selective prevention approaches. These strategies seek to persuade members of a target audience as well as promote well-being.

Universal direct prevention interventions are often based on the premise that knowledge impacts attitudes and that attitudes affect behavior. This more traditional concept is based on the assumption that the messaging, such as with campaigns, will improve understanding about the topic, and that this newly acquired knowledge will lead to changes in attitudes and, ultimately, behavior.

Universal direct campaigns must identify a target audience and an intervention strategy. The expressive nature of these universal direct campaigns requires being persuasive without appearing judgmental—without shaming or creating or supporting existing stigma. Expressive leadership (see Chapter 2) builds on collaboration to foster mutual support for adopting new health or safety behaviors.

One example of prevention campaigns includes those *aimed at youth*, which often focus on the legal and health risks of alcohol use, vaping, prescription drug misuse, and driving under the influence. Campaigns *geared to adults or parents* range from setting behavioral expectations such as with "Talk They Hear You" (Substance Abuse and Mental Health Services Administration, 2019a) to encouraging family time with children and teens. A campaign may emphasize the acceptability or desirability of a particular type of conversation (consider the "See Something, Say Something" messaging or signage that says "Feel Confident to Ask for Soda or Water" at a bar).

By design, universal direct prevention strategies encompass high-risk and low-risk populations. Campaign planners must understand that the campaign's effect may be disproportional; those efforts aimed at stemming texting and driving may be less effective with older drivers because of their lower engagement in this behavior. Challenges may also be found with younger drivers, who may believe they can text and drive safely, even though they possess much less experience with driving. Thus, campaign planners must attend to audience segmentation and differential messaging (see Chapter 12), and they should incorporate some members of the target audience into their planning efforts, as Case Study 5.1 makes clear.

Universal indirect strategies primarily focus on the environment, with attention paid to policies and procedures. Advocating for policy changes requires a clear target audience and a credible threat to community well-being. Historically, laws, ordinances, and policies have been enacted to eliminate or reduce problematic drug and alcohol behaviors. For example, to curb impaired driving, blood alcohol concentration limits became more restrictive. Concerns about youth and alcohol brought about minimum purchase ages—first enacted by states and then made universal with the National Minimum Drinking Age Act in 1984. Standards are established for items such as hours of operation, on-premise and off-premise sales, special events licenses, food sales, places for public possession, public intoxication, trained servers, and advertising. A review of state standards considers criteria that are typically overseen by a state's and/or locality's liquor control agency or alcoholic beverage control commission. Campus policies, whether they complement these sources or stand alone, are other universal indirect approaches.

When considering law and policy changes, broad support is essential. Successful policy does not overreach. For example, restrictions on drink specials (e.g., prohibiting alcohol sales below wholesale costs) are more likely to appeal to policymakers and community members than the elimination of all drink specials. Restaurant owners may push back on regulations that negatively impact their business. Clear differences exist, for example, between a "two for one" drink with a meal and an "all you can drink with a cover charge" drink special found at a bar near campus.

With policy changes it is likewise important to identify the threat to community well-being. Individuals may view health risks as "no big deal" until they or someone they love is affected by them. Similarly, those who do not live near a college may not see the risk some college bars pose to the community; however, if data are compiled and disseminated to the community about the incidence of alcohol-related injuries, fatalities, and DUIs near bars that feature regular drink specials, then residents may find more reason to support change. Sometimes advocacy requires raising awareness of health and safety risks, the consequence of inaction, and the potential consequences of varied types of a proposed action.

With all universal interventions, it is essential to identify ways to measure the impact of health behavior appeals. In terms of universal direct campaigns, this effort may include assessing whether the specified audiences were aware of the campaign, what they thought of it, whether it was credible and persuasive, and whether any desired outcomes took place (such as increased knowledge about the issue at hand, a shift in attitudes, enhanced confidence, improved conversation skills, and actual behavioral changes). For universal indirect approaches, the impact of a law or policy change can examine immediate as well as longer term results. Monitoring results will be critical for gaining support for sustaining and enhancing the strategies used.

Finally, many initiatives may include a blend of both indirect and direct interventions. One example is the Click It or Ticket campaign. The indirect intervention changed the law to allow police to stop and ticket drivers who did not comply with the existing seat belt law. The complementary media campaign (a direct intervention) communicated the importance of using seat belts and the risk of getting ticketed. The overall result was increased compliance with seat belt laws—the outcome sought. The Click it or Ticket campaign identified a clear risk (getting a ticket) and how to avoid a ticket (click the seat belt). Use of both direct and indirect approaches, performed within the systems approach context, helped promote the behavioral outcomes sought.

CASE STUDY 5.1

Engaging Students in Behavioral Pledge Campaign Development

Susie Bruce, MEd
Director
The Gordie Center
University of Virginia

Aditya Nàrayan, BS
Former Education and Outreach Coordinator
The Gordie Center
University of Virginia

Behavioral pledges, as part of health promotion campaigns, can be an effective tool to address hazardous drinking. These pledges invite students to sign a statement regarding future actions. However—and this is a large caveat—this efficacy is secured only if students from the target populations are engaged throughout campaign development. Signing a pledge to engage in protective strategies or to refrain from hazardous drinking practices employs the change process of "self-liberation" (i.e., by publicly stating a commitment to change; McKenzie-Mohr, 2011; Prochaska et al., 2015). When individuals state a behavioral intention in advance (e.g., sign a pledge), they increase the likelihood of attaining their goal (Costa et al., 2018; Gollwitzer, 1999; Koessler, 2019).

Student-led data collection methods, including Web-based surveys and focus groups of students in the target population, should guide the campaign. Pledges should offer specific, reasonable action steps that the target population would consider taking. Focusing on positive actions likely to minimize harm, instead of listing actions to eliminate (i.e., "use safe ride" instead of "don't drink and drive") can be more effective, as they point toward the desired behavior. Peer educators can lead focus groups with students recruited from heavier-drinking clusters to review draft pledge language and ensure that proposed goals are, in fact, attainable.

Visible pledge-related gear (e.g., T-shirts, cups, water bottles, laptop stickers, phone stickers), including examples used when drinking (i.e., bottle openers), can increase campaign reach and promote healthier social norms, particularly if the items display alcohol safety messages. If budgets are limited, consider holding a drawing for unique experiences such as dinner with a campus "celebrity," concert tickets, or a month of free parking. Students are unlikely to participate in the campaign if the pledge incentives are not desirable. Peer educators should gather ideas about appropriate incentives through surveys and focus groups, as their own friends or student leaders may not be representative of diverse populations or those with risky behaviors.

Marketing of pledge campaigns should involve partnering with organizations from the target populations (e.g., fraternities, sororities, athletics). This collaboration increases participation and ensures students receive consistent and customized information.

THEORETICAL UNDERPINNINGS OF UNIVERSAL PREVENTION STRATEGIES

As one component of a comprehensive campus effort, universal prevention strategies are essential. To be effective, however, they must be grounded in prevention science. Although some approaches, particularly the campaigns, may appear engaging and fun, their sophistication is embedded in this prevention science. Further, prevention science is clearly distinguished from marketing—prevention specialists choose interventions based on public health and community well-being.

Universal prevention is built on four pillars: research, epidemiology, intervention, and evaluation. The *research* pillar is vital for determining which interventions are most appropriate for addressing the health or safety risk, enhanced resiliency, or promotion of human potential. Prevention research relies on both evidence (e.g., evidence-based practices) as well as theories that explain change as a result of specific interventions. A symbiotic relationship exists between research and practice: Research informs prevention practices, and evaluation creates opportunities to improve research outcomes. Research informs and grounds decision makers with choices about the most suitable interventions.

The second pillar—*epidemiology*—supports universal prevention by fostering an understanding of the prevalence of substance misuse and the underlying factors that contribute to the initiation and continued use of substances. Epidemiologic factors that influence substance use include income disparities, health disparities, crime, peer affiliation, biological influences, family history of a substance use disorder, adverse childhood experiences, trauma, and mental health history. Knowing the context or pretext of substance use helps researchers and prevention specialists as they formulate hypotheses that can be empirically tested, and then plan interventions.

Within this context, prevention specialists identify the *intervention*, making decisions about what is necessary, reasonable, and appropriate. Epidemiology is particularly useful when considering the effect of a new or existing policy or law intervention, as it can guide planning decisions. The use of evidence-based practices (EBPs) grounds choices for locally appropriate interventions. When based on research, EBPs can be manualized and replicated across different settings. If based on sound theory, EBPs can result in interventions that will have the desired efforts; they can also yield approaches that go beyond reasonable or popular opinion. Also worthy of consideration is the role of peers and peer groups; Dolores Cimini's segment in Lessons From the Field 5.1 offers insight in this regard.

Evaluation, the fourth pillar, ties back to research. Interventions need to be consistently evaluated when implemented across settings. This is especially important when EBPs cannot be implemented in the same way they were researched. Implementing an EBP and maintaining the model integrity is challenging. Few settings are able to replicate research studies as they were designed and implemented. Successfully implementing EBPs relies on understanding their core components and controlling for differences between the population receiving the EBP, the training or expertise of the staff implementing the intervention, and the degree to which adequate funding is available to execute the intervention. Evaluation allows for consideration of factors that may diminish the effect of an EBP. Evaluation leads to new knowledge about the efficacy of these interventions, whether they were adapted from EBPs or grounded in theory. Post-intervention evaluation results should incorporate a feedback loop, mainly if efforts do not result in desired outcomes; this evaluation can determine if specific epidemiologic factors or lack of model integrity influenced the response.

These four pillars of prevention science undergird universal direct and universal indirect approaches. Although significant effort goes into designing and implementing those strategies identified, they are ultimately cost effective. Despite concerns that population-level interventions are costly and the outcome of the effort is difficult to quantify, universal strategies often lead to changes in perception of a risk or protective behavior. A population-level approach distributes consistent messaging across groups. For example, a message directed primarily for youth is heard by adults and parents, who subsequently reinforce that message. Overall, the prevention science behind universal prevention grounds these efforts and, ultimately, makes them more effective.

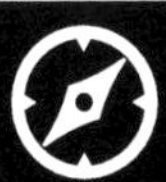

LESSONS FROM THE FIELD 5.1

Peer Education Reconsidered: Weighing the Benefits and Costs

M. Dolores Cimini, PhD
Psychologist and Director
University at Albany

I have gleaned so many insights from having led for over half of its 50 years of existence a pioneering peer assistance program that delivers hotline, education, and prevention services. Although I was initially aware of the many benefits of peer education—to both the students who delivered the services and the students who received them—I never could have imagined some of the important considerations and potential costs associated with administering peer education services on a college campus. Here are some of the unexpected lessons I learned:

- Keep in mind that students are arriving to campus with increasingly complex substance use backgrounds and associated concerns about physical and mental health, financial and food insecurity, and other challenges. Training about campus resources can address these general issues in addition to the ones in your primary program focus area.
- Leading a peer education program requires time and resources. Ensure that your job description incorporates

your supervisory and training role, that necessary financial and other resources are provided to operate the program safely, and that departmental commitment to peer education efforts exists.

- Be sure you develop a clear, detailed, and grounded training curriculum, and design evaluations to assess important learning outcomes. Continue with ongoing professional supervision so that peer educators' work will sustain quality and consistency.
- Students have many competing demands, so be clear about the benefits of serving as peer educators. Seek nominations for potential peer educators from faculty colleagues and share with potential peer educators that they have been nominated for this important role by a valued instructor. To motivate them to offer their best, ensure that they are rewarded for their work.
- Remain current regarding communication methods and platforms students use; be nimble regarding the strategies you use to convey prevention content.
- To address potential liability concerns, establish a formal documented relationship with each peer educator, either through an instructor–student relationship within an academic credit-bearing course or via a formal appointment letter and work/volunteer contract in place. For hotline or coaching services, ensure that peer educators are working under a licensed professional or that you have a supervisory agreement in place with a local mental health or substance use agency.
- Evaluation is important. Routinely collect data on peer education efforts, create an "organizational résumé" that summarizes program accomplishments, and use data to apply for campus, regional, and national awards.

> Additional information regarding peer education best practices may be found through the NASPA Peer Education Initiatives (https://www.naspa.org/project/peer-education-initiatives).

UNIVERSAL PREVENTION: INFORMATION DISSEMINATION

One core and widely used strategy with universal prevention is information dissemination. This approach is one-way communication that passively shares knowledge. It may include knowledge, opinions, examples, results, or other messages. Often referred to as "the 3 *P*s of Information Dissemination," the approach consists of posters, presentations, and papers.

Information dissemination addresses risk and protective factors associated with a known health threat. It identifies the effects of health threats on community members and includes information on available resources that promote and improve well-being. For example, a tobacco information campaign may highlight the physical harms associated with tobacco products and identify local smoking cessation services. Because the directionality of information dissemination is one way, the content may include third-party contact information for follow-up by the audience. Standard tactics include developing awareness of new or emerging health threats, identifying resources, and giving referrals to resources. Tavis Glassman provides insights on health communication strategies in Lessons From the Field 5.2. Also helpful is Worksheet 5.1: Communication Results, which emphasizes considerations to be made by prevention specialists as they orchestrate their efforts. The worksheet highlights the types of messages planners wish to change, to reinforce, or to introduce with their audiences.

Sound planning processes undergird successful efforts. Prevention specialists start with clarity about who their audience is and what they want the audience to know, feel, or do. This specificity guides planners' messages and strategies. Prevention specialists must also frame the messaging: Is it intended to *reinforce, change, or introduce* the desired outcome? With a knowledge focus, for example, is the aim one of providing support for something the audience would likely have already heard of or known (i.e., *reinforce*), providing updated information (i.e., *change*), or advertising new laws (i.e., *introduce*)? This framing makes the messaging, and thus its receptivity, more effective. These considerations are essential with such issues as revised guidelines about the safe, appropriate quantity of alcohol consumption; dangers of vaping; changes in enforcement; or information about hazards associated with specific substances.

Prevention specialists must inform the planning efforts by a relevant theory, specifically identify target norms or misperceptions to challenge, and spell out the consequences of a specific behavior (Campello et al., 2014). Prevention specialists can be guided by theories such as the health belief model, the precaution adoption process model, or the stages of change model. These and other factors serve to inform and guide the prevention specialists with the design of information dissemination efforts. Equally important is including self-efficacy messaging with any threat appeals. When fear overcomes individuals, they tend to retreat; thus, a mix of threat appeals (to get the attention of the audience) and a strong self-efficacy message (specifying what can be done to avoid the danger posed by the messaging) is recommended.

Information dissemination efforts can address varied desired outcomes, such as the following:

- **Attitude:** the desirability or appropriateness of getting involved with others' behavior (e.g., bystander intervention); the value or propriety of a particular law (e.g., minimum drinking age, cannabis sales).
- **Intention:** plans to limit drinks, use a designated driver, or not use illicit drugs.
- **Belief**: feelings of susceptibility, the severity of consequences of inaction, benefits of action, barriers, and self-efficacy.
- **Skills:** appropriate strategies for intervention (e.g., talking with a friend about concerns with their substance use).
- **Knowledge:** awareness of a crisis helpline, helpful resources, or an engaging website.

By considering these types of outcomes, prevention specialists determine whether the aim is to change an unwanted behavior, reinforce a wanted one, or introduce the desired result. Further, the approach may blend more than a single desired outcome.

Consider, for example, that the aim of the information dissemination strategy is to increase the likelihood that students will engage in difficult conversations about drugs or alcohol; the approach may be to provide conversation starters. The foundation blends skills (sample scenarios and suggested wording) with belief (benefits of acting on information coupled with increased confidence). The information campaign's content may suggest an action, provide permission or encouragement, and offer tools to the audience, all in preparation for more meaningful conversations.

A skill-building outcome is also reasonable for universal prevention. Because skill building is interactive between a facilitator and an audience, it is typically associated with selective prevention. Because universal prevention focuses on populations not designated as "at risk," attention to life-skill training is appropriate. Universal intervention skill-building strategies often include training manuals delivered to an audience by a professional. Increasingly implemented are interactive, digital skill-building programs that are designed by subject matter experts and accessed online.

A wide range of strategies can be used to disseminate information. Basic approaches include brochures, posters, and fliers; they may also include billboards, rotating electronic signs, signage on public transportation (bus, taxi, subway), and advertising wrapping on buses and garbage trucks. The signage may be at waiting areas for public transportation (bus stops) as well as on trash cans. Information may be included in various print media, whether newspapers, magazines, or programs provided at events. Messages are included in swag, such as T-shirts, tote bags, coffee cups, pens, and other promotional items.

Messaging should be formulated to provide ample opportunities for broad coverage. Messaging may be limited to a specific topic or a compilation of different topics as part of a campaign. Information may be included on websites, social media, text messages, mass emails, and blogs. Other content may be disseminated in news releases and on radio or television stations, as well as at movie theaters, athletic and concert venues, and other community settings. Today, more than ever, multiple avenues exist to get the message out. Information dissemination messaging that reinforces self-efficacy is vital to prevention efforts.

As an example, consider prescription drug misuse and its varied issues. Clarity regarding the facts that information dissemination efforts might address is essential, and these facts will be informed by local and external needs assessment activities. Potential topics for a prescription drug information dissemination campaign include the following:

- how to read prescription drug labels;
- understanding interactions and potential side effects;
- identifying risks associated with mixing prescription and nonprescription drugs (e.g., using Xanax with alcohol may be fatal);
- raising awareness about counterfeit pills (e.g., a drug labeled as Xanax may be fentanyl);
- identifying signs and symptoms of an overdose or a withdrawal; and
- training to intervene as a bystander.

Prior to launching the campaign, planning efforts would assess whether the information dissemination efforts seek to address one, more, or all of these topics.

LESSONS FROM THE FIELD 5.2

Health Communication Strategies in College Health

Tavis Glassman, PhD
Professor
School of Population Health
University of Toledo

At most universities, there are tens of thousands of students and only a small number, if any, of prevention specialists, so the need to implement cost-effective interventions is paramount. An often underutilized and poorly understood intervention strategy is health communication. A witty, theory-based health communication campaign can reach large numbers of students quickly. The media channels on campus are relatively inexpensive and provide tremendous visibility for health-related messages.

For example, posters could be hung in the residence halls, at the recreation center, at the student union, and in classroom buildings; they can also be placed in restrooms at the "stall seat," targeting captive audiences who are likely to read the messages repeatedly. Table tents could be placed in high-traffic areas, such as restaurants, dining halls, and seating areas throughout the university. Screensavers are another inexpensive way to reach large numbers of students, faculty, and staff with prevention information. Messages can also be sent electronically to students' email accounts and/or through social media.

Many prevention messages and materials already exist and can be obtained from the local health department, the Centers for Disease Control and Prevention, and other reputable nonprofit and government organizations (National Cancer

Institute, 2002, 2011). Although most efforts focus on prevention, crisis communication strategies can be used to respond quickly to events such as a public health pandemic or an opioid overdose fatality crisis among others (Substance Abuse and Mental Health Services Administration, 2019b). With proper supervision, students can prepare messages, graphics, designs, and materials. The university's marketing and communication department may be willing to create and disseminate prevention messages. Before designing messages, review the scientific literature as well as conduct a thorough needs assessment. Health messages should also be pilot tested (sometimes referred to as *message testing*) before dissemination to ensure that priority audiences understand and find the message(s) credible. Moreover, assessment with health communication interventions needs to occur before, during, and after the campaign; this evaluation helps with future planning (Drug Enforcement Administration, 2020).

UNIVERSAL PREVENTION: ENVIRONMENTAL STRATEGIES

Another central area within universal prevention concerns environmental strategies. Although they are commonly subsumed within the scope of universal indirect strategies, their primary aim is to affect the context within which individuals and groups operate. The social-ecological model's constructs of public policy and community form the theoretical foundations of environmental strategies. Public policy addresses prevailing norms and policies and their enforcement in the larger society; community efforts advocate for change within more discrete settings, such as schools, worksites, neighborhoods, and other places where individuals gather.

Environmental prevention creates or modifies written community standards and codes. It opens a dialog about existing attitudes and beliefs in an attempt to garner support for policy interventions. Environmental prevention includes advocacy initiatives that raise awareness of risk and protective factors and creates opportunities for community mobilization in response to specific health threats. Chapter 4 goes into greater detail on policies and procedures.

Just as with the information dissemination approaches, prevention specialists benefit from determining whether the aim is to *reinforce, change, or introduce* a policy, procedure, or protocol; this determination will be based on issues or gaps identified through needs assessments. For example, if the policy needs some refinement or clarification, or if enforcement needs enhancement, this would be *reinforcement*. Separately, *change* may be required because the policy may have had some unintended consequences, it may no longer be needed, or laws may have been updated with implications for policy change. New legislation (e.g., vaping or marijuana laws) or changed needs (e.g., heightened awareness of specific issues) may necessitate the *introduction* of policy.

These adjustments may be called for because of any of a variety of circumstances:

- a specific situation, such as a tragedy
- increased levels of problems, documented by needs assessment data, incident reports, or archival data
- new substances or behaviors documented locally or externally
- growing intolerance with continued behaviors, attitudes, or issues
- new leadership wanting a revised focus
- scheduled time (e.g., biennial review or systematic review)

Useful environmental strategies for college campuses include those developed by the campus for their settings. They can also include advocacy by campus personnel for policies, procedures, and enforcement activities in local venues; thus, city, town, or countywide ordinances may be helpful, as would statewide laws. Regardless of the location or sponsor, many environmental strategies exist; the following are some examples:

- limitations on drink specials
- limited vendor hours of operation
- campus-sponsored traditions that discourage misuse of alcohol
- increased enforcement of existing laws, such as minimum legal drinking age, impaired driving, public intoxication, and possession
- enforcement of campus policies prohibiting the use of illicit substances
- vendor practices promoting safer behavior
- nonpermissibility or settings for various substances (e.g., tobacco-free)
- settings where alcohol may be used (e.g., sporting events, special activities)
- responsible beverage service training
- increasing the availability of food and nonalcoholic beverages
- socially responsible marketing and advertising
- increased surcharges or other fees to offset negative externalities associated with alcohol abuse

As part of the overall systems approach, these environmental strategies are complemented by information dissemination, which helps the targeted audience learn about changes in policies and procedures, thus reinforcing their effectiveness. Information dissemination can be a means to an end—reducing risk and promoting health.

Coalitions enhance environmental strategies and are central to a comprehensive campus approach with its focus on group cohesion and ongoing work among diverse community stakeholders. These strategies also benefit from collaboration with students and campus police, though in different ways. Ryan Snow's Case Study 5.2 highlights an interesting approach. Also, Chapter 11's discussion of coalitions details the importance of and strategies for effective partnerships. Campus and community coalitions provide opportunities to improve the reach of existing service agencies as well as support interagency collaboration.

CASE STUDY 5.2

Walk as One: Community Building Messages With Peer Focus

Ryan Snow, MEd
Instructor
Preventionleaders.com

An event that began to educate the student population on policy and rules grew to become one of the largest educational missions in the campus community: "Walk as One" (https://www.champaigncommunitycoalition.org/initiatives/walk-as-one) was created to get members of the community together to pass out educational material about an unsanctioned event held every year. This event had led to several drug- and alcohol-related medical emergencies and, sadly, even a few deaths.

To pull in different areas of the community, recognizable members of the university (dean, counselor, police chief, president, coach, athletic director) would each team up with a group of students (fraternities and sororities, student organizations, athletic teams) and walk the campus and hand out information. This effort not only brought together students to speak to other students on campus but also demonstrated that the goal of safety is shared by the entire community—and is, in fact, a partnership between students, student groups, and campus officials.

After 8 years, the "Walk as One" event at the University of Illinois at Urbana–Champaign has enjoyed such popularity that some volunteers have been asked to participate in other events due to the overwhelming turnout on campus. Although the initial purpose of this event was to educate students on one particular matter, "Walk as One" has much greater potential. Getting students, staff, and faculty to come together and send a unified message about safety issues, especially those related to substance misuse, can be a very powerful tool for campus communities. It is helpful to highlight—collaboratively—what is important to the students, staff, and faculty as a campus community rather than what the administration alone thinks is important.

CRITICISMS OF UNIVERSAL PREVENTION STRATEGIES

Although universal prevention strategies are essential for a campus's comprehensive prevention effort, they must be seen as one part of this overall plan and be firmly rooted in science. These universal prevention strategies may provide the requisite foundations or groundwork for the other initiatives to be effective.

Critics of universal prevention strategies primarily cite a lack of quantitative research showing a direct link between information dissemination and behavior change; additional criticisms include the breadth of reach of universal prevention interventions. It is difficult to isolate the change effect within a universal intervention because of the many variables that may account for a behavior change. Similar criticisms may be relevant for the efforts of a community coalition. Despite these and other criticisms, universal strategies are essential to creating and maintaining community well-being.

Motivational enhancement theory may be helpful for understanding the vital role of universal prevention strategies. This theory suggests that individuals change when they have sufficient motivation to do so. Prevention specialists cannot predict when someone will move into an "action" state of readiness to change (i.e., stages of change model). Schulenberg et al.'s (2020) Monitoring the Future study showed that high-risk binge drinking in the previous 2 weeks declined among college students from 43.9% in 1980 to 32.7% in 2019. Similar reductions among high school students also took place. These changes are too broad to be a result of selective or indicated prevention strategies. Something changed in the environment of students, both in high school and in college. Widespread information dissemination targeted elementary, middle, and high school students from 1997 to 2019; similarly, many efforts increased on college campuses over this time. While it is difficult to prove what, precisely, accounts for binge drinking reduction, it is clear that it did happen. Perhaps information dissemination strategies, or policy approaches, with marginal empirical support can explain these changes. Universal prevention should not be discounted simply because a straightforward cause–effect relationship cannot be demonstrated; increased diligence to sound planning, execution, and review and evaluation will gather needed documentation.

It is also noteworthy that universal prevention relies on tipping points to create a new level of health or civic awareness and thereby dispel previous beliefs and behaviors (Gladwell, 2000). Cigarette use was not stigmatized in the 1960s, but it was accepted as a public health threat a decade later. Although seat belts were required in automobiles in the 1960s, it was not until the 1990s that virtually all states had laws requiring their use; current usage rates are above 90% (National Highway Traffic Safety Administration, 2019). Information dissemination helped convince large groups of people to change their behavior. The stages of change model credits the initiation of doubt as a precursor to the motivation to change. It is likely that universal prevention interventions—information dissemination and environmental or community-based processes—led to increased doubt about the safety of smoking tobacco. The same is true for injuries related to motor vehicle crashes. While these strategies are not yet labeled as evidence-based practices, it is clear that behavior changes occur in the context of community mobilization; this is particularly important for prevention specialists planning a community forum, health fair, or awareness day/month program. The impact of these efforts may be more focused on changing the culture, promoting general awareness, making issues more visible, promoting the permissibility of discussion or action, and perhaps initiating doubt—the first step on the path to behavior change.

The redundancy of the message, with increased dosage for an individual, helps change behavior. Behavior change is aided by framing messages in different ways or repeating them in different contexts (e.g., radio ad, print ad, social media post, news coverage). Also important is acknowledging that the expressive function of appealing to or raising community consciousness does not provide a quick fix; universal direct campaigns take time and effort to reach and influence a general audience. These strategies are long-term investments in mobilizing community health.

Finally, targeted universal prevention addresses the fact that people have varying behavior change needs. Individuals who are low risk are not engaged by campaigns that address high-risk behaviors, and very high-risk subpopulations dismiss protective messages because of their frame of reference—such as "all of my friends act as I do, and we are all OK." Although a reasonable criticism, this thinking highlights the importance of vetting messages with members of subgroups within a target population through pilot testing; this process finds the intersection where all groups meet. The stages of change model explains why some people respond favorably to a message (i.e., they are in a preparation or action change stage) and others react less favorably. Overall, universal prevention messages can be useful in creating ambivalence among those at-risk individuals who are precontemplative. In contrast, these same messages may validate the behavioral choices of low-risk individuals who are already engaged in protective strategies.

Michael McNeil, who has blended innovation within theoretical and experience-based frameworks on various health promotion issues, has instructive perspectives in Innovator 5.1.

INNOVATOR 5.1

Beyond Universal

Michael P. McNeil, EdD
Chief of Administration, Columbia Health
Adjunct Assistant Professor, Sociomedical Sciences, Mailman School of Public Health
Columbia University

For decades, colleges and universities have taken a "one-size-fits-all" approach to addressing alcohol and other drugs. Using a variety of tools (including canned online programs that do not account for unique institutional characteristics), schools have assumed that all students are the same in terms of drinking and drug use. Despite so many population-level data collections (e.g., the American College Health Association's [2020] National College Health Assessment, Core Survey [Core Institute, 2020]) and the availability of institutional data (e.g., policy violations, emergency room transports, medical service or hospital data), campuses have not embraced the reality that not every student needs the same message. In fact, the prevention field needs to recognize that students are not the same. As a colleague once noted, "College students are the most diverse homogenous population."

When institutions work only from a one-size approach, it tends to be more about checking a box than creating a culture where lower risk drinking or drug use is the norm. These cookie-cutter approaches also contribute to reinforcing the false norms on alcohol and other drugs that many of us have worked for decades to change. Higher education cannot simultaneously try to change the norm while reinforcing it. This type of thinking has the substance abuse prevention field trapped in a cycle—without a chance of achieving the change the prevention field claims to seek.

Let's consider the nondrinker group. These students get the message that most of their peers drink and experience a range of related consequences. Although this message is technically true on the consumption level, most students drink in a smart, safe, and responsible manner. Consider, though, that when campuses do this education, they are typically using the stories of the extreme. These nondrinking students (and even the majority of other responsible students) can easily come to believe that the campus alcohol culture is one of excess; then, their desire to conform could create a problem drinker. The alternative, and preferred, approach is to support nondrinking as an equal option that is openly valued on the campus. While this narrative illustrates alcohol consumption, similar scenarios play out with marijuana, other illicit drugs, and nonmedical use of prescription medication (e.g., "study aids").

Interestingly, several campuses have tried to update the narrative by focusing on the following principles:

- Not everyone drinks/uses drugs—and that's supported as a valid option.
- Those who do consume drugs/alcohol tend to do so in a smart, safe, and responsible manner.
- Extra focus is put on populations for which drug/alcohol use rates are higher or behaviors are more concerning (these groups vary by campus, so local data are the key to understanding them):
    - Fraternities and sororities
    - Athletics

- Marching band
- "Party" residence halls

Across these campuses, there have been real and lasting changes. Reductions in higher risk drinking measures (quantity, frequency, and consequence) have been reported and sustained after using the local data to move to selective and indicated prevention. The changes are happening across years and in places where the numbers were stable, but they are not reflective of the healthier drinking goals previously professed.

Let's also not be fooled into thinking this is just an undergraduate problem. Subgroups of graduate students may engage in these behaviors at levels equal to or greater than some undergraduates. For example, it's not a secret in higher education that drinking parties occur in graduate-level business and law programs. Why are campus leaders not recognizing the need for selective and indicated prevention with these groups? And how might these graduate groups be reinforcing the campus culture that has historically been defined by undergraduate behaviors?

If the prevention field is really dedicated to changing individual and group behaviors, then it must be data driven. Further, practitioners must use the available tools (or create some) to identify populations where indicated or selective prevention efforts would actually speak to the alcohol and other drug use and related consequences that our institutions claim to care so much about. Each campus leader has (or has access to) the information needed to break this busy, but unsuccessful, cycle. The question is whether the prevention field actually has the political will to truly create positive change.

CONCLUSION

Universal prevention strategies address public safety risks, promote risk reduction, and support self-efficacy. Leveraging the four pillars of universal prevention grounds campus efforts in the core components of change management. With attention to direct and indirect frameworks, universal prevention plays a vital and cost-effective role within the comprehensive campus initiative. Both information-focused strategies and environmental approaches offer significant opportunities for prevention specialists and their partners to be innovative. Prevention specialists are best positioned to orchestrate locally relevant initiatives that can enhance student health and well-being.

REFERENCES

American College Health Association. (2020). *National college health assessment.* http://www.acha-ncha.org

Campello, G., Sloboda, Z., Heikkil, H., & Brotherhood, A. (2014). International standards on drug use prevention: The future of drug use prevention world-wide. *International Journal of Prevention and Treatment of Substance Use Disorders, 2*, 6–27.

Core Institute. (2020). *Core alcohol and drug survey.* Southern Illinois University. http://www.core.siu.edu

Costa, M., Schaffner, B. F., & Prevost, A. (2018). Walking the walk? Experiments on the effect of pledging to vote on youth turnout. *PloS One, 13*(5), e0197066. https://doi.org/10.1371/journal.pone.0197066

Drug Enforcement Administration. (2020). *Prevention with a purpose: A strategic planning guide for preventing drug misuse among college students.* https://www.campusdrugprevention.gov/sites/default/files/Strategic%20Planning%20Guide%20%28Final-Online%29%20%281%29.pdf

Gladwell, M. (2000). *The tipping point: How little things can make a big difference.* Little, Brown and Company.

Gollwitzer, P. M. (1999). Implementation intentions: Strong effects of simple plans. *American Psychology, 54*(7), 493–503. doi:10.1037/0003-066X.54.7.493

Koessler, A.-K. (2019). *Setting new behavioral standards: Sustainabilty pledges and how conformity impacts their outreach.* SSRN. https://dx.doi.org/10.2139/ssrn.3369557

McKenzie-Mohr, D. (2011). *Fostering sustainable behavior* (3rd ed.). New Society Publishers.

National Cancer Institute. (2002). *Making health communication programs work: A planner's guide.* https://www.cancer.gov/publications/health-communication/pink-book.pdf

National Cancer Institute. (2011). *Making data talk: A workbook.* https://www.cancer.gov/publications/health-communication/making-data-talk.pdf

National Highway Traffic Safety Administration. (2019). *Seat belt use in 2019—Overall results.* https://crashstats.nhtsa.dot.gov/Api/Public/ViewPublication/812875

Prochaska, J. O., Redding, C. A., & Evers, K. E. (2015). The transtheoretical model and stages of change. In K. Glanz, B. K. Rimer, & K. Viswanath (Eds.), *Health behavior: Theory, research, and practice* (5th ed., pp. 125–148). Jossey-Bass.

Schulenberg, J. E., Johnston, L. D., O'Malley, P. M., Bachman, J. G., Miech, R. A., & Patrick, M. E. (2020). *Monitoring the future: National survey results on drug use, 1975–2019: Volume II, college students and adults ages 19–60.* Institute for Social Research, The University of Michigan.

Springer, J. R., & Phillips, J. (2007). *The Institute of Medicine framework and its implication for the advancement of prevention policy, programs and practice* (SMA-4205). U.S. Department of Health and Human Services. http://ca sdfsc.org/docs/resources/SDFSC_IOM_Policy.pdf

Substance Abuse and Mental Health Services Administration. (2019a). *Parent-focused national media campaign backgrounder.* https://store.samhsa.gov/product/talk-they-hear-you-campaign-backgrounder/PEP18-TTHY-BACKGRD

Substance Abuse and Mental Health Services Administration. (2019b). *Communicating in a crisis: Risk communication guidelines for public officials.* https://store.samhsa.gov/product/communicating-crisis-risk-communication-guidelines-public-officials/pep19-01-01-005

CHAPTER 6

Selective Prevention Strategies

"Prior to my first day on campus, I had a preconceived notion that my university was a party school. With a family history of alcoholism, this reputation lingered over my first impressions of the campus, and I knew my studies had to take priority. After engaging in an alcohol abuse prevention program that utilized a social norming approach, I realized the importance of reducing the discrepancy between perceived and actual alcohol-related behaviors among college students, and in giving students the real facts about alcohol!"

—Senior at a large public Southern university

Selective prevention approaches, the second of three parts of the Institute of Medicine's (IOM's) prevention model, fall between universal and indicated strategies (Springer & Phillips, 2007). These targeted measures focus on prevention efforts with groups or groupings of people who share specified characteristics. Selective prevention initiatives adapt overall campus prevention messages and strategies in ways that speak to and engage more effectively with the identified audience.

Typically, selective prevention focuses on groups with demonstrated higher levels of substance misuse, such as first-year students, fraternity or sorority members, and student-athletes. Selective prevention also reaches out to those whose group affiliation brings the potential for the heightened risk of substance misuse; in addition to the last three groups, this includes student-veterans, LGBTQIA+ students, and children of alcoholics. Selective prevention can also engage groups and affiliated individuals to harness their potential for positive engagement—for example, student leaders, honors programs, and service organizations.

Selective approaches are essential for a comprehensive campus prevention effort. They provide opportunities for more effective messaging, individual engagement, collective ownership, group norms, and enhanced evaluation. Selective strategies focus attention on the unique challenges and opportunities for working with specific populations or groups. Information sharing, skill building, and alternative activities are components of interventions that target selective populations.

Highlighted in the five segments provided by a range of prevention professionals are various practical approaches relevant to prevention specialists. Three Lessons From the Field are offered; two address specific higher risk groups and one presents a broader perspective on social norms efforts. The Innovator segment, prepared by H. Wesley Perkins and Jessica Perkins, provides exemplary perspectives about social norms strategies as part of a comprehensive campus strategy.

DEFINING SELECTIVE POPULATIONS

The general focus of selective prevention is to organize and orchestrate strategies with groupings of individuals. Each of them has some common, unifying characteristics that make opportunities for consistent and focused interventions and messaging reasonable. Three overall constructs define this perspective.

1. Selective prevention creates *parameters to target groups* rather than individuals. It is the only IOM category of prevention that identifies specific risks or issues to be addressed by an intervention—universal prevention promotes health, and indicated prevention uses diagnostic criteria to rule out behavioral health disorders. Selective strategies target a population subgroup,

regardless of the degree of risk of any individual within the group, and with no individual risk factor assessment.

2. Participants' inclusion is based on *group membership or group affiliation*. After a target group is identified, the next step for prevention and health promotion specialists is to determine ways to access and recruit group members to participate in the specific interventions.
3. The selective group designation is based on one of three factors:
   - *membership* resulting from joining a club or organization (e.g., student-athletics, fraternity, sorority, student organization)
   - *specified affiliation* based on demographics or identifying characteristics (e.g., first-year students, graduate students, military-connected students) or behavior (e.g., those with campus disciplinary charges, those convicted of an impaired driving offense)
   - *self-identified affiliation*, which may or may not include group membership (e.g., an LGBTQIA+ student, a first-generation student, a child of an alcoholic, a person in recovery)

Selective prevention promotes targeted messaging for individuals with common characteristics, based solely on their group membership or affiliation. Individuals with shared interests and needs are more likely to connect with messaging relevant to them, based on that affiliation. For example, student-athletes (as well as members of specific sports) will likely connect with messaging linked to athletic performance, endurance, and unique stressors.

When looking at selective prevention efforts historically, the primary work has been done with groups with higher risk behaviors. Peer-reviewed research over the past 25 years has identified the following groups as "at risk": fraternity and sorority members, student-athletes, and first-year students. Although overall trends of student consumption demonstrate reductions in alcohol use, the usage patterns of these populations remain differentially higher, thus warranting attention. That said, it is important to note that contemporary students' consumption levels are the lowest in decades (Schulenberg et al., 2020).

Among fraternity and sorority members, it is unclear whether individual risk-taking is an impact of group norms or self-selection on the part of individuals who already engage in risky behavior. It is a "chicken or egg" (which comes first) dilemma. Regardless of the cause, the rationale for greater attention being paid to these groups is due to the face validity of higher risk behaviors and related problems associated with membership into these groups (Capone et al., 2007).

Similarly, student-athletes have a higher risk of substance-using behaviors. As documented by the National Collegiate Athletic Association's data collection over many years with its NCAA Student-Athlete Substance Use Survey, student-athletes have higher substance-using behaviors than those who are not student-athletes (National Collegiate Athletic Association, 2018b). Also, members of some athletic teams have higher usage rates than those in other teams; for example, men's lacrosse, ice hockey, wrestling, and football report higher use of pain medication than other sports; for women, highest are gymnastics, softball, ice hockey and lacrosse (National Collegiate Athletic Association, 2018a). This information makes clear that there are needs and opportunities for selective interventions at varying levels.

For students entering college, this transition—and especially the residential component—involves students' expectations and self-responsibility; it has historically resulted in higher risk behaviors (Brower et al., 2003). Emerging risk considerations may include the lack of viable sober social options and an environment that promotes rather than eschews high-risk behavior. That said, heavy (binge) drinking behavior is trending downward among first-year students. Recent data indicate high-intensity drinking (HID; having 10 or more drinks in a row) is shifting from the late teens to the low- to mid-20s (Patrick & Terry-McElrath, 2019). These data indicate the importance of prevention efforts for young adults throughout their 20s and demonstrate a shift in the traditional wisdom of first-year college students having a greater risk of high-risk drinking than students in general. These data also indicate alcohol, tobacco, and other drug abuse prevention strategies should not exclude traditional graduate students.

Beyond the traditional three higher risk groups are other audiences that warrant consideration. Substance misuse concerns pertaining to LGBTQIA+ students have been documented and relate to factors such as discrimination, isolation, shame, and personal uncertainties (Green & Feinstein, 2012). With veterans, another higher risk group, adjustment, age differences, and post-traumatic stress disorder may be factors (Teeters et al., 2017).

These data attest to the importance of staging prevention efforts for young adults throughout their 20s. Also, selective prevention approaches are appropriate for students in recovery or according to the medical model "in remission" from substance use disorders as well as other behavioral health disorders. Although often seen as outside of traditional prevention methodologies, selective prevention is deemed appropriate because it seeks to prevent harm and impede the progression of a substance use disorder. This approach is consistent with the expanded role of health promotion and well-being on campus. Attention to recovery and support services, and a supportive campus environment, are applicable within selective prevention. Chapter 7 goes into more detail about recovery services within the context of a comprehensive campus program.

Other higher risk audiences do exist, and prevention specialists are encouraged to examine data from national and local sources to identify factors most relevant and appropriate for their campuses. Relevant, well-sourced data are the foundation of targeted efforts. Applying prevention science strategies heightens the likelihood of positive and lasting impact. Social norms marketing is a popular approach to target selective audiences; in Lessons From the Field 6.1, Michael Haines provides some contextual observations.

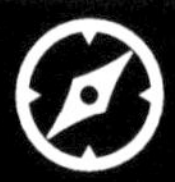

LESSONS FROM THE FIELD 6.1

Social Norms Approaches: More Than Meets the Eye

Michael P. Haines, MS
Director (former)
National Social Norms Resource Center

Applying the social norms approach to select populations is not as straightforward as it might seem. It may be that the greatest chance for success in applying the social norms approach to select populations is likely when a universal (campuswide) effort is combined with an effort aimed at a select population.

Although there have been some successes—most notably with student-athletes (Perkins & Craig, 2006) and with sequential small group classes or online interventions (Baer et al, 2001; Lewis & Neighbors, 2007; Neighbors et al, 2004, 2009)—the literature describes occasional failures. Some of these ineffective efforts may stem from the usual implementation flaws: poor messaging, inadequate message exposure, no fidelity to the norm approach. Other unsuccessful efforts may be the result of the *social identity error*; this occurs when a social norms marketing intervention fails to select the peer group most influential to a select population.

A college student has multiple social identities. For instance, a male Latino freshman student-athlete is influenced by his perception of overall college student norms, Latinx/a/o norms, freshman norms, student-athlete norms, and male norms. It is not always easy to identify which norm perception is most salient for this student. To reduce the likelihood of a social identity error, consider simply implementing a marketing campaign using the universal *college student* identity.

First-year students are identified in the literature as high risk for heavy drinking and alcohol-related harms. A common example of the social identity error is seen when an intervention chooses first-year students as a select population and uses first-year student norms for a social norms project. The intervention may fail to influence first-year students' heavy drinking behavior because these students do not identify strongly as first-year students; they aspire to be *college students,* not first-year students. So, an intervention using the campuswide student norm may be more effective.

Another pitfall of choosing a select group for a social norm intervention is underestimating the powerful influence of the campus social norm. An effort may correct norm misperceptions and behaviors of the select group while having no impact on the misperceptions of the campus in general (universal norm). As the select group is subsequently exposed to a widespread campus misperception, the gains made with the select group may be diminished or even reversed altogether.

It should also be noted that some select populations (e.g., Greek-letter organization members, LGBTQIA+ students, student-athletes) may have higher rates of "risk" behaviors than does the campus in general. In such cases, care must be taken not to shame or stigmatize the select population. This can be accomplished by developing efforts that expose *only* the select population to its peer norms while simultaneously marketing the campus norm to everyone.

WHY SELECTIVE PREVENTION IS APPROPRIATE

The rationale undergirding selective prevention is based on access, relevant approaches, and cost-effectiveness. With localized attention and content for specific groups and affiliations, campus prevention efforts are more likely to be customized—based on local factors instead of "cut and paste" programs. The implicit message of using a "one size fits all" approach is that local expertise is unnecessary. The opposite is true; prevention strategies work best when they are customized to account for different student populations. The reach of prevention efforts is greater in number than is found with efforts aimed at specific individuals within a population. Whether with group members, affiliation based on identifying characteristics, or self-identified affiliation as noted earlier, efforts at the intentional, micro level have a greater chance for reach, success, and sustainability.

Selective prevention's value is drawn from the fact that different audiences have different needs and issues, and will likely respond better to approaches relevant to them. Group members are more apt to believe and react positively to strategies and messages when they perceive the content and style as relevant and credible; they are more likely to engage when the approach is deemed pertinent to their needs and seen as "speaking to them." Some examples include the following:

- Appeal to leadership qualities and a service orientation for fraternity and sorority members.
- Cite stressors faced by student-athletes, including juggling academics and workouts, demands for high performance, and behavioral expectations as a model student.
- Acknowledge challenges faced by military-connected students particularly those with combat experience or who may be older.
- Target specific approaches to those with substance misuse judicial sanctions or with impaired driving convictions.
- Plan directed efforts for those transported to the emergency room for a drug- or alcohol-involved incident.
- Organize messages for those in recovery from a substance use disorder or for students living with (on campus or at home) someone with drug/alcohol issues.

Selective prevention also allows for opportunities to build shared experiences. Pointed prevention approaches encourage students to reflect on and discuss the messages. Particularly for those in an intact group, conversations about group norms, standards, and expectations may emerge. These discussions may focus on individual behavioral choices and normative expectations of group membership, the group's vision, protocols, operational guidelines, and consequences appropriate for those acting outside agreed-upon standards. Selective prevention promotes open conversation, shared decision making, and community building—all of which lead toward a positive and healthy living and learning environment.

Similarly, when individuals with shared characteristics hear messages that resonate with them, such stimulus can act as a conversation starter. Even with self-affiliated individuals (such as first-generation students or LGBTQIA+ students), focused messages may resonate individually, and discussions may emerge that help with sharing experiences and insights.

A final benefit with selective prevention relates to assessment and evaluation. Measuring the effectiveness of a selective strategy is more manageable than measuring that of a universal one. Intact groups, such as membership organizations that offer in-person meetings as well as a roster of members, offer straightforward access to evaluation—whether pretest/posttest, follow-up assessments, qualitative approaches, or targeted inquiries. Other audiences, such as those based on demographics (e.g., first-year, graduating, first-generation, military-connected students), may also provide opportunities for periodic needs assessments, monitoring, and evaluation to determine the impact of a strategic intervention. As Susie Bruce highlights in Case Study 6.1, community service sanctions can create learning opportunities directly and indirectly related to students' substance use.

Community Service Sanctions

Susie Bruce, MEd
Director, Gordie Center
University of Virginia

For 2 decades, the University of Virginia's Gordie Center has partnered with the University Judiciary Committee (UJC) to host community service students with alcohol or other drug policy violations. The UJC may assign community service hours as part of the sanction for students' behavior, with the intent of linking sanctions with violations, providing an opportunity for restitution to the community, promoting reflection on the effects of substance misuse, and reducing recidivism (Asher, 2008; Emerson, 1992; Kompalla & McCarthy, 2001). Because the UJC is student run, staff reach out annually to the newly elected officers to remind them of the program, explain how staff can support students in finding motivation to make healthier decisions, and address any concerns around confidentiality or the types of projects assigned.

The administrative assistant coordinates student schedules and manages project flow; having a warm, empathic personality is essential for setting students at ease and is key for the program's success. Students complete a personal skills checklist to determine which projects would be appropriate and engaging; a weekly schedule ensures someone with knowledge of the project is available.

Potential projects are identified and updated throughout the year. Examples include data entry, updating PowerPoint slide formatting, reviewing educational materials for clarity, conducting literature reviews, and checking website hyperlinks. Some students assist peer educators by setting up booths, posting flyers, and sorting materials.

Through this work, students gain office skills and learn about the effects of alcohol and other drugs. The accepting, collaborative office environment encourages many students to confidentially initiate conversations about their lives and drinking choices. Some participants self-reported making healthy changes, a few became alcohol peer educators, and several remain in touch after graduation.

Although not all students put forth their best effort, the vast majority perform a valuable service. This frees up staff time and yields insights on how to reach students with high-risk drinking patterns. Most students gain as much from the experience as the office gains from their service.

IMPLEMENTING SELECTIVE PREVENTION STRATEGIES

With selective prevention, the target audience will be based on common needs, interests, or issues. Interventions will be tailored to the common interests or needs of the group and show an understanding of the audience's shared values. For example, as illustrated in Phil McCabe's Lessons From the Field 6.2, attention to the unique issues faced by students who identify as LGBTQIA+ is an important component of selective approaches.

Once the audience is identified, the initial question is how to access group members. This is relatively straightforward with *intact and membership-based* groups, as they have a recognized memberships and are typically registered student organizations with rosters (e.g., fraternities and sororities, student-athletes). With organized groups, opportunities abound for targeted outreach, meetings, training, engagement, and follow-up; the national affiliation of many of them offers additional motivation or expectations for engagement, such as those entailed with selective prevention efforts. Groups based on *identifying characteristics* may have database-linked items (e.g., first-year students, graduate students, transfer students, military-connected students); other groups may include off-campus students, those with a registered automobile, financial aid recipients, service organization members, and students in leadership positions. Also included would be those with a court conviction or with a substance-related incident involving the emergency room. Harder-to-reach groups are those whose affiliation is based on other factors; these individuals may self-identify or begin to do so, based on messaging, strategies, and campaigns. For example, those who identify as LGBTQIA+ or as children of alcoholics may gain a heightened awareness of their unique susceptibility vis-à-vis drugs and alcohol. Selective prevention efforts may promote services and resources, with messages that offer support and champion self-efficacy for personal enhancement and success.

The tailoring of messages, within the context of overall campus outreach, allows for selective prevention strategies to resonate with identified audiences. With student-athletes, for example, attention to their athletic performance is paramount; thus, framing prevention strategies within that context works well (e.g., how alcohol use affects athletic performance). Similarly, strategies for fraternity and sorority members may appeal to their leadership and service aims (e.g., how drug/alcohol use harms these opportunities) as well as reputational aspirations (e.g., identifying strategies to reduce individual and chapter risk taking).

Information dissemination and skill building are common selective prevention strategies. Although information dissemination is primarily a universal prevention strategy, Selective prevention enhances information dissemination with the addition of skill-building strategies to support self-efficacy. Building skills equates with learning, and deciding which skills to address is influenced by both pragmatic considerations and aspirational goals. Pragmatic considerations often include recognizing the negative outcomes of policy and law violations; aspirational goals, or values clarification, encompass a review of the norms related to membership in a group. Skill building, thus, is a two-way communication strategy, distinguished from information dissemination by the interaction between the educator/facilitator and the participants. Activities under this strategy seek to impart critical life and social skills and incorporate protective and resiliency factors, such as decision making, refusal skills, critical analysis (e.g., of media messages), and systematic judgment abilities.

The example of new students transitioning to college illustrates an important skill-building tactic. Campus programs and staff assist students in navigating this transition with information dissemination about time management, substance-use refusal skills, social engagement, and finding supportive peer groups; similar adaptations can be made for transfer students. Some campuses have all first-year and transfer students complete online curriculum-based programs designed to educate them about success strategies and to develop the skills needed to thrive on campus.

Another example is found with residence hall students, where programs offer instrumental skill building via activities and meetings. Prevention specialists work with campus activities staff to create opportunities for safer community activities and group events. Students with academic struggles, whether based on substance misuse or not, often come to the attention of student affairs professionals, as do faculty members. Appropriate skill-building strategies include study skills, time management, goal setting, and decision making.

Selective prevention has the benefit of *cultivating coping skills* within a subpopulation as opposed to within an individual. Selective prevention often uses "strengths-based" interventions—tactics that promote healthy behavior versus tactics that focus on identifying and preventing disease and substance use disorder.

Specific groups such as fraternity and sorority members, scholarship student-athletes, and intramural sports team members have a higher profile on campus than do other groups. This recognition is often coupled with behavioral expectations related to group membership and may create conflict between individual behavior and expectations of group affiliation. Skill building related to bystander intervention is an example of aspirational goals or values clarification. Group decision-making norms related to intervention to protect the safety of another is the heart of bystander intervention.

A recent bystander intervention is one that addresses opioid overdoses and targets the Generation Z age cohort. Using active learning strategies, the curriculum-based intervention program explains how bystanders can respond to acute intoxication. Social media influencers become engaged to identify and recruit known opinion leaders/influencers committed to moving their community toward optimal health, and students design all message content and actively participate in implementing a project. The campaign—"When in Doubt, ACT Like a Friend"—emphasizes ACT: Ask questions, Care, and Take action. The first step, "A – Ask questions," means checking in on people you care about and asking if they are OK or if they need anything, thus creating an opportunity to instill hope. This step supports those who are socially isolated or whose behavior is stigmatized such that they believe they are not worth the trouble to help. The second step, "C – Care," involves reaching out with genuine concern, which validates the worth of another. Caring also consists of responding to a vulnerable person. An acutely intoxicated person, if left alone, may be at risk for sexual assault, physical injury, or death. The act of caring is a safety net for persons who are risk-takers. The acutely intoxicated person may not be aware of danger, but a compassionate, caring bystander can. The final step, "T – Take Action," results in risk reduction and a call for intervention by professionals. The campaign is a selective strategy that focuses on training specific groups to respond to individuals who appear to need help.

Implementing selective prevention efforts requires an assessment of who the target audience is and what attributes set them apart from other groups. Understanding group norms, and risk and protective factors is important for pairing an effective strategy with a selective group. Additional thought must be given to new public health initiatives, greater awareness of social justice matters and disparities, and the resulting changes in societal norms. Prevention specialists are often ahead of the institutional change management learning curve, as their work is founded on engaging with and being relevant to students within the various target audiences. By staying current with emerging science and building relevant approaches, prevention specialists orchestrate appropriate change management measures. Effective prevention specialists are adept in developing criteria to identify at-risk and problematic populations and communicate the importance of the campus intervention in ways that support, rather than stigmatize, these communities. Interventions that build community trust and engagement are more effective than punitive policies.

The application of these data to selective prevention has implications for environmental strategies. Consistent with the themes of expressive leadership (see Chapter 2), creating a community is a function of bottom-up change. Instrumental leaders (the top-down influencers) are also needed for diverse communities to grow. Because different audiences have different needs and issues, designing and selecting prevention programming can become complicated. Seek assistance from subject matter experts before implementing new, untested selective prevention strategies.

Another application of selective prevention to environmental strategies involves residential campuses that have a high concentration of bars nearby. When few on-campus social venues are open after 10 p.m., students who choose not to drink may feel alienated with the limited options for socialization. Having a designated sober "coffee house" or entertainment space on campus that appeals to multiple groups (e.g., first-time in college students, students in remission from behavioral health disorders, students who prefer not to drink) is a selective prevention intervention that creates community.

Finally, attention to the campus culture as a whole can be subsumed within the selective prevention approach. Meaningful engagement of individuals and groups helps selective prevention efforts become an integral part of promoting well-being. Complementing skill building and information dissemination is attention to community building—with an emphasis on quality relationships. These relationship skills—focusing on respect, conflict resolution, and leadership—affect both drug and alcohol issues and general community culture concerns.

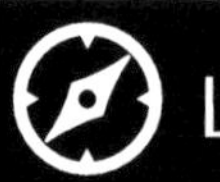

LESSONS FROM THE FIELD 6.2

Prevention of Substance Use Disorders and Other Behavioral Health Issues With Sexual Minorities/LGBTQIA+ Individuals

Philip T. McCabe, CSW, CAS, DRCC

Rutgers University

People who identify as lesbian, gay, bisexual, transgender, queer, questioning, intersex, or asexual (LGBTQIA+) often face social stigma, discrimination, and other challenges not encountered by people who identify as heterosexual. They also face a greater risk of harassment and violence. As a result of these and other stressors, sexual minorities are at increased risk for various behavioral health issues (Medley et al., 2015). Additionally, the Substance Abuse and Mental Health Services Administration (2016) reported serious mental illness and major depressive episodes significantly increased in LGBTQIA+ young adults between 2015 and 2018.

To give needed specialized attention to LGBTQIA+ individuals, the National Association of Lesbian and Gay Alcoholism Professionals (NALGAP) was formed in 1979. The original charter's goals emphasized advocacy for quality, nonhomophobic treatment; understanding of alcoholism/addiction; and professional networking (NALGAP, 2020). Now known as NALGAP–The Association of Lesbian, Gay, Bisexual, Transgender Addiction Professionals and Their Allies, the group continues its mission to ensure the health and well-being of all sexual minorities. NALGAP recognizes that the complexity of substance misuse and addiction calls for increased prevention efforts.

It is incumbent upon all college and university staff and faculty to be proactive and provide necessary support for members of the LGBTQIA+ community (Institute of Medicine, 2011; The Joint Commission, 2011). Specifically, the institution should provide a safe and supportive environment; it should be free from all forms of oppression, homophobia, heterosexism, and transphobia for any LGBTQIA+ person.

A university can demonstrate affirmation for LGBTQIA+ individuals in various ways:

- Ensure health education and institutional marketing materials show images representative of LGBTQIA+ individuals, same-sex couples, and families.
- Display LGBTQIA+-specific signs, stickers, and brochures in common areas.
- Include postings for LGBTQIA+ people on community bulletin boards, websites, and social media.
- In waiting areas (e.g., student center, student health center, campus offices), have reading materials (e.g., newsletters, magazines) that appeal to LGBTQIA+ people.
- Provide restrooms that conform to all genders.
- With intake and enrollment forms, specifically indicate sexual orientation and gender identities reflective of that individual.
- Ask students which name and pronouns they use.
- Ensure that all faculty, staff, students, and clients respect the person's gender identity.
- Take corrective action when a student is misgendered.
- Provide ongoing awareness and skills training for staff, faculty, student leaders, and students (NALGAP, 2020).

In summary, acknowledging, recognizing, and affirming LGBTQIA+ individuals is accomplished through a range of approaches that make a campus more visible as an ally and a safe space to all members of the LGBTQIA+ community. These approaches, in turn, alleviate the stigma, discrimination, and other challenges faced by LGBTQIA+ young adults and, ultimately, reduce factors leading to substance misuse and a substance use disorder.

SPECIAL CONSIDERATIONS FOR GENERATION Z STUDENTS

A National Academies of Sciences, Engineering, and Medicine (2019) report identifies peer relationships, as well as the media that youth consume, as critical in creating interventions designed to promote "optimal health." The report defines optimal health as "a dynamic balance of physical, emotional, social, spiritual, and intellectual health" (p. S2). The report recommends more work in the area of utilizing social media to promote adolescent health—specifically, students should be involved in creating and distributing messages.

Overall, Generation Z students (those born 1997 to present) are drinking less alcohol than the millennials who preceded them, in part due to the implementation of effective selective interventions over many years. The contemporary risk may be from a lack of sober social options within an environment that promotes rather than prevents high-risk behavior. Based on current and emerging data, appropriate strategies would emphasize leveraging the protective characteristics of these Generation Z students.

Offering well-designed alcohol-free venues for first-year students is more consistent with their current norms and beliefs; these students appear willing to reject the stereotype that drinking in college is a rite of passage. The challenge for prevention specialists may be less about changing the misperceived alcohol-use norms of first-year students and more about changing the static conceptions that faculty, staff, and administrators hold about alcohol use.

Further, today's Generation Z students were born into a world of technological innovation that shapes their social and emotional development. A challenge—and an opportunity—for prevention strategies is how to leverage technology to promote well-being. Keeping pace with technology to improve optimal health includes designing, implementing, and evaluating health programs, inclusive of drug and alcohol misuse prevention. Social media and virtual environments often distort perceptions and shape unrealistic perceptions of what is "normal." Expressive leaders or "influencers" represent a type of independent third-party endorser who shapes audience attitudes through the use of interpersonal relationships. Expressive leaders can be helpful, through the use of social media, with supporting current and appropriate well-being practices; they can also challenge unhealthy norms often portrayed by groups with vested economic interests. The effect of social media on promoting wellness and identity development is unclear, but because early adulthood is a critical phase of development in which individuals acquire skills that will carry them through life, selective prevention strategies at this stage are essential.

Prevention messaging for Generation Z youth and young adults through relevant social media platforms is an untapped, novel strategy. Self-management, social awareness, and responsible decision making are core components of evidence-based programs (Springer & Phillips, 2007). *Self-management* is defined as the ability to manage thoughts, emotions, stress, and behaviors in various situations. *Social awareness* is defined by knowledge of behavioral norms and recognition of social support. *Responsible decision making* takes into account multiple options, safety concerns, and consequences when making decisions. There is a gap between what was known to be evidence-based prevention outcomes with millennials and the rapidly evolving contemporary use of social media in health communication. Selective prevention programs benefit from using core components to inform social media strategies that teach skills and impact youths' lives and assist them in making healthy decisions.

Collaboration between faculty and prevention specialists is vital to sustaining dynamic selective prevention initiatives. Qualitative research methods (e.g., a "snowball" sample) can be used to identify expressive student leaders. A snowball sample consists of asking group members to identify peers they believe are influential. Each time the question is asked, the sample increases—just like a snowball rolling downhill. Focus groups help to identify common themes within a group. Messaging can be prepared in conjunction with faculty and students specializing in marketing, and then tailored to make project interventions as relevant as possible. Student leaders and other influencers identify which technology platforms allow optimal exposure to selected messages and what format the posts should take on each platform (whether text, picture, video, or other).

By involving students with collaborating faculty specialists—and allowing students creative control over selective health and safety messaging, language, and dissemination—student connection and relevance is enhanced. Students are inspired to encourage each other's positive self-development. In Lessons From the Field 6.3, Heather Kovanic describes the important role of orientation, transition, and retention efforts in general as well as those focused on drug and alcohol issues.

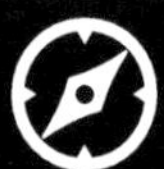

LESSONS FROM THE FIELD 6.3

Orientation, Transition, and Retention

Heather Kovanic, MEd

Director, Orientation and Transition Programs

University of Delaware

Orientation and transition programs are often students' first impression of their new college environment, so it is critical that drug and alcohol prevention be incorporated into these efforts. As students begin college, they seek a sense of belonging; thus, it is imperative for institutions to provide experiences that maximize opportunities for students to create authentic relationships, combating any preconceived notions and popular media images that suggest finding a sense of belonging in college is centered around a culture of alcohol and drug use. The aim, as specified by Wiese and Wheeler (2019), is to promote belonging by "providing opportunities for students to develop their individual academic and social identities grounded in their institution's values, norms, and expectations" (p. 41).

In his research on improving student persistence and completion rates, Vincent Tinto (2016) asserted that "students who perceive themselves as belonging are more likely to persist because it leads not only to enhanced motivation but also [to] a willingness to become involved with others in ways that further promote persistence" (para. 10). Orientation and transition programs are essential for laying the foundation of this belonging; as such, they should not only include education about the impact of alcohol and drug use on the academic and social experience, but also create space for students to begin building healthy relationships with their peers. This goal can be achieved through programmatic initiatives such as small-group facilitated dialogue on values and how the choices students make reflect those values; late-night social events as alternatives to substance use; and social norming campaigns to share accurate data about how students choose to engage in campus life—which often challenge new students' assumptions about how many of their peers partake of alcohol and drugs. Utilizing peer mentors in orientation, first-year seminars, or other facilitated programs allows students to see positive examples of student behaviors and shows them how to create meaningful relationships by seeking out campus activities and opportunities that align with their values. By fostering this type of holistic approach—that is, incorporating drug and alcohol issues honestly, throughout students' first-year experience—orientation and transition programs play an integral role in students' engagement and, ultimately, their success.

REFRAMING SELECTIVE PREVENTION

Selective prevention, all-too-often based on a problem-oriented approach, warrants reconsideration as a proactive, engaging strategy within a comprehensive campus prevention initiative. Because of its power and promise with intact, identified, or unidentified groups, for whom shared issues and needs exist, it can serve as the foundation for strategies with likely positive outcomes on individual and group behavior.

Attention has been paid primarily to those groups with higher drug and alcohol usage and/or incident rates and those with a higher risk for drug and alcohol problems; that is, the actual prevalence of or potential for drug/alcohol problems is the primary focus. Selective prevention efforts include information-based, skills-oriented, and policy-driven approaches designed to reduce or halt the progression or to minimize problematic behaviors.

An exciting and most promising approach with selective prevention revolves around the *opportunity to be proactive, positive, and aspirational.* Engaging groups in appropriate ways can have significant outcomes for the campus prevention effort. Whether the outreach is based on the previous groups identified (e.g., first-year students, military-connected students, those with judicial sanctions) or merely some other convenience-oriented approach (e.g., based on living in a specific residence hall or part of town), this selective prevention approach attends to the future. This is not a problem- or issue-oriented strategy; it is aspirational and proactive. It is opportunistic, and it seeks to draw upon the dreams and visions of students in ways that have the added benefit of reducing drug and alcohol problems and supporting health and well-being.

The combination of these reasons for using selective prevention—problem amelioration, risk reduction, and personal growth—allows for many opportunities to reframe and reshape the overall campus prevention effort. With strategic planning (see Chapter 10) and the engagement of collaborators and coalitions (see Chapter 11), the potential for impact in meaningful and long-term ways can be realized.

Pulling together the various considerations surrounding selective prevention efforts, Innovator 6.1 gives grounded views for a central strategy with students and for affecting the campus culture. H. Wesley Perkins, with his decades of experience and practical applications in this field of study, is joined by Jessica Perkins to provide insight about influencing the norms on campus. Prevention specialists and campus leaders will appreciate the rich views and extensive bibliography of substantive resources.

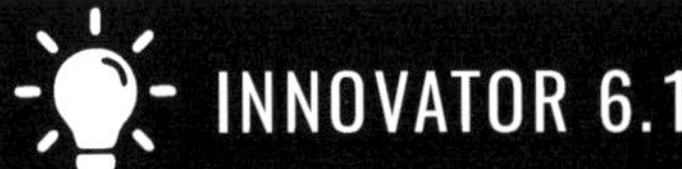

The Social Norms Approach: Confronting the "Reign of Error" as a Successful Strategy to Reduce Harmful Drinking and Drug Use in College

H. Wesley Perkins, PhD
Professor
Hobart & William Smith Colleges

Jessica M. Perkins, PhD
Assistant Professor
Vanderbilt University

Decades of effort to prevent harmful alcohol consumption and drug use among college students have shown that simply trying to educate students about pharmacological effects or to "scare the health" into them by dramatizing extreme tragedies have clearly failed. Even the creation of more policy restrictions on the purchase and possession of alcohol and drugs, and campus amnesty policies for seeking help, though somewhat beneficial, have not markedly reduced the problem levels observed at most colleges. Common explanations include greater risk taking in youth and young adulthood as an inevitable developmental phenomenon; problem behavior not frequently ending in immediate punishments by authorities or in the horrific unintended consequences portrayed by scare messages; and predominant exposure to peer influence in relatively unsupervised peer-intensive environments.

The influence of social norms among peers is undeniably powerful for youth and young adults who commonly want (or feel pressured) to conform to peer expectations and actions, regardless of what the larger culture stipulates. However, Perkins and Berkowitz's seminal 1986 study surprisingly documented that college students frequently misperceive their peer norms about drinking attitudes and behavior. Students tended to believe that peers drink more heavily and are more permissive about alcohol consumption than was the case. Subsequent research on harmful alcohol consumption and other substance use in higher education contexts has widely demonstrated gross overestimation, as students mistakenly think that heavy alcohol consumption and drug use reflect most peer behavior (Borsari & Carey, 2003; Miller & Prentice, 2016; Perkins, 1997, 2003, 2014; Perkins & Perkins, 2018). This pattern is well documented throughout the United States and found in other countries as well. (For an extensive listing of research studies supporting this claim and subsequent claims about the social norms approach, see Appendix B of this book).

As students myopically focus on, talk about, and "normalize" their perceptions of harmful drinking and other substance use, they lose sight of peers' predominantly healthy attitudes and behaviors. Misperceptions of widespread exaggerated alcohol consumption and drug use then become students' beliefs about the peer norm, a process starting in secondary schools and continuing through college. News, entertainment, social media, and even health advocacy campaigns typically sensationalize high-risk consumption behavior to gain greater reader or viewer attention, all contributing to incorrect beliefs about permissive peer attitudinal and behavioral norms. These norm misperceptions give students license to consume alcohol, tobacco, and other drugs, including nonmedical use of prescription medications, in problematic ways if they are so predisposed. These misperceptions may also nudge other students to engage in occasional harmful behavior as well as make passive bystanders of yet others who fail to intervene or speak up. Believing "everyone does it" also hinders compliance with protective institutional policies as a "reign of error" takes control (DeJong, 2003).

In almost all circumstances, the actual norms of a student population represent healthy, positive, or low-risk attitudes and behaviors. Numerous studies have now demonstrated the benefit of broadly communicating these actual behavioral and attitudinal norms to counter students' misperceptions about their peers' alcohol- and drug-related behaviors and attitudes. By communicating actual student norms based on credible data, through media campaigns, personalized normative feedback in counseling and online programs, focus group discussions, curriculum infusion, orientation programs, and text or other social media messaging, norm misperceptions about alcohol consumption and other substance use have been reduced.

Moreover, bringing students' perceptions more in line with the actual positive peer norms has cut harmful drinking and drug use and improved student health and well-being. This "social norms approach" can effectively intervene with both a broad population as well as selective groups such as student-athletes and members of Greek-letter organizations. The design requires (a) collecting or culling available data about how the majority exhibits protective behaviors, holds positive or healthy attitudes, and exhibits low-risk behavior; and then (b) promoting this information in high-dosage levels and sustained time spans.

Fundamentally, adopting this approach requires a paradigm shift. The goal is to move away from traditional approaches that so consistently and problematically highlight problem behaviors as if they were typical of most students—when they are not—and instead harness the power of positive norms that are already present in young adult populations.

CONCLUSION

The emphasis of selective prevention with specific groups provides opportunities for meaningful impact with these membership or affiliation constituents. Reframing selective prevention from a problem-oriented approach to one that is more proactive provides opportunities for innovation as well as a greater likelihood of appealing to and connecting with these audiences. The movement beyond the traditional higher risk groups propels prevention specialists in ways that match the unique features of the local campus culture and its members. Thoughtful planning sessions that include a range of stakeholders create a strong foundation for practical evaluative approaches. These approaches inform how to document outcomes and the return on investment of selective strategies.

REFERENCES

Asher, K. (2008). *Educating college students through judicial response: Examining the effectiveness of judicial sanctions for alcohol-related violations* [Unpublished doctoral dissertation]. University of Pittsburgh.

Baer, J. S., Kivlahan, D. R., Blume, A. W., McKnight, P., & Marlatt, G. A. (2001). Brief intervention for heavy-drinking college students: 4-year follow-up and natural history. *American Journal of Public Health, 91*, 1310–1316.

Borsari, B., & Carey, K. B. (2003). Descriptive and injunctive norms in college drinking: A meta-analytic integration. *Journal of Studies on Alcohol and Drugs, 64*(3), 331–341.

Brower, A. M., Golde, C. M., & Allen, C. (2003). Residential learning communities positively affect college binge drinking. *NASPA Journal, 40*(3), 132–152. https://doi.org/10.2202/1949-6605.1260

Capone, C., Wood, M., Borsari, B., & Laird, R. (2007). Fraternity and sorority involvement, social influences, and alcohol use among college students: A prospective examination. *Psychology of Addictive Behaviors, 21*(3), 316–327.

DeJong, W. (2003). A social norms approach to building campus support for policy change. In H. W. Perkins (Ed.), *The social norms approach to preventing school and college age substance abuse: A handbook for educators, counselors, and clinicians* (pp. 154–170). Jossey-Bass.

Emerson, D. (1992). Combining community service and judicial sanctions: Not an administrative nightmare. *Journal of College Student Development, 33*, 280.

Green, K. E., & Feinstein, B. A. (2012). Substance use in lesbian, gay, and bisexual populations: An update on empirical research and implications for treatment. *Psychology of Addictive Behaviors, 26*(2), 265–278. https://doi.org/10.1037/a0025424

Institute of Medicine. (2011). *The health of lesbian, gay, bisexual, and transgender people: Building a foundation for better understanding.* The National Academies Press.

The Joint Commission. (2011). *Advancing effective communication, cultural competence, and patient- and family-centered care for the lesbian, gay, bisexual, and transgender (LGBT) community: A field guide.* https://www.jointcommission.org/-/media/tjc/documents/resources/patient-safety-topics/health-equity/lgbtfieldguide_web_linked_verpdf.pdf?db=web&hash=FD725DC02CFE6E4F21A35EBD839BBE97

Kompalla, S. L., & McCarthy, M. C. (2001). The effect of judicial sanctions on recidivism and retention. *College Student Journal, 35*(2), 223.

Lewis, M. A., & Neighbors, C. (2007). Optimizing personalized normative feedback: The use of gender-specific referents. *Journal of Studies on Alcohol and Drugs, 68*, 228–237.

Medley, G., Lipari, R., Bose, J., Cribb, D., Kroutil, L., & McHenry, G. (2015). *Sexual orientation and estimates of adult substance use and mental health: Results from the 2015 national survey on drug use and health.* https://www.samhsa.gov/data/sites/default/files/NSDUH-SexualOrientation-2015/NSDUH-SexualOrientation-2015/NSDUH-SexualOrientation-2015.htm

Miller, D. T., & Prentice, D. A. (2016). Changing norms to change behavior. *Annual Review of Psychology, 67*(1), 339–361.

National Academies of Sciences, Engineering, and Medicine. (2019). *Promoting positive adolescent health behaviors and outcomes: Thriving in the 21st century.* National Academies Press. https://doi.org/10.17226/25552

National Association of Lesbian and Gay Alcoholism Professionals. (2020). *Homepage.* http://www.nalgap.org.

National Collegiate Athletic Association. (2018a). *NCAA national study on substance use habits of college student-athletes.* http://www.ncaa.org/sites/default/files/2018RES_Substance_Use_Final_Report_FINAL_20180611.pdf

National Collegiate Athletic Association. (2018b). *NCAA national study on substance use habits of college student-athletes: Executive summary June 2018.* https://www.ncaa.org/sites/default/files/2017RES_Substance_Use_Executive_Summary_FINAL_20180611.pdf

Neighbors, C., Larimer, M. E., & Lewis, M. A. (2004). Targeting misperceptions of descriptive drinking norms: Efficacy of a computer-delivered personalized normative feedback intervention. *Journal of Consulting and Clinical Psychology, 72,* 434–447.

Neighbors, C., Lee, C. M., Lewis, M. A., Fossos, N., & Walter, T. (2009). Internet-based personalized feedback to reduce 21st-birthday drinking: A randomized controlled trial of an event-specific prevention intervention. *Journal of Consulting and Clinical Psychology, 77,* 51–63.

Patrick, M. E., & Terry-McElrath, Y. M. (2019). Prevalence of high-intensity drinking from adolescence through young adulthood: National data from 2016–2017. *Substance Abuse: Research and Treatment,* 13. https://doi.org/10.1177/1178221818822976

Perkins, H. W. (1997). College student misperceptions of alcohol and other drug norms among peers: Exploring causes, consequences, and implications for prevention programs. In *Designing alcohol and other drug prevention programs in higher education: Bringing theory into practice* (pp. 177–206). Higher Education Center for Alcohol and Other Drug Prevention.

Perkins, H. W. (Ed.). (2003). *The social norms approach to preventing school and college age substance abuse: A Handbook for educators, counselors, and clinicians.* Jossey-Bass.

Perkins, H. W. (2014). Misperception is reality: The "reign of error" about peer risk behaviour norms among youth and young adults. In M. Xenitidou & B. Edmonds (Eds.), *The complexity of social norms* (pp. 11–36). Springer International Publishing.

Perkins, H. W., & Berkowitz, A. D. (1986). Perceiving the community norms of alcohol use among students: Some research implications for campus alcohol education programming. *International Journal of the Addictions, 21*(9–10), 961–976.

Perkins, H. W., & Craig, D. W. (2006). A successful social norms campaign to reduce alcohol misuse among college student-athletes. *Journal of Studies on Alcohol and Drugs, 67,* 880–889.

Perkins, H. W., & Perkins, J. M. (2018). Using the social norms approach to promote health and reduce risk among college students. In M. D. Cimini & E. M. Rivero (Eds.), *Promoting behavioral health and reducing risk among college students: A comprehensive approach* (pp.127–144). Routledge.

Schulenberg, J. E., Johnston, L. D., O'Malley, P. M., Bachman, J. G., Miech, R. A., & Patrick, M. E. (2020). *Monitoring the future national survey results on drug use, 1975–2019: Volume II: college students and adults ages 19–60.* Institute for Social Research, The University of Michigan.

Springer, J. R., & Phillips, J. (2007). *The Institute of Medicine framework and its implication for the advancement of prevention policy, programs and practice* (SMA-4205). U.S. Department of Health and Human Services. http://ca-sdfsc.org/docs/resources/SDFSC_IOM_Policy.pdf

Substance Abuse and Mental Health Services Administration. (2016). *Sexual orientation and estimates of adult substance use and mental health: Results from the 2015 National Survey on Drug Use and Health.* https://www.samhsa.gov/data/sites/default/files/NSDUH-SexualOrientation-2015/NSDUH-SexualOrientation-2015/NSDUH-SexualOrientation-2015.htm

Teeters, J. B., Lancaster, C. L., Brown, D. G., & Back, S. E. (2017). Substance use disorders in military veterans: Prevalence and treatment challenges. *Substance Abuse and Rehabilitation*, *8*, 69–77. https://doi.org/10.2147/SAR.S116720

Tinto, V. (2016, September 26). *From retention to persistence. Inside Higher Ed.* https://www.insidehighered.com/views/2016/09/26/how-improve-student-persistence-and-completion-essay

Wiese, D., & Wheeler, E. (2019). A theoretical grounding for orientation, transition, and retention practice: A dynamic three-part heuristic. In J. Ward-Roof & J. M. Mastrogiovanni (Eds.), *Building successful foundations: Best practices in orientation, transition, and retention* (pp. 38–49). NODA–Association for Orientation, Transition, and Retention in Higher Education.

CHAPTER 7

Indicated Prevention Strategies

"One of the biggest benefits to being a college student in recovery is a heightened sense of self-responsibility. While recovery is collaborative, it promotes being accountable both to oneself and to one's commitments. I was, honestly, incredibly shocked by how much easier going to class made college."

—Graduate student at a large public university

Indicated prevention approaches, the third of three parts of the Institute of Medicine's (IOM's) prevention model, fall after universal and selective strategies (Springer & Phillips, 2007). Indicated prevention focuses on individuals with risky drug and/or alcohol use patterns as well as those individuals at risk for developing a substance use disorder (SUD). Prevention with these groups addresses reducing current harm and problematic behaviors and working to halt the potential progression of a SUD.

Within a supportive campus environment, effective indicated prevention requires the breadth of knowledge and appropriate skills held by prevention specialists. Equally important is the promotion of this knowledge among campus decision makers, intermediaries, faculty, staff, and students.

As illustrated in the IOM continuum of care protractor (see Figure 3.1 in Chapter 3), indicated prevention borders treatment (Mrazek &

Haggerty, 1994). Although campus prevention specialists emphasize universal, selective, and indicated components, they may also benefit from acknowledging the full range of the continuum of care from prevention, through treatment, to maintenance. The IOM's broad conceptual grounding has practical campus applications. Thus, this chapter considers how campuses address a range of students with varying needs. The chapter includes discussion of what is an appropriate range of services for campus personnel to implement. Because the availability of on-campus addiction recovery services is crucial, with attention to staffing, support, and resources, the associated role of self-help and mutual aid services is also covered, as are issues of stigma.

This third prevention component has several practical applications for many individuals. Although some of the five contributions in this chapter have clinical or counseling foundations, the content of all of them is relevant for anyone working with prevention specialists and campus leaders. The two case studies provide insights for conversation and collaboration. The two Lessons From the Field help in different ways; one highlights early intervention efforts, and the other addresses recovery as a social justice issue. The chapter culminates with empowering perspectives from Michael Dunn, an Innovator, who discusses SUDs.

THE CONTEXT FOR ADDRESSING INDICATED POPULATIONS

Among institutions of higher education, an overarching demonstration of care anchors the various systems and services for indicated prevention. The well-being and human potential of all students is a key concern for higher education professionals, who typically spend a disproportionate amount of time with students in need of indicated prevention. More attention to these students is warranted because of their substance abuse, engagement in the campus judicial system, participation with counseling, health service's needs, poor academic performance, or a combination of these factors. The axiom that "an ounce of prevention is worth a pound of cure" still applies here, but several ounces of indicated prevention may be needed.

Two contexts are crucial for indicated prevention efforts. One is incident based; here, intervention by others is vital to attempts to halt SUD behavior and its harmful consequences. In such cases, the individuals are impaired and planning to drive, using prescription drugs and consuming alcohol, at risk for sexual exploitation, or at risk for overdose. Immediate intervention is critical; however, those who learn about these situations later should also try to prevent a recurrence of that problematic behavior, or the individuals themselves may elect self-referral to a professional.

The second context for indicated prevention incorporates a focus on SUD and, thus, takes a longer term approach. The recurrence of various individual harmful incidents may demonstrate a pattern and therefore warrant more focused attention. Previously referred to by the terms *dependence* or *addiction*, the SUD classification is the professional designation of this disease—with the diagnosis made by a clinician.

The *Diagnostic and Statistical Manual* (*DSM-5*), prepared by the American Psychiatric Association, combines the previous *DSM-4* categories of substance abuse and substance dependence into a single disorder measured on a continuum from mild to severe. Specific diagnostic criteria are used to determine if a SUD is present. Nine classes of drugs are identified within the spectrum of SUDs (e.g., alcohol use disorder, opioid use disorder, cannabis use disorder). Caffeine is not included as a disorder. However, caffeine intoxication and caffeine withdrawal criteria are identified (American Psychiatric Association, 2013). So, a SUD is viewed along a continuum, with both progression and regression. Prevention science offers campus health and wellness professionals the opportunity to act versus react—that is, to prevent the onset of SUDs, via early intervention. In other words, students do not have to hit rock bottom before learning new coping skills. However, it is important to note that the stages of change allow for both progression and regression. While a student may not progress to a substance use disorder, the student's use of protective behaviors is dynamic.

When campuses create pathways for a referral before an acute incident, students benefit from a harm reduction approach. Personnel at all levels—from student affairs professionals to undergraduate residence hall staff, to faculty—can play an essential role. Whether it is an acute situation or a series of them, what is important is assisting the student in accessing appropriate campus resources. This does not mean an automatic referral to treatment. On the contrary, treatment should remain in the purview of trained behavioral health professionals. Instead, the cadre of caring individuals on campus should demonstrate a level of concern so that, when they encounter a problematic situation, they get involved. Likely actions would be halting the problematic situation and making a referral to a suitable source; ideally, campus leaders create pathways for a referral.

Indicated prevention does not prevent the initiation of substance use—risky use patterns develop over time. Indicated prevention is typically offered to students who have come to the attention of peers, law enforcement, academic advisors, residence hall directors, faculty members, or the dean of students. Some seek help voluntarily after a life event that shakes their confidence. The referral path is less important than identifying the skill set of the prevention professional.

The essential skill set for prevention counseling within the indicated prevention area includes two tactics: (1) prevention counseling, and (2) problem identification and referral. Prevention counseling consists of teaching skill-building techniques, providing personalized normative feedback, and giving nonjudgmental brief advice. Problem identification and referral uses screening tools to determine if the assessment for a substance use disorder is indicated. Prevention counseling, problem identification, and referral to treatment can be carried out in multiple domains. Indicated prevention is not limited to the campus counseling or health center. Academic advisors, residence life staff, faculty, student conduct personnel, and student leaders can learn specific skills to respond to students in all types of emotional distress, including sadness, worry, and substance misuse. Karen Moses, in Case Study 7.1, offers perspectives about screening and intervention.

CASE STUDY 7.1

C3: Compassion, Communication, and Connection to Improve Student Outcomes

Karen S. Moses, EdD
Director, Wellness and Health Promotion
Arizona State University

Compassion, communication, and connection are core principles that guide the C3 program at Arizona State University (ASU). C3 was established to facilitate the implementation of Screening, Brief Intervention, and Referral to Treatment (SBIRT) in ASU Health and Counseling Services. Further, it was designed to train and support staff working in student-facing positions across ASU's four Phoenix-area campuses in engaging in motivational interviewing (MI). Initial funding was provided by a grant through the Arizona Governor's Office of Youth, Faith and Family; costs to sustain ongoing efforts have been incorporated into regular annual budgets. The C3 staff include health educators and leaders within the Live Well @ ASU Network, which organizes ASU Health and Counseling Services, Sun Devil Fitness and Wellness, and Sexual and Relationship Violence Prevention departments for planning, implementing, and evaluating student health and well-being efforts.

SBIRT and MI are evidence-based strategies for substance abuse prevention (McCambridge & Strang, 2004; Patton et al., 2014). To establish SBIRT, C3 staff convened a team of health and counseling staff. This multidisciplinary partnership resulted in nearly all clinical and counseling staff participating in trainings to build capacity in MI and brief interventions, select screening tools, and develop a system for SBIRT that meets the needs of the health and counseling staff.

MI training prepares faculty, staff, and student leaders to identify and support the needs of students who may be struggling with substance use or other personal challenges that can hinder academic and personal success. Training and adoption of MI across ASU is facilitated through relationship building with departmental leaders, who commit both to using MI when communicating with students and to referring students to ASU clinical settings for screening, when appropriate. C3 offers ongoing training, technical support, and materials to strengthen MI capacity across ASU.

Initially, C3 instruction was delivered by consultants who worked in university health (for medical staff), university counseling (for counseling staff), university policing (for ASU police), and student affairs (for remaining staff). Discipline-specific experts were used to ensure relatability with the audience, facilitate ongoing technical support by C3 staff, and build capacity among the C3 staff for post-grant sustainability.

PREVENTION COUNSELING STRATEGIES

For students who may be harmfully involved with drugs and/or alcohol yet who do not meet *DSM-5* criteria for a SUD, prevention counseling is appropriate. Because prevention counseling focuses primarily on preventing the progression of misuse to SUD, it is distinguished from treatment and recovery. Prevention counseling is an appropriate strategy for students to build skills and confidence. Successfully navigating challenges and resolving ambivalence about risky behaviors is the intended outcome of prevention counseling; further, it does not carry the real or perceived stigma of being "sick" or "a patient."

What is appropriate with prevention counseling is working with students who are not managing their sadness, worry, or substance misuse. Students at risk for developing a SUD may benefit from social and emotional support. Prevention counseling may also help students in recovery from a SUD clarify values or learn how to deal with difficult people or situations.

Although intervention at this level does not require professional licensure, it does require a specific skill set. Prevention counseling skill sets include being nonjudgmental; listening well; showing empathy; and being able to teach resilience, communication, and coping strategies. The simple acts of listening, offering solutions, and withholding judgment are key to engaging students struggling with academic or campus life. An important aspect of prevention counseling is confidentiality. Staff who do not hold clinical licensure may be mandated reporters. Nonclinicians need to know their limits of confidentiality, advise students before intervening, and remind students often of the legal limits of confidentiality.

The motivational interviewing (MI) approach (Miller & Rollnick, 2012) and the stages of change, or transtheoretical, model (Prochaska et al., 1994) are helpful strategies in prevention counseling. The blend of the two provides a useful framework for understanding students' willingness to change and for devising strategies that facilitate this change. The aim is to assist a student with transitioning from harmful and potentially dangerous behavior and move toward, with personal ownership, healthier decision making; a supportive campus environment, with appropriate systems and services, makes the achievement of these outcomes more likely.

Underlying the stages of change/transtheoretical model is the assumption that no single strategy exists to alter behavior. People choose their path based on the perceived benefits of changing versus not changing. While it may sound strange to think about the *benefits* of substance misuse (like the benefits of anxiety and depression), for many it will be apparent that little benefit exists in staying in a situation that negatively affects quality of life or educational and career goals. Change is a process that involves introspection and self-awareness. For some people, the anxiety aroused by the idea of change—even altering a harmful behavior—is enough to make them resist change. An individual's beliefs block change. Beliefs are embraced when all doubt is resolved—believing terminates inquiry. Ambivalence or doubt is the only motive for change. This concept is essential in prevention counseling, problem identification, and referral to treatment. Caring and compassionate others cannot will individuals to change. Adept prevention counseling relies on seizing opportunities to create doubt about risky behaviors, and creating a space for individuals to process their ambivalence.

It is within this context that challenging fixed beliefs depends on creating ambivalence or doubt about the meaning or symbols associated with "normal." The motivation to change involves reformulating how one feels about something. A person's perception of the value or benefit of choosing something unfamiliar over something familiar gets challenged. The tension between changing and not changing becomes more intense until the ambivalence gets resolved. When it is evident to family or friends that a loved one needs to change, and the loved one chooses not to change, some people label that nonchanging behavior as "denial." But denial is a powerful way for a person to resolve ambivalence and return to their state of "normal." It is frustrating for both the helper and the person who is experiencing ambivalence when change is coerced or forced. A surefire way to engage resistance to change is to use the threat of punishment or guilt to foster change. These tactics will encourage someone who is not ready to change to resist change at all costs.

As a related example, consider healthy diet and exercise. People often vacillate between embracing them and not embracing them. The health benefits of diet and exercise are clear, but if a person doesn't believe they can change their behavior, or does not feel the importance of changing their behavior, they are unlikely to make a reasoned decision to do something different.

The stages of change model/transtheoretical model describes a construct of dynamic stages people pass through on their way to making a behavior change. This model has five stages: precontemplation, contemplation, preparation, action, and maintenance. Although the steps are ordered, in practice people may skip a step or move back from one stage to another. An important aspect of change management is understanding that change is not simple and that a person may perceive benefits to not changing even when it seems clear that they should change.

The first stage, *precontemplation,* describes a state in which a person sees no reason for, need to, or benefit from changing a pattern of thought or behavior. Precontemplation is a stage that frustrates parents, caregivers, partners, and friends who see the need for someone to change; however, the individual is steadfast in this decision not to change. Negotiating, presenting facts, and using guilt or shame will not move a precontemplative person toward change. Coercing or forcing someone to change may do more harm than good. The "righting reflex" (Prochaska et al., 1994) is described as a paradoxical effect of coerced change—coercion may strengthen one's resolve not to change. Supporting the autonomy of people whom others think may benefit from change strategies does not mean that they must agree with the choices made; people can honor another's right to choose without supporting their choice. The skill of "rolling with resistance" is the process of not engaging the righting reflex.

The next stage, *contemplation,* is like a seed that germinates in the nutrients of doubt or ambivalence. An individual who begins to question their beliefs or actions is moving toward change. The act of talking about and imagining change is the beginning of this stage. Contemplation is a time when a person thinking about change can benefit from the availability of social support to change. If help and support are not present, or if the righting reflex or resistance to change is activated, the individual may retreat to precontemplation.

The process of imagining change or talking about change leads to preparing for change—seen as the *preparation* stage of change. Ambivalence is intense at the onset of making plans for change. Change is seen as balancing between moving forward or falling back, with mental lists of reasons to change or not change often considered. A person may seek out others to help decide how to proceed, but onlookers are advised to stay neutral, offer support, and remember the importance of self-determination in the change process. It is essential for the individual to own the decision; thus, if unanticipated challenges arise, a reason to retreat to the familiar is less likely to occur.

If the ambivalence is resolved, a new belief grows from the seeds fertilized by doubt, and change is realized—the *action* stage. The action stage is marked by creating a new "normal." Because change is a seismic shift in a belief, the action stage is, for many, exciting and terrifying at the same time. The energy generated by the action stage can cause distress or worry for friends and family. There will be those who question the sincerity of change or duration of change ("You can't keep this going in the long run"). Support, not judgment, is vital at this point.

The fifth stage is the *maintenance* stage; this is a time when relapse into previous behaviors may occur. Moving back and forth between stages is not a sign of failure; an individual moving between stages of change is advancing. Change is possible wherever ambivalence is present.

A mnemonic device for remembering the stages of change is **I WANT TO** change.

Irritation—the irritation of doubt or ambivalence (precontemplative).
Willingness—the willingness to think about change (contemplative).
Ability—the belief in ability to change (preparation).
Necessary—the possession of necessary skills needed to change (preparation).
Taking—taking steps toward change (action).
Taking—taking action to change (action).
Ongoing—ongoing follow-up (maintenance).

MI is vital to engaging students and communicating respect and caring. MI is founded on four basic principles: learning how to express empathy, learning how to roll with resistance, learning how to support self-efficacy, and teaching others how to develop discrepancy (Miller et al., 1992). The process of learning to express empathy starts with suspending judgment and bias. The interviewer assumes the person's viewpoints are logical, clear, and valid; empathy communicates acceptance and lays the groundwork for mutual respect of each person's perspectives, feelings, and values. Basic interviewer skills include eye contact, self-awareness of sending nonverbal cues, reflective listening, and withholding judgment. Learning how to roll with resistance involves avoiding arguments. Giving advice leads to resistance and undermines the principles of expressing empathy. Reflecting—instead of reacting—is an essential lesson for prevention specialists to learn. When resistance and reaction are present, individuals may retreat to an emotional place of safety where beliefs about the benefits of not changing are nurtured.

Supporting self-efficacy means recognizing the right of self-determination. Listening is the key to facilitating behavior change. Most people know what they need to do to change; however, their beliefs about self and others obscure their view and reinforce not changing. A powerful tool is allowing others to voice the benefits, drawbacks, and energy or resources regarding change. The process of learning these basic MI skills enables prevention specialists to effectively teach others how to develop discrepancy—that is, to question if there is another way. Doubt activates a conversation about the impact of current behavior on future goals. Resolving doubt is the only immediate motive to change. Developing discrepancy opens the door to challenging those beliefs that limit personal growth and achievement. Insightful and practical approaches consistent with these perspectives are noted by Robert Chapman in Case Study 7.2.

The positive psychology literature offers guidance on sustaining change (Seligman, 2002). Skill-building topics relate to communication, compassion, coping, caring, forgiveness, gratitude, and mindfulness. Questionnaires let prevention professionals measure the degree of social support individuals think is present in their network. The positive youth development (PYD) literature is useful in developing prevention counseling strategies. PYD focuses on the five *Cs*: connection, confidence, competence, character, and caring. Mastery of skills in these areas correlates with decreased substance misuse, anxiety, and sadness (Bowers et al., 2010; Li & Lerner, 2013).

The use of the stages of change/transtheoretical model in conjunction with MI techniques and positive psychology strategies are helpful in prevention counseling. They act as a useful framework for individual and group work on campus. In addition to residence life staff, counseling staff, and prevention specialists, others on campus (e.g., physicians, nurses, law enforcement officers, faculty members, academic advisors) benefit from learning how to express empathy, roll with resistance, and support self-efficacy. Worksheet 7.1: Motivational Interviewing Checklist is designed to prepare campus professionals to embody appropriate MI techniques.

CASE STUDY 7.2

Salting the Oats

Robert J. Chapman, PhD
Alcohol and Other Drug Program Coordinator (former)
LaSalle University

Although you can lead a horse to water but not make it drink, you can make it thirsty—at least, that is what I told myself when I engaged a particularly reluctant student who sat across from me in a mandated alcohol or other drug assessment. This student had recently had a drinking episode that resulted in him vandalizing his residence hall.

"Michael" sat defiantly—arms crossed, legs outstretched and crossed at the ankles—as if to say, "I dare you to make a difference in my life." He was expecting the "Dad Talk" and ready to engage in a verbal tug-of-war, so he was surprised when I said that I wanted to hear his account of what happened.

As Michael shared without interruption his view of the events, we reached a point when it occurred to him that he would not be getting the expected "Dad Talk," and he agreed to expand on his story, sharing his pattern of consuming "8 cups"—those red cups that hold 16 ounces—of beer in 3 hours as somewhat routine. With permission, I asked him the following series of questions:

"Which seems larger to you: 8 cups of beer or 8 pints?"

"Pints," he responded.

"Which seems larger: 8 pints or 4 quarts?"

"4 quarts," he replied.

"Which seems larger: 4 quarts or *a gallon*?"

"A gallon," he said.

"And when was the last time you drank a gallon of water or whatever in 3 hours?"

"I never drank a gallon of anything in 3 hours" was his reply.

"Interesting," I mused. "Because you just told me a moment ago that you routinely drink a gallon of beer in 3 hours."

He looked confused and said, "No, I didn't."

To which I added: "Yes . . . 8 cups . . . 8 pints . . . 4 quarts . . . a gallon," pausing slightly after each quantity for effect.

Michael's reticence in our interview waned as his ambivalence regarding his consumption blossomed. It would seem that salting the oats can at least start the process of motivating a change in perspective.

PROBLEM IDENTIFICATION AND REFERRAL

Complementing the tactic of prevention counseling is that of problem identification and referral to treatment. On the IOM's continuum of care, treatment encompasses "case identification" and "standard treatment for known disorders." Screening tools help professionals assess whether a SUD exists. Noting the signs of a problem, choosing ways of responding or intervening, and determining appropriate roles (i.e., who should do what) are fundamental aspects of problem identification and referral to treatment.

Problem identification and referral services are typically handled by campus health centers, counseling centers, and wellness centers. Primary care physicians frequently include screening for SUDs in office visits. The Screening Brief Intervention and Referral to Treatment (SBIRT) has documented benefits with screening for SUDs with asymptomatic patients (Babor, 2007). Those interventions that prevent the onset of a mental disorder and a SUD are associated with increased resilience and problem-solving skills (Dimeff et al., 1999). Screening tools are important considerations; they include AUDIT (Babor et al., 1989; Saunders et al., 1993), CUDIT-R (Adamson et al., 2010), DUDIT (Berman et al., 2005), PHQ 9 (Kroenke et al., 2001), and GAD 7 (Spitzer et al., 2006). Also important are the settings where screenings take place (e.g., primary care, academic advising, student activities, residential life, judicial affairs). Various campus personnel benefit from using concise tools as part of their routine assessment work, and these screening tools can be used to determine if a referral for treatment is indicated.

The *DSM-5* SUD identifies 11 criteria that indicate whether a diagnosis of a SUD is likely (American Psychiatric Association, 2013). The criteria are simple and straightforward, yet critical nuances must be to be taken into account by a behavioral health specialist before ruling out a SUD. Prevention specialists should err on the side of caution and make a referral to treatment for further evaluation if any of the SUD criteria are met.

A problematic pattern of alcohol or other drug use leading to clinically significant impairment or distress, as manifested by at least two of the criteria occurring within a 12-month period, is the *DSM-5* definition of a SUD. A mnemonic device for remembering these 11 criteria is **MUST CUT DOWN.**

Managing—not managing to do what you should at work, home, or school because of substance.

Urge—craving or a strong desire or urge to use the substance.

Sustained—use continues despite knowledge of having a persistent or recurrent physical or psychological problem that is likely to have been caused or exacerbated by substance use.

Taking—taking the substance in larger amounts or over a longer period than was intended.

Continuing—continued use despite having persistent or recurrent social or interpersonal problems caused by or exacerbated by the effects of alcohol.
Unable to control—a persistent desire or unsuccessful efforts to cut down or control use.
Time—a great deal of time is spent on activities necessary to obtain, use, or recover from the effects of the substance.

Danger—recurrent use in situations where use is physically hazardous.
Occupational—important social, occupational, or recreational activities are given up or reduced because of substance use.
Withdrawal—the substance is used to relieve or avoid withdrawal symptoms.
Need—tolerance, as defined by either a need for markedly increased amounts to achieve intoxication or desired effect, or a markedly diminished effect with continued use of the same amount.

The screening tools and the *DSM-5* criteria help determine the level of intervention that is appropriate. Any intervention must be based on a set of predetermined risk levels. Risk levels are intended to rule out the presence of disorder, not to diagnose a disorder. A *stepped care approach* describes screening guidelines and sets parameters for intervention and referral. Indicated prevention can be viewed with four classifications: (1) Low to moderate risk; (2) high risk; (3) very high risk yet not *DSM-5* criteria; and (4) indications of *DSM-5* criteria and the need for a referral to treatment. Empirically supported screening tools are useful for determining risk levels. Worksheet 7.2: Alcohol Risk Reduction Scale serves as one example of a screening tool.

Students categorized as *low to moderate risk* on the screening instrument may benefit from a small group intervention. The goal of the single-session small group (8 to 10 members) intervention is to provide students with information and feedback related to substance use. For example, students may be provided the mean blood alcohol concentration (BAC), as well as peak BAC for students referred to the group. A comparison between the group and mean and peak BACs for the campus in general is discussed. The goal is to challenge misperceived norms. Harm-reduction strategies may be included, with participants asked to identify specific tactics they can implement to reduce the likelihood of experiencing negative consequences in the future.

Students who meet the criteria for *high risk* on the screening instrument (such as the AUDIT or CUDIT) may receive, at minimum, a two-session brief intervention. The intervention includes personalized feedback and skills training given in a one-on-one session format informed by best practices. The goals of this intervention are similar to the goals of the group intervention, though there is a brief psychosocial interview during the first session here. This component allows the provider to gather additional information about the student's lifestyle and assess the role that substance use plays in it. Other goals of this initial session are to build rapport with the student and gain the student's commitment to participate actively in the intervention. An additional difference between the group and individual intervention is that each student is asked to monitor their substance use for the next 10 to 14 days using provided monitoring cards. These interventions may be extended for an additional session if concerns arise or if the student requests extra time.

When students meet criteria for *very high risk* on the screening instrument but do not meet *DSM-5* criteria for a SUD, a three- to six-session brief intervention is warranted. This intervention builds on the session content of the previous intervention levels, with the initial sessions similar to those of the two-session intervention for high-risk clients and the focus on building rapport while gathering information. Students receiving this protocol are asked to monitor their substance use from one session to the next; they are provided with personalized feedback, taught to calculate BAC, and asked which tactics they will utilize to reduce their risk of experiencing substance misuse–related harms. An additional component includes completing a cost-benefit analysis exercise geared toward a greater understanding of the antecedents and consequences of substance misuse and thus toward better decision making.

The final grouping includes those for whom the screening indicates *a need for referral to treatment.* Provided are resources to aid in this process, including information regarding appropriate treatment providers. It is fitting to explore treatment services, such as residential treatment, outpatient treatment, and assistance that focuses specifically on college students or young adults. A referral to treatment may come directly from the screening, or it may also occur at any time during a stepped care approach intervention. A referral may be appropriate after the first session, after several sessions into care, or at the outcome of participation.

The Brief Alcohol Screening and Intervention for College Students (BASICS) program is an SBIRT-type intervention that uses the MI/transtheoretical model (Dimeff et al., 1999). BASICS was designed to incorporate a brief screening, provide face-to-face psychoeducational information, and give personalized feedback based on client responses to the initial screening. Traditionally, BASICS is a two-session intervention. Counseling and wellness centers often use BASICS, and many campuses require students who have violated campus alcohol use policies to complete a BASICS protocol. Designed as an individual intervention, BASICS gathers information to determine if a referral to treatment is warranted. Also, skill-building strategies are discussed to highlight protective tactics and minimize risk behaviors, with students asked to monitor alcohol use after the first session. The second session gives advice on the use of protective strategies, discusses normative feedback, and sets goals. A BASICS intervention is consistent with a stepped care approach of problem identification and referral to treatment. Training on these intervention approaches is widely employed; Jason Kilmer shares some enlightening perspectives in this regard in Lessons From the Field 7.1.

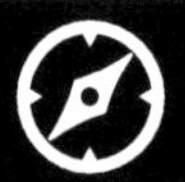

LESSONS FROM THE FIELD 7.1

Screening and Brief Intervention Efforts

Jason R. Kilmer, PhD
Associate Professor
University of Washington

In brief interventions addressing alcohol use by college students, strategies that use Miller & Rollnick's (2012) motivational interviewing (MI) are among the approaches deemed most effective in reducing alcohol use and any drinking-related consequences (National Institute on Alcohol Abuse and Alcoholism, 2019). Prevention and intervention strategies that employ MI typically attempt to prompt contemplation of or commitment to change while remaining nonjudgmental and nonconfrontational. One of my favorite articles related to MI and brief interventions comes from the two developers of MI: "Ten Things That Motivational Interviewing Is Not" (Miller & Rollnick, 2009). As a fan of top 10 lists since first seeing them on *Late Night with David Letterman*, I was excited to see this incarnation, and number 8 ("MI is not easy") has always stuck with me. The authors noted that they are often invited to teach MI during a 2-hour workshop or a lunch with pizza provided (always a good call if you can provide pizza at a training, by the way). They concluded, "Think of a similar invitation to teach the viola, or tennis, or for that matter psychoanalysis, over lunch" (Miller & Rollnick, 2009, p. 135).

I fully understand people's schedules are very busy on campus. And, among the things I appreciate about the basic strategies of MI is that they are good communication strategies that can be used outside of clinical contexts; in other words, the strategies can be helpful for anyone trying to be a better communicator. However, if intended to be used in a clinical setting or as part of an intervention delivered with fidelity, it is a really challenging situation when well-intended people expect that it can be taught or learned in a short meeting. If it is worth doing, it is worth doing well—and worth doing correctly. And that means an appropriate investment in time. Becoming proficient in MI can be an ongoing process that can take practice, so being open to "boosters" or follow-up trainings is also important. Brief interventions can be powerful, but getting someone trained to deliver an effective intervention in a brief window should be, ironically, a lengthier process.

RECOVERY AND SUPPORT SERVICES

Services designed to aid students with their ongoing recovery are essential for a comprehensive drug and alcohol abuse prevention effort. Although generally not subsumed in the IOM's view of indicated prevention, recovery and related support services support and sustain individuals after treatment for a SUD. These services are viewed as prevention oriented, as they serve to prevent relapse, prevent experimentation with preferred substances or other substances, and prevent harm. Recovery services also promote resiliency, foster self-esteem, and create a support network for students recovering from an addiction.

The presence of organized recovery services has grown dramatically on college campuses over recent decades. Group counseling for problem drinkers was found on 33% of college campuses in 1979 and peaked with 72% in 1991; however, campus recovery programs are presently found on only half of 4-year institutions (Anderson & Santos, 2018). Just over one third (38%) of campuses offer group counseling for students who have problems with marijuana, and 36% offer this service for students who struggle with other drugs (Anderson & Santos, 2018).

Organized recovery services, reported with the most recent data available, are found on nearly half (47%) of campuses, an increase from 36% reported 3 years earlier (Anderson & Santos, 2018). This research shows that these organized services are comprised of student group involvement (31%), social events for recovering students (28%), a designated coordinator or leader (23%), dedicated space (21%), funding (21%), sober housing options (16%), and faculty involvement (9%). Most significant is the presence of a designated coordinator or leader; these 2018 results doubled from the previous triennial survey administration in 2015, growing from 9% to 23%. Specific components of organized recovery services are based on the campus's particular needs and interests.

Related to campus recovery efforts are self-help groups, such as Alcoholics Anonymous (AA), Narcotics Anonymous (NA), and SMART Recovery. These regularly scheduled meetings offer significant support for participants, as demonstrated by their widespread adoption around the world and AA's status as a model for more than 100 types of support groups. Although participants in these groups often view them as essential (i.e., a "lifeline"), campus leaders often question whether these sessions will generate enough attendance to provide the necessary support for individual students. If AA and NA meetings are located far from campus, students may have trouble finding transportation or feel uncomfortable attending meetings with individuals of varying backgrounds and ages. SMART Recovery has held virtual meetings for several years, and in a post-COVID-19 environment, virtual 12-step meetings are more common than ever. The support provided by these and other mutual aid groups is worthy of exploration by campus leaders.

The nature of recovery and support services appropriate for a campus is based on local needs and priorities of the campus leadership. The issues surrounding recovery, including the social justice context of its components and services, is an essential and growing component of comprehensive campus prevention efforts. Stepping beyond the identification of appropriate resources for campus, attention to recovery as a social justice issue is an important perspective. Ahmed Hosni addresses this matter in Lessons From the Field 7.2.

LESSONS FROM THE FIELD 7.2

Recovery as a Social Justice Issue

Ahmed Hosni, MSW
Director of Recovery
The Higher Education Center for Alcohol and Drug Misuse Prevention and Recovery
The Ohio State University

Collegiate recovery programs (CRPs) play a pivotal role for students who decide to change their maladaptive relationship with substances. These campus programs help current students—undergraduate, graduate, and professional—to develop the necessary recovery capital to succeed academically and thrive personally. CRPs are also an important resource for individuals in recovery hoping to come to college and pursue a degree. Entering and sustaining recovery is difficult for anyone, due to the lack of affordable, accessible, effective, and culturally relevant resources. For decades CRPs have supported emerging adults in recovery or those seeking it, by providing a continuum of services that meet their social, emotional, physical, and recovery needs. These affordable, developmentally appropriate, and lifesaving services, such as those highlighted by the Association of Recovery in Higher Education (2020), allow students to discover their sense of purpose, graduate, and create the life they want.

To understand why recovery is a social justice issue, just look at the vastly different outcomes someone might experience based on their race, gender identity/expression, sexual orientation, socioeconomic status, veteran status, previous criminal justice interaction, or ability when trying to initiate recovery

(Substance Abuse and Mental Health Services Administration, 2014). People face stigma and get other negative responses from having been part of the criminal justice system, and they suffer health inequities. These social factors prevent many of them from ever receiving the treatment, recovery support, or social services they need. Additional stigma, associated with substance misuse, stems from decades of intentional vilification of people of color dating back to the "War on Drugs" that led to the incarceration and exploitation of millions of Black and Brown drug users, a form of legalized slavery (Drug Policy Alliance, 2020; Stevenson, 2019). These harmful and unjust practices disrupt the lives of entire families and communities—and are merely one of many forms of systemic racism and White supremacy. These same practices have created serious gaps in higher education enrollment and graduation rates for students of color.

CRPs can act as an avenue to higher education and graduation for individuals of marginalized identities who have a SUD; CRPs can particularly help those students who have been justice involved, through advocacy and utilization of culturally competent and sensitive practices. Campuses must address all levels of their ecology, the physical setting or place, the human aggregate or characteristics of the people, the organizational and social climate, and the characteristics of the surrounding community that have made campuses an unwelcoming, unsupportive environment for many individuals' recovery and identity. A campus is "recovery hostile" when its climates and norms make being a student or staff/faculty a threat to maintaining one's recovery; similarly, a campus is "identity hostile" if its policies and practices create a threatening climate for those who are not cisgender and White. It is incumbent upon campus leaders to create a just and equitable environment for all people in or seeking recovery from a SUD. Social justice must be the means *and* the end.

REFLECTIONS ON INDICATED PREVENTION SERVICES

Indicated prevention efforts, particularly surrounding SUDs, often raise questions about their relevance and appropriateness on the college campus. Although couched within the full continuum of prevention approaches, indicated prevention is designed around individualized, and sometimes small group, approaches. Further, these efforts focus on students who have experience with substance misuse, at varying levels of harm to self, others, and the institution as a whole. It is thus appropriate to address harm reduction, priorities, and stigma.

The phrase *harm reduction* often conjures up worst-case scenarios; however, harm reduction, as an overall risk mitigation strategy, is found with many societal issues. Automobile safety, seat belts, airbags, and crumple zones all reduce the harm associated with driving. Safety caps on medication bottles protect children from an accidental overdose, and vaccines protect from population-level viruses. The same kind of safety measures can be applied to alcohol use, such as limiting the availability of alcohol (e.g., when and where), specifying the number or size of drinks, providing nonalcoholic beverages and food, and mandating responsible beverage service training. Education campaigns may encourage individuals to alternate between alcoholic beverages and water, not mix alcohol with prescription medications, and designate a sober driver before going out. Other substance-related harm reduction strategies include needle exchange programs, medication for opioid use disorder, and free nasal Narcan—an opioid overdose antidote.

Overall, substance use harm reduction strategies, such as those highlighted within indicated prevention, are often quite successful in halting the progression from substance use to misuse, and then to SUD. It may be beneficial to reframe these tactics as policies and practices that support the use of protective strategies and reduce risk factors.

Indicated prevention strategies can also be challenged due to the risks associated with these efforts. Campus leaders may be risk-averse based on the institution's reputation or image, sense of responsibility, and even liability. Campuses with a low risk tolerance may respond to hazardous behavior by having the student seek services off campus, including taking medical leave to seek treatment in the community. The risk of this kind of response is prescribing a treatment intervention when a prevention intervention is indicated; thus, campuses are encouraged to give attention to prevention counseling to arrest the progression of substance misuse to disorder.

Some campuses may address perceived risk by avoiding students' admission or readmission if a SUD diagnosis, or completion of treatment, is revealed. This standard to consider a student for admission or readmission who is a labeled "drug addict" will likely be different than the standard for someone who has had cancer treatment or who is recovering from an automobile crash. Students who have witnessed how "druggies" are dealt with may delay seeking early help because of the fear of being labeled with a mental or substance use disorder.

Another aspect of the campus response vis-à-vis indicated prevention deals with cost. When considering the staff-to-student ratio as well as return on investment, campus administrators may prioritize funding for universal and selective prevention efforts. The risk of identifying students in recovery or students in need of treatment may be too high for the institution. Some campuses may worry about brand management; this encompasses whether the campus leaders are willing to recruit students in recovery, and whether alumni will support eliminating traditions that do not foster recovery. A safer option for some institutions may be print and digital media campaigns (e.g., posters and coasters), online prevention education portals, and swag promoting health behavior targeting "universal or selective" student populations (Springer & Phillips, 2007).

Stigma at both the institutional and individual levels is a final consideration with indicated prevention. There may be "stigma" for the institution and its reputation associated with having well-developed indicated prevention and recovery and support services. This stigma may affect funding and priority decisions. More important, however, is stigma related to students, particularly those in recovery. When asked about their campus experience, students in recovery often cite accounts of navigating an inhospitable environment. Examples include faculty who feel unprepared to respond to a student sharing their recovery in class, or student health center medical providers' preconceptions of "medication-seeking addicts." Also cited is campus resistance to hosting NA meetings on campus due to the perception that other students will be "at risk" because "addicts" from the community may attend on-campus meetings. If the aim is to reduce stigma and have SUDs viewed not as a behavioral or moral shortcoming, then prevention specialists must advocate for a kinder, gentler approach—one that offers the same kind of social support as that given to students managing other acute or chronic illnesses.

Finally, understanding perspectives about indicated prevention is helpful for assessing institutional readiness for change. What are the prevailing institutional or senior leadership views about indicated prevention strategies? Is indicated prevention seen on par with student counseling services or support for vulnerable student groups? Is there support to expand prevention beyond universal and selective strategies? Although the prevention specialist may advocate for appropriate services, this can be challenging if such a person doesn't exist on a campus, or if the decision makers do not share the vision regarding the need for or appropriateness of these services. The forward-thinking, assertive work by Michael Dunn on a specific initiative is highlighted in the Innovator 7.1 segment; it brings indicated prevention local and makes it practical for all campuses.

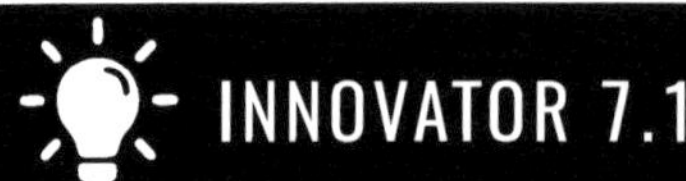

Making Progress When Decision Makers Are Predisposed to Say "No"

Michael E. Dunn, PhD

Director, Health, Expectancy & Addiction Laboratory

University of Central Florida

Over the course of 20 years, my university went from having virtually no resources for drug and alcohol use and associated problems to having a full-service SUD clinic for assessment and treatment, prevention programming, and services for students in recovery. Those of us who recognized the need had to fight tirelessly for support—and we risked losing ground every year. Dealing with student drinking and drug use is not in my job description as a faculty member, but I have unintentionally been involved with indicated prevention since I decided to become a clinical psychologist. I was fortunate to work for Alan Marlatt, best known in higher education for developing BASICS (Brief Alcohol Screening and Intervention for College Students; Dimeff et al., 1999). My good fortune continued by training with another renowned scientist, Mark Goldman, the future co-chair of the National Advisory Council on Alcohol Abuse and Alcoholism task force that produced the report *A Call to Action: Changing the Culture of Drinking at U.S. Colleges* (National Institute on Alcohol Abuse and Alcoholism, 2002).

As a new faculty member with a background in alcohol research on college students, I enjoyed early support from a university vice president, who saw the connection between student success and addressing alcohol use in a scientific and compassionate manner. I had the opportunity to screen all incoming students during orientation for risky drinking. I was also provided finances to build a "Bar Lab" (a research laboratory that looks and functions like an actual bar) and conduct expectancy challenge groups as an indicated prevention program (Darkes & Goldman, 1993, 1998). That support ended abruptly after 2 years when the vice president moved to another position; 20 years of struggle with administrators predisposed to say "no" followed. A new vice president believed involvement with faculty was a potential liability. At the time, my university had nearly 30,000 students, no professional prevention personnel, and our counseling center referred all students with alcohol and drug-related issues to off-campus treatment. Although the new vice president wanted nothing to do with me, I was determined to identify a way to create an alcohol and other drug (AOD) office to address these issues. Fortunately, an opportunity presented itself with an invitation to serve on a presidential task force on student alcohol use. I pushed hard for the creation of a comprehensive, professionally run AOD office, and we hired a visionary director who was up to the challenge.

It was never easy, but working together with the director of AOD programming, we were ultimately successful in creating an award-winning SUD assessment and treatment clinic, in addition to offering prevention programming and services for students in recovery. Senior administrators within student affairs denied almost every request (hence the title of this piece). But we persevered and garnered support from colleagues in various places on campus and in the community.

While there are many lessons learned, I offer the following three: First, don't take "no" for an answer when you know a problem exists and you have an effective solution. Because I supported the AOD director with my help and with graduate students from the clinical program, we were usually able to launch new services without additional support—and after proving their value, we eventually received administration support. Second, reach out to faculty with relevant expertise and forge partnerships. By working together, the AOD director and I received more than a million dollars in external funding for student services and research. We were able to open our first clinic because I supervised clinical doctoral students who wanted the experience and our AOD director was able to secure space and get students referred for screening and indicated prevention. Third, creative thinking is essential. It is important to think beyond "what has always been done" and try new things (with good scientific grounding, of course, as well as a quality evaluation design to assess what works). Perseverance, partnerships, and creative thinking are the components of ultimate success in implementing strategies, programs, and services that work.

CONCLUSION

Strategies associated with indicated prevention are best employed at institutions that value caring for and avoid judgment of those students affected by a SUD. The institution, through its personnel, resources, and support, can send a clear message of its willingness to assist students who may have a SUD. By using validated screening tools and two resourceful mnemonic devices ("I WANT TO" and "MUST CUT DOWN"), prevention specialists can orchestrate assistance for those with risky drug/alcohol use patterns as well as those at risk for developing a SUD. Attention to problem identification and referral, as well as prevention counseling, provides insight to appropriate campus processes within a stepped care approach. Grounding with the stages of change model and MI provides foundations for campus personnel to organize appropriate strategies. Further attention to recovery services and other support services helps with designing campus-based resources.

REFERENCES

Adamson, S. J., Kay-Lambkin, F. J., Baker, A. L., Lewin, T. J., Thornton, L., Kelly, B. J., & Sellman, J. D. (2010). An improved brief measure of cannabis misuse: the Cannabis Use Disorders Identification Test-Revised (CUDIT-R). *Drug and Alcohol Dependence, 110*(1-2), 137–143. https://doi.org/10.1016/j.drugalcdep.2010.02.017

American Psychiatric Association. (2013). *Diagnostic and statistical manual of mental disorders* (5th ed.). https://doi.org/10.1176/appi.books.9780890425596

Anderson, D. S., & Santos, G. M. (2018). *College alcohol survey: The national longitudinal survey on alcohol, tobacco, other drug and violence issues at institutions of higher education*. George Mason University.

Association of Recovery in Higher Education. (2020). *Homepage*. https://collegiaterecovery.org

Babor, T. F., de la Fuente, J. R., Saunders, J., & Grant, M. (1989). *AUDIT: The alcohol use disorders identification test; Guidelines for use in primary health care* (Document No. WHO/MNH/DAT/89.4). World Health Organization.

Babor, T. F. (2007). Screening, brief intervention, and referral to treatment (SBIRT): Toward a public health approach to the management of substance abuse. *Substance Abuse, 28*(3), 7–30. https://doi.org/10.1300/J465v28n03_03

Berman, A. H., Bergman, H., Palmstierna, T., & Schlyter, F. (2005). Evaluation of the drug use disorders identification test (DUDIT) in criminal justice and detoxification settings in a Swedish population sample. *European Addiction Research, 11*(10), 22–31.

Bowers, E., Li, Y., Kiely, M., Brittian, A., Lerner, J., & Lerner, R. (2010). The five Cs model of positive youth development: A longitudinal analysis of confirmatory factor structure and measurement invariance. *Journal of Youth and Adolescence, 39*, 720–735. https://doi.org/10.1007/s10964-010-9530-9

Darkes, J., & Goldman, M. (1993). Expectancy challenge and drinking reduction: Experimental evidence for a mediational process. *Journal of Consulting and Clinical Psychology, 61*, 344–353.

Darkes, J., & Goldman, M. (1998). Expectancy challenge and drinking reduction: Process and structure in the alcohol expectancy network. *Experimental and Clinical Psychopharmacology, 6*, 64–76.

Dimeff, L., Baer, J., Kivlahan, D., & Marlatt, G. (1999). *Brief alcohol screening and intervention for college students (BASICS): A harm reduction approach*. Guilford.

Drug Policy Alliance. (2020). *Race and the drug war*. https://www.drugpolicy.org/issues/race-and-drug-war

Kroenke, K., Spitzer, R. L., & Williams, J. B. (2001). The PHQ-9: Validity of a brief depression severity measure. *Journal of General Internal Medicine, 16*(9), 606–613. https://doi.org/10.1046/j.1525-1497.2001.016009606.x

Li, Y., & Lerner, R. M. (2013). Interrelations of behavioral, emotional, and cognitive school engagement in high school students. *J Youth Adolescence, 42*, 20–32. https://doi.org/10.1007/s10964-012-9857-5

McCambridge, J., & Strang, J. (2004). The efficacy of single-session motivational interviewing in reducing drug consumption and perceptions of drug-related risk and harm among young people: Results from a multi-site cluster randomized trial. *Addiction, 99*(1), 39–52. https://doi.org/10.1111/j.1360-0443.2004.00564.x

Miller, W. R., & Rollnick, S. (2009). Ten things that motivational interviewing is not. *Behavioural and Cognitive Psychotherapy, 37*, 129–140.

Miller, W. R., & Rollnick, S. (2012). *Motivational interviewing: Helping people change*. Guilford.

Miller, W. R., Zweben, A., DiClemente, C. C., & Rychtarik, R. G. (1992). *Motivational enhancement therapy manual: A clinical research guide for therapists treating individuals with alcohol abuse and dependence*. National Institute on Alcohol Abuse and Alcoholism.

Mrazek, P. J., & Haggerty, R. J. (1994). *Institute of Medicine (IOM), Reducing risks for mental disorders: Frontiers for preventive intervention research*. National Academy Press.

National Institute on Alcohol Abuse and Alcoholism. (2002). *A call to action: Changing the culture of drinking at U.S. colleges* (Publication No. 02-5010). U.S. Department of Health and Human Services, National Institutes of Health.

National Institute on Alcohol Abuse and Alcoholism. (2019). *Planning alcohol interventions using NIAAA's CollegeAIM alcohol intervention matrix* (Publication No. 19-AA-8017). U.S. Department of Health and Human Services, National Institutes of Health. https://www.collegedrinkingprevention.gov/CollegeAIM/Resources/NIAAA_College_Matrix_Booklet.pdf

Patton, R., Deluca, P., Kaner, E., Newbury-Birch, D., Phillips, T., & Drummond, C. (2014). Alcohol screening and brief intervention for adolescents: The how, what and where of reducing alcohol consumption and related harm among young people. *Alcohol and Alcoholism, 49*(2), 207–212.

Prochaska, J. O., Norcross, J. C., & DiClemente, C. C. (1994). *Changing for good*. William Morrow.

Saunders, J. B., Aasland, O. G., Babor, T. F., de la Fuente, J. R., & Grant, M. (1993). Development of the alcohol use disorders identification test (AUDIT): WHO collaborative project on early detection of persons with harmful alcohol consumption—II. *Addiction (Abingdon, England), 88*(6), 791–804. https://doi.org/10.1111/j.1360-0443.1993.tb02093.x

Seligman, M. (2002). *Authentic happiness: Using the new positive psychology to realize your potential for lasting fulfillment*. Free Press.

Spitzer, R. L., Kroenke, K., Williams, J. B., & Löwe, B. (2006). A brief measure for assessing generalized anxiety disorder: The GAD-7. *Archives of Internal Medicine, 166*(10), 1092–1097. https://doi.org/10.1001/archinte.166.10.1092

Springer, J. R., & Phillips, J. (2007). *The Institute of Medicine framework and its implication for the advancement of prevention policy, programs and practice* (SMA-4205). U.S. Department of Health and Human Services. http://ca-sdfsc.org/docs/resources/SDFSC_IOM_Policy.pdf

Stevenson, B. (2019, August 18). Why American prisons owe their cruelty to slavery. *The New York Times*. https://www.nytimes.com/interactive/2019/08/14/magazine/prison-industrial-complex-slavery-racism.html

Substance Abuse and Mental Health Services Administration. (2014). *Results from the 2013 national survey on drug use and health: Summary of national findings* (Publication No. SMA 14-4863). https://www.samhsa.gov/data/sites/default/files/NSDUHresultsPDFWHTML2013/Web/NSDUHresults2013.pdf

CHAPTER 8

Staff, Student, and Student Leader Training

"My relationship with alcohol has not served me well in the past. It has affected my grades, contributed to the loss of a few friendships, and made me feel like I was worthless. I am proud to say that I have finally graduated, and I am now enrolled in graduate school. My current job on campus is providing consultations to students who get in trouble with the university for alcohol-related circumstances. I provide guidance to those individuals for self-reflection on their drinking habits."

—Senior at a 4-year public university

Institutions of higher education prepare students with knowledge, critical thinking abilities, interpersonal skills, values-based considerations, and much more both to help them succeed on campus and to prepare them to thrive for the rest of their lives. These same attributes emphasized generally by the college or university are relevant and appropriate for prevention specialists guiding the campus prevention effort. Specifically, prevention specialists must learn current best practices, engagement strategies, theoretical constructs, implementation approaches and innovative considerations, and also do this within an evolving societal climate and changing student needs. Professionals and paraprofessionals handle the widespread training efforts of key campus personnel.

The underlying premise of training is that everyone can improve. Training is not limited to those dealing directly with drug and alcohol misuse prevention; in fact, training is appropriate for faculty, staff, paraprofessionals, student leaders, and students in general. The vast majority of individuals on campus do not have current knowledge about drugs and alcohol; while they are typically aware of some facets surrounding drugs and alcohol, they are generally not aware of the range of consequences of drug or alcohol misuse, the signs of problems, the appropriate role for engagement on drug or alcohol issues, and much of the context surrounding drugs and alcohol. Although most faculty, staff, and students have experiences that inform their worldview, they typically do not see the larger picture of issues, needs, opportunities, and shared responsibilities regarding needed and desired prevention efforts.

This chapter highlights a range of professional development opportunities for campus personnel and pays particular attention to the wide variety of intermediaries who reach students. It also addresses training for students and ongoing training needs of prevention specialists. The importance of such instruction is continual improvement, with more people learning about how they can contribute, positively, to the campus culture.

Because prevention specialists must take the lead on a range of drug and alcohol issues, training necessarily becomes a large part of their work. Three contributions in this chapter offer very practical approaches for campus professionals. Case Study 8.1 sheds light on the importance of student engagement; Lessons From the Field 8.1 offers suggestions about implementing a course on peer education; and in the Innovator segment, Jason Kilmer gives an insightful view, based on dedicated work over decades, about how to connect with a wide range of audiences.

THE RATIONALE FOR TRAINING

In terms of the overall comprehensive campus prevention effort, training is instrumental for getting the myriad individuals and offices on the same page. Training drives the systems approach (see Chapter 4), in which the emphasis is on all engaged groups speaking the same language, having consistent messaging, and moving in the same direction even though they occupy varied yet complementary roles on campus. Because police officers, nurses, student affairs professionals, faculty, and others have different professional standards and codes of ethics, it is essential that these different groups and individuals collaborate and gain consensus about issues such as direction, areas of emphasis, and messaging.

Training is also essential for keeping key individuals current on the latest science. Scientific discoveries on issues such as brain health and plasticity over recent decades, as well as the evolution of diagnosis of substance use disorders, mean that key constituencies must be updated on these matters. These personnel also must be kept aware of the emergence of new substances and the changes in usage patterns of existing ones. Novel evidence-informed strategies, best practices, and cost-effective approaches provide opportunities to update campus strategies.

An important aspect of training is the "unlearning" of previously held knowledge and beliefs. This is vital as new scientific information and new technologies become available; it is even more essential to correct any misperceptions held by stakeholders. Attitudes that are neither helpful nor supportive likewise warrant attention (see Chapter 7's segment on stigma). The aim is for key campus personnel—the intermediaries and the decision makers—to be understanding, supportive, and respectful of those prevention professionals who have knowledge and experience with drug and alcohol issues.

Just as faculty members, nurses, police officers, and other professionals are respected for their expertise in their fields, so should campus prevention specialists be esteemed for theirs. It is particularly incumbent on these specialists to educate others on campus about up-to-date science-backed approaches. With drug and alcohol issues omnipresent in society, everyone has some exposure to, experience with, and personal knowledge of them; however personally valid, these perspectives are not necessarily complete or grounded in current science. For this reason, most campus personnel need their understanding and attitudes about drugs and alcohol "reshaped."

Further, training is crucial to keep key personnel up to date about changes in the student population, including their needs, interests, lifestyles, and learning modalities. Related to this is learning ways of matching current and relevant technological approaches with what is most appropriate for engaging students in meaningful ways.

Another training issue surrounds renewals and refreshers for personnel. These "booster shots" affirm earlier learning; they may also emphasize "continual improvement" and program modifications based on appropriate refinements. With the turnover of personnel, training explains the campus priorities and educates individuals on strategies as well as protocols. It also helps to promote consistent messaging—essential for healthy conversations and engagement.

Overall, ongoing training builds a collaborative, team approach (consistent with the systems approach). Maintaining training initiatives fosters higher level culture change (see Chapter 2) and shapes the conversation vis-à-vis substance issues. The shared experiences that come with training activities allow participants to bond over the shared aims of student success. Whether the training is live or digital, self-directed or participatory, asynchronous or synchronous, it creates shared understanding and shared vision.

GENERAL TRAINING CONSIDERATIONS

Some brief overall perspectives anchor training within the context of the campus and its needs. The training opportunities described here highlight key issues for drug and alcohol prevention.

First, *training incorporates a wide variety of approaches*. Often, when people hear the word *training,* they think of a face-to-face, 2-hour or full-day seminar; maybe they think of a particular format or of an expert "doing" the training. Training, however, encompasses diverse approaches and can have varying duration, delivery, design, and content. It may be self-directed, include practice, incorporate reading, or involve face-to-face interaction. Training is an overall mindset and reflects continuous improvement.

Second, *training is integral to a successful campus prevention effort*. It must be based on current local needs and issues. Training approaches will need to be implemented widely and updated regularly. Due to the general lack of awareness about drug and alcohol issues and appropriate intervention strategies, training of a varied nature is warranted on an ongoing basis. Further, with the turnover of faculty, staff, and particularly students, training warrants being conducted regularly. Whether the training is brief or more specialized and detailed, continual outreach and updates will be necessary to promote core competencies as well as consistency throughout the campus.

Third, *training should be framed within the overall prevention mission and goals.* Because comprehensive campus prevention efforts are grounded in sound theory and evidence-informed practices, the training activity should be promoted and implemented within that context. The training method selected should be consistent with the Institute of Medicine (IOM) model of universal, selective, and indicated strategies (Springer & Phillips, 2007), and it should remind participants of their particular roles within the context of a shared responsibility for success.

Fourth, *training approaches should vary based on different audience needs.* Some topics and strategies may be identified for all members of the campus community (e.g., policy awareness, emergency response for overdose) and may be taught via a brief, self-directed email blast linking to a timely video. Other topics may be more directed, such as an orientation for new faculty or staff members, or a session for student leaders. Based on their role, some intermediaries may need more in-depth training on a topic; examples may include health professionals, residence hall student staff, advisors, faculty members, or peer educators.

Fifth, *training can be envisioned as an introduction to a topic or issue.* Because "unlearning" is likely needed, training can be orchestrated to be foundational and sequential. Subsequent training can renew, refresh, and build on earlier practice, gradually leading to competence and understanding. Such "booster shots" are helpful for regular student programming and are likewise appropriate to enhance skills, knowledge, and attitudes among intermediaries and other staff members.

Sixth, *training content can be varied.* While some efforts can emphasize drug and alcohol issues, others can address what underlies drug/alcohol use and misuse, such as risk and resiliency factors. Training content can easily emanate from the IOM framework, with topics related to individuals' functions and needs. Training may also address process-oriented concerns such as leadership, communication, group dynamics, and workshop preparation and delivery.

Seventh, *training should be reasonably focused and narrow.* Various individuals and groups, based on their roles, warrant training on specific topics and issues. Just as sharing confidential information is often based on a "need-to-know" basis, training can focus on what is helpful and/or necessary to know.

Finally, *training is warranted for the campus prevention personnel themselves.* These prevention professionals, leading the campus effort, should be kept up to date on data and strategies. They also warrant learning about new technologies, trends, evidence-based approaches, promising directions, and resources. They may also learn how to address the various challenges of implementing the campus strategies; these new skills can help these individuals overcome obstacles and resistance to implementing the campus strategies. This ongoing professional development not only provides new content for these professionals but also renews their dedication.

TRAINING CONTENT

Many topics and issues are appropriate training content. Frequent training is essential to remain informed and professionally certified. Overall, training can be organized within five broad categories: Alcohol and Drug Specific, Indirect Strategies, Leadership, Helping Skills, and Group Facilitation. Each is integral to the successful implementation of a comprehensive campus prevention effort, mainly because prevention efforts focus on the overall campus culture.

The *Alcohol and Drug Specific* category incorporates several topics and subtopics. Examples may include short-term and long-term effects, health and safety considerations, medical use, legal aspects, dependence potential, signs of use, and overdose potential. Also included may be new formulations available, changes in usage patterns, and effects of using multiple substances at once.

This category may also include topics such as BASICS, bystander intervention, impaired driving, the amnesty policy, and the Good Samaritan policy. Training may address policies and procedures, enforcement, event planning, and program development. Topics may cover issues surrounding emergencies (e.g., drug overdose, alcohol poisoning), problematic substance use, intervention, and referral. In addition, training can guide attendees with the most current and appropriate language relevant to drug and alcohol issues. Some examples include "recovering alcoholic" (versus "recovered alcoholic"); "impaired driving" (to include marijuana and other illicit drugs); "substance use disorder" (versus "addiction" or "dependence"), and "alcohol and other drugs" or "drugs and alcohol" (to communicate the drug properties of beverage alcohol). Helping students set guidelines or standards for themselves and their peers allows them to address drug and alcohol misuse issues. Also relevant is the context of the social-ecological model as well as reasons for individuals' use or misuse of substances (see Chapter 1 for each of these items).

Indirect Strategies address the range of factors that contribute to substance use and misuse. Consider attention to risk and protective factors, as managing them are essential for practical prevention efforts with drug and alcohol issues, as well as just being valuable on their own and independent of drugs and alcohol. Topics include life skills such as stress management, sleep, time management, and study skills; competence in these areas is valuable for reducing drug and alcohol misuse. Similarly, helping individuals improve their skills with interpersonal relationships, communication, conflict management, and related social skills promotes health and well-being, and thus serves as protective factors. Skills development for intermediaries, as well as for students, ultimately addresses the promotion of healthy choices among students.

Leadership training is a distinct component for consideration by prevention specialists. Specifically, many division leaders, department chairs, student organization leaders, and others in elected or appointed leadership positions will benefit from training. Training on an ongoing basis helps these individuals improve their leadership skills, as these individuals in positions of designated responsibility have influential or indirect roles with persuading and guiding others within their organizations or groups. These skills incorporate quality planning and organization, meeting management, group dynamics and collaboration, listening and communication, and documentation. Leadership incorporates visionary and practical perspectives, as well as values and ethical grounding. Having more effective leadership skills can thus help them infuse important content and concepts regarding various drug and alcohol issues. Worksheet 8.1: Leadership Guide for Student Staff and Volunteers provides details about the value of leadership training for paraprofessionals and volunteers, with attention to benefits and strategies.

A fourth training category is *Helping Skills*. This training assists those individuals whose roles are, for example, peer helper, peer educator, and peer advisor. Appropriate skills include effective listening, reflection, support, and referral; these skills allow caring, accessible, and skilled individuals to meet specific student needs, particularly for those students who may not feel comfortable contacting a professional. Training emphasizes the limits of prevention and knowing when and how to provide appropriate referrals for professional assistance. Noteworthy is that this type of training is documented to have positive effects on the helper, through the "helper therapy principle" (Reissman, 1965). Susie Bruce in Lessons From the Field 8.1 gives specific details about offering a course for peer educators.

Group Facilitation is a final training category, as it is essential for effective delivery. With educational sessions, whether conducted by professionals or peer educators, skills can be enhanced for planning and running a workshop or other activity. Topics may include appropriate materials, techniques, participant engagement, quality learning environments, and time and discussion management. It may also involve balancing content and process, staying focused, being respectful, handling questions, and evaluating strategies.

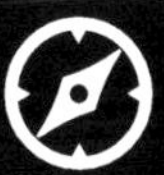

LESSONS FROM THE FIELD 8.1

Peer Education Training Courses

Susie Bruce, MEd
Director, The Gordie Center
University of Virginia

The *Peer Alcohol Education* class is a three-credit peer-educator training course that addresses alcohol and other drug misuse, facilitation skills, and cultural competence. Students learn brain chemistry basics, the progression of substance use disorders, the fundamentals of motivational interviewing (Miller & Rollnick, 2013), the social norms approach (Perkins, 2003), and the transtheoretical model of behavior change (Prochaska et al., 2015). Students are selected by current peer educators through a competitive application and interview process.

Panel discussions provide students with information about campus resources and combat common myths. The dean of students, a campus police officer, and an emergency department physician explain campus policy and response protocols concerning alcohol- or other drug-related emergencies. Staff from the Student Disability Access Center and from Multicultural Student Services (which includes multicultural, Latinx/a/o, LGBTQIA+, and interfaith centers), help students explore implicit bias and how to promote the inclusion of diverse populations and learning styles in their peer presentations. Students also attend a recovery-focused self-help group meeting.

Students develop facilitation skills by creating and delivering several in-class presentations. Each student completes a self-assessment of their presentation skills and receives peer and instructor feedback on both strengths and areas for improvement. This structured feedback format increases student confidence and trust.

For the final project, student pairs create an educational program, including an evaluation, and present it to an outside audience. Students submit learning outcomes, a draft script, and planned activities. The instructor attends the presentation to assess students' delivery of an engaging, respectful, and interactive program. Students consistently rate this class requirement as essential to their later success as peer educators.

Evaluation found that students made significant gains in knowledge, helping skills, and comfort level in giving presentations. In the final reflection paper, students reported learning how to be "a more compassionate friend" and feeling increased confidence "in [their] abilities to keep [their] peers safe," and that the class "helped [them] find [themselves] in helping others." One student summed it up this way: "I could very concretely see where my areas of improvements were, and this itself was extremely rewarding."

TRAINING APPROACHES

Training incorporates a wide range of strategies; the important thing is for facilitators to know ahead of time the needs and learning style of their audience members. The facilitators start with clearly defined outcomes they seek to achieve as a result of the training. Within this context, the facilitators can then create appropriate training content and incorporate a variety of approaches and strategies.

The face-to-face workshop is the classic training approach. Providing a rich opportunity for learning and direct engagement with the facilitator, this training typically blends lecture, guided discussion, reflection, small group interaction, skill building (perhaps with role playing), visioning, and strategic planning. Group size, space, and time limits determine the specific components.

Gaining popularity is asynchronous training, with the learner becoming engaged at their own time and place. Examples may include reading, reviewing case studies, working through examples, watching videos, listening to situations, engaging in reflection, writing, and more.

Self-directed training lacks formal organization. There may or may not be a specified curriculum; the focus is based on an individual's desire to guide the research and reading. This approach may include a reference list, including articles, books, videos, or webinars that an individual can review. Such self-directed inquiry can be very rewarding and can take as much or as little time as desired.

It is important to note that blending approaches is not uncommon. For example, self-direction can be organized so individuals discuss their instruction, discuss controversies, raise questions, and identify new directions for examination. Another example is that face-to-face training can incorporate more than the interpersonal time together; attendees can be asked to do some reading, exercises, activities or reflection prior to the face-to-face time, to maximize the quality and efficiency of the training experience. With thoughtful planning, particularly when implemented over a long period of time, a healthy variety of approaches can result in greater engagement and ownership—and, ideally, greater impact.

TRAINING TECHNIQUES AND TIPS

Quality training is an art. No single approach or formula is best, whether for a solo event, a single topic, or a particular audience. The key to effective training is quality planning, which incorporates the audience, the content, the desired outcomes, and the delivery. Many resources exist to assist with shaping grounded and engaging messages (Anderson & Miller, 2017). The overarching mantra of the Seven *P*s is relevant: Proper Prior Planning Prevents Pathetically Poor Performance. In Case Study 8.1, Whitney Boroski discusses the important role of students in planning and implementing efforts.

Prevention specialists must consider the *audience*, so clarity is needed regarding audience needs, interests, learning styles, and expectations. They should also make certain that there is consistency between what is advertised and what is delivered. Useful for preparation is information gathered before the training, such as queries or self-assessments conducted with email, print, or online polling. Such data collection can also be performed at the beginning or throughout the training; live polling with or without technology helps with this effort.

The training *content,* the central factor, derives from the specific learning outcomes. Topic areas include knowledge, attitudes, skills, and self-confidence, and can focus on content as well as process. Attention is best focused on basic knowledge, areas of controversy, new and future learning, and resources. Training facilitators should try to develop an ability to explain often difficult concepts in easily understood ways, thus generating personal "ownership" of the material.

Coupled with content are *desired outcomes*. Facilitators should be clear about what is expected of the audience—that is, what the audience should know, feel, or do—as a result of the training. Blending desired outcomes with content is critical for a focused and ultimately successful training. It is important for prevention specialists to specify these outcomes regardless of the training approach(es) used—whether webinars, short training events, daylong sessions, self-directed courses, readings, or other types. This clarity also aids with preparing the training evaluation, allowing reviewers to see the links among the objectives, content, and measures. Even quick polling at the beginning and end of training can document results.

The *delivery* of the training is where the preparation comes together. Having a robust toolbox of strategies allows facilitators to select the most appropriate and relevant approaches, examples, and illustrations. Relevant techniques include lectures, small group discussions, data, research findings, slides, verbal summaries of group discussions, case studies, role playing, audience polling ("clickers"), video clips, Q&As, readings, sample materials, worksheets, scenarios, resources, testimonials, simulations with audience observations, and practice sessions. On a practical level, instructors should blend approaches and manage time well to maintain session flow and engagement. To help the training content resonate with audience members comprising diverse learning styles, facilitators are encouraged to appeal to three different factors: *logos* (for intellect and logic), *pathos* (to engage emotions and interests), and *ethos* (to connect to values and character) (see Anderson & Miller, 2017).

From preparation through delivery, constant attention to content and process is essential. Clarity on desired outcomes and timeframes helps to determine appropriate approaches. Training is most effective when the blend of content and process works well with the trainer's style and comfort level. Because trainers, by being facilitators, are engaging in ongoing professional development, they benefit from many resources, including guidance about presentation of visuals, group facilitation, participants' engagement, and other tips.

CASE STUDY 8.1

Getting Learnt on Being Turnt: Student Engagement Makes the Difference

Whitney M. Boroski
Manager of Student Health and Wellness
Michigan Technological University

In the world of higher education, it is common to have regular discussions focused on integrating alcohol and other drug prevention programming on college campuses. However, when the student community is asked for their input on how this message can be shared more effectively, the response is often something to the tune of "You mean you want to have *more* alcohol and other drug education?" This case study highlights engagement strategies based on work with peer ambassadors focused on health and well-being prevention strategies.

THE STRENGTH OF THE STUDENT VOICE

Although listening to students can be time consuming, it is empowering. I started to engage student leaders when my institution was awarded a grant that emphasized empowering students to make legal, healthy, safe, and appropriate choices about alcohol (Ansari, 2010). I listened to their thoughts and opinions about drugs and alcohol, along with their experiences and the suggestions on improvement to education and prevention outreach.

I called upon student groups, asked the same set of questions, and listened. One comment I heard was, "If I hear another drug or alcohol presentation from professional staff, I'm going to explode." I said, "Then, make me something that you'd want to hear." That's when the *Getting Learnt on Being Turnt* workshop was created. When I first saw the workshop draft, I was shocked that topics professional staff typically covered were also addressed by the student; the difference was that these areas now had a student perspective.

COLLABORATIONS TAKE TIME

The next few years brought even more conversations about drug and alcohol prevention—with slight, but noticeable, changes. Greek life students had a strong interest in the workshop, but they wanted to know more about how they could impact their peers with the alcohol and other drug prevention education that was most timely and valuable to them; this local finding was consistent with Sloane and Zimmer's (1993) research. Greek life leaders wanted information specifically about the Good Samaritan provision and how their community could use it to stay safe. In response, my student board recommended "just ask Public Safety."

BEING NOTICED

The chief of police was very supportive and requested to be the point of contact, wanting to foster a stronger connection between his officers and the student community; he shared this initiative with his groups and so did others in leadership positions. From there, the workshop received more attention, requests, and feedback.

As professionals at institutions of higher education, we continue updating and improving our messaging; these little changes capture the student voice and ownership. Our aim of helping students "get learnt" continues!

AUDIENCES

Additional, detailed attention is warranted regarding four audiences: staff members, faculty members, peer helpers and educators, and student organizations. Such attention will help facilitators better connect with these groups and thus achieve the desired outcomes.

To maximize engagement with and consistency of the comprehensive campus prevention effort, training of *staff members* is essential—and, again, is in line with a systems approach. According to their areas of specialization, staff members (e.g., police, medical, counseling, student affairs) have their professional preparation and codes of conduct. Training is important for consistency among these areas. For example, law enforcement personnel have roles beyond enforcement, such as with education, support services, and policy development. Similarly, those working with student activities, judicial affairs, resident life, and academic support services will benefit from instruction on active listening, problem identification, referral, and support; this training will aid issues related directly or indirectly to drugs or alcohol.

More extensive training may be warranted, based on staff members' areas of responsibility. Residence hall personnel, for example, benefit from training on conflict resolution, emergency response, referral, program delivery, and support for recovery. Those in health care settings, as well as those in varied student affairs settings, will gain from appropriate training on problem identification and referral to those personnel with expertise on substance use disorders.

For *faculty members*, issues surrounding drugs and alcohol are widely present in their academic and advising roles. Multiple challenges exist with faculty members, as they typically are not prepared to identify these issues, often believe that attending to such personal behaviors are not their responsibility, do not feel comfortable with this type of personal conversation, and are unaware of available resources and referral options. Further, faculty members (as well as others) may unintentionally say something that is not accurate according to current science, make comments inconsistent with the desired prevention messaging, or not be supportive of those challenged with drug or alcohol issues (e.g., students in recovery).

Because of their regular engagement with students, faculty members have a vital and important role and benefit from applicable insights on how they can help and support student success. They can infuse supportive and accurate messages within courses, including lecture or discussion content, readings, assignments, or mentoring. Their role with enforcement, problem identification, and referral can shape the campus climate in positive ways. Further, faculty members will benefit from a healthier learning environment if students who have problems with drugs or alcohol, or who have faced negative consequences with their drug or alcohol use (e.g., class absence, low class participation, poor academic preparation) have these issues dealt with in constructive ways. As the campus culture does a better job with addressing drug and alcohol issues and concerns, students as a whole are more likely to demonstrate positive outcomes in academic performance, class participation, and engagement.

Peer helpers and educators have training needs based on their specific roles (e.g., advising, presentations, activities, policy review). Because students often look to other students for advice and support, peer helpers have important roles in shaping the campus environment in positive ways, promoting affirmative, supportive, and empowering messages. Peer helpers serve as a type of "first responder" and constitute a network of interested and capable individuals, thus aiding campus decision makers with shaping the campus culture. Training can be embedded in an academic course or in noncredit options. Those completing training can have a designation as an "approved" peer educator.

Finally, training with specific *student organizations* or other groups is important. While there may be overlap with other groups cited in this section, there may also be some unique features. With groups such as student-athlete mentors, some of their roles may overlap with those of a peer helper, and thus warrant some shared training efforts. The paraprofessional residence hall staff, such as resident advisors, will have training commensurate with their responsibilities faced in a residence hall. Some student leaders, such as orientation staff or advisors, may warrant similar, though less intense, training. Other organizations benefit from leadership training; among them are leaders in student government leaders, officers in other student organizations, leaders of fraternities and sororities, athletic team captains, and members of the student athlete advisory council. Their specific roles on campus are important for inclusion, such as awareness of the range of drug and alcohol issues, signs of use or impairment, intervention strategies, helpful support, and constructive language. The training can blend topics directly related to drugs and alcohol as well as those of a more general nature.

FINAL CONSIDERATIONS

Several remaining issues warrant attention. Training is viewed as an ongoing process with multiple audiences who have varied needs. Because of the significant amount of learning and unlearning that permeates drug and alcohol misuse prevention, training must be viewed with a systematic and long-term perspective. Having a broad range of campus personnel adequately prepared—and working in sync with one another—is a colossal enterprise. Because of staff turnover, the changing landscape of knowledge about drugs and alcohol, and the shifting nature of students' needs, issues, and engagement styles, ongoing training is vitally important.

A related concern is that those planning the overall training efforts must maintain an attitude of constructive risk taking. There is a need to push the boundaries of campus personnel. Prevention planners and campus leaders must acknowledge that training will not result in perfection. Although their efforts should highlight the audience and topics that will result in the most significant impact for the campus, at that specific point in time, training is an ongoing process. Its planners are encouraged to continue to move forward—to "stretch"—in order to change knowledge, attitudes, and behaviors.

Training of trainers is another way of expanding the reach of the campus effort. Multiple benefits result from preparing a cadre of individuals to do the training. One advantage is the cost savings of having local personnel skilled for conducting local training—a clear return on investment. Another result is the trainers become acquainted with local issues. The ongoing presence of the trainers means that follow-on clarifications, booster sessions, and ongoing support can be accommodated relatively easily. Although conducting training of trainers requires attention to skills beyond drug- and alcohol-related content, the focus on "how to train" issues can also be helpful for application with group facilitation, lecture, and presentation skills.

Finally, training can be seen as an opportunity for collaboration and mentoring. With the wide range of specialty areas on campus, prevention specialists can seek out individuals with relevant expertise and ask them to share it with others—whether as a sole presenter or a keynote speaker, as a co-presenter, or in another opportunity. Training allows individuals to mentor and to be mentored—engaging in the ongoing learning that is central to the mission of higher education. When personnel from different parts of campus assist directly with training objectives, they can be instrumental in furthering support for the campus prevention effort itself.

In the Innovator 8.1 segment, Jason Kilmer imparts some succinct and germane views on training. These tips are helpful for prevention specialists and for those trained by them.

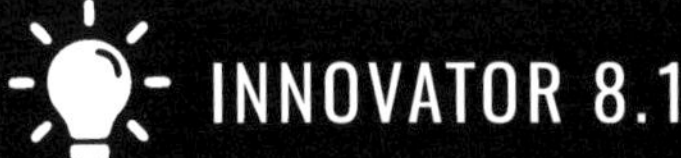

"Make 'em Laugh": The Role of Humor in Presenting and Teaching

Jason R. Kilmer, PhD
Associate Professor
University of Washington

"Make 'em laugh, make 'em laugh, make 'em laugh . . ."
—Donald O'Connor, *Singin' in the Rain*, 1952

I love working in the field of alcohol and other drug (AOD) prevention, and I only hope that my passion and commitment shines in my interactions with those I work with.

Prevention professionals are often asked to provide trainings about AOD for our colleagues (staff, faculty, and/or administrators), student leaders, or students on campus. Too often, when something is offered for professionals (e.g., an on-campus conference presentation, an in-service training), I hear people choose not to attend a training opportunity—even when it is free and not very lengthy—because they "can't miss work to participate." In my eyes, knowing how to address alcohol and other drug issues *is* part of the work of staff and faculty on college campuses! It is a shared responsibility across departments and divisions as college professionals work to support student success. How can the field address this seeming disconnect between what people see as the job of AOD prevention professionals and something in which they also play a part? It is essential to make clear that what is done on college campuses about AOD issues will pay dividends elsewhere, including academic outcomes and mental health.

There is over a decade of compelling research that shows that substance use is associated with everything from lower GPA to less engagement with faculty and less likelihood of graduating on time. If administrators proudly announce and promote that they are champions for student success, then they should, truthfully, also be champions for AOD prevention and intervention. Further, there is clear research that shows that AOD use can exacerbate or even cause the very issues that students often seek help for in counseling and health settings. Similarly, what campus faculty, staff, and administrators do about substance use also will impact mental health, suicide, and other health behaviors.

Yet, despite its importance, even the topic of AOD can make some people anxious. They may think about their own behavior in a way that brings up discomfort, worry that the presenters are there to change those who are participating in a program, or have some long-standing beliefs challenged by more recent research. I believe there is something that can be done about that.

In the early 1970s, researchers showed that exposure to humor in a test reduced anxiety, and this anxiety reduction enhanced test performance (Smith et al., 1971). Exposure to funny cartoons boosted performance on a math test, and it seemed to be the same pathway of reduced anxiety that led to better performance (Ford et al., 2012). Even having humorous cartoons in a textbook increased comprehension—although it is important to use humor in the right place (Piaw, 2014). *And that is the key.* The AOD field has a lot of heavy content, including some material that doesn't often lend itself to humor; however, we can reduce anxiety and open people up to learning by interspersing humor that is appropriate to the content. Get the audience laughing, then introduce important or poignant information. Always remember that humor should never be at someone's expense, and should be used thoughtfully.

As the scene with the lyrics referenced above comes to an end, the character asks, "Don't you know everyone wants to laugh?" They very well might, and incorporating humor into training and presenting efforts can be more than just refreshing; it can keep people open to, and increase the likelihood of, learning about this amazing field.

CONCLUSION

Regular improvement of campus-based strategies is a central theme of ongoing training efforts. Having a robust training initiative as part of the prevention effort is helpful for the range of training activities with the variety of intermediaries such as faculty, staff, and student leaders, who will ultimately be affecting students on campus. In addition, substantive and up-to-date training is essential for the prevention specialists themselves. The collaborative nature of training, with shared content and language, ultimately gets all audiences on the same page. Using both established and creative approaches, as well as varied content and style, instruction can be tailored to emerging needs as well as the diverse constituency of audiences. Topics may range from drug and alcohol–specific concerns and indirect strategies to leadership and helping skills. Incorporating this breadth of efforts is essential for the campus prevention effort to be evidence-informed, and thus more likely for having the desired impact.

REFERENCES

Anderson, D. S., & Miller, R. E. (2017). *Health and safety communication: A practical guide forward*. Routledge.

Ansari, W. E. (2010). Is the health and wellbeing of university students associated with the academic performance? Cross sectional findings from the United Kingdom. *International Journal of Environmental Research and Public Health, 7*(2), 509–527.

Ford, T. E., Ford, B. L., Boxer, C. F., & Armstrong, J. (2012). Effect of humor on state anxiety and math performance. *Humor: International Journal of Humor Research, 25*(1), 59–74.

Miller, W. R., & Rollnick, S. (2013). *Motivational interviewing: Helping people to change* (3rd ed.). Guilford.

Perkins, H. W. (Ed.). (2003). *The social norms approach to preventing school and college age substance abuse: A handbook for educators, counselors, and clinicians*. Jossey-Bass.

Piaw, C.Y. (2014). The effects of humor cartoons in a series of bestselling academic books. *Humor: International Journal of Humor Research, 27*(3), 499–520.

Prochaska, J. O., Redding, C. A., & Evers, K. E. (2015). The transtheoretical model and stages of change. In K. Glanz, B. K. Rimer, & K. Viswanath (Eds.), *Health behavior: Theory, research, and practice* (5th ed., pp. 125–148). Jossey-Bass.

Reissman, F. (1965). The "helper" therapy principle. *Social Work, 10*(2), 27–32. https://doi.org/10.1093/sw/10.2.27

Sloane, B. C., & Zimmer, C. G. (1993). The power of peer health education. *Journal of American College Health, 41*(6), 241–245.

Smith, R. E., Ascough, J. C., Ettinger, R. F., & Nelson, D. A. (1971). Humor, anxiety, and task performance. *Journal of Personality and Social Psychology, 19*(2), 243–246.

Springer, J. R., & Phillips, J. (2007). *The Institute of Medicine framework and its implication for the advancement of prevention policy, programs and practice* (SMA-4205). U.S. Department of Health and Human Services. http://ca-sdfsc.org/docs/resources/SDFSC_IOM_Policy.pdf

CHAPTER 9

Measuring the Impact of Prevention Efforts

"As I entered my freshman year, I was not unfamiliar with the effects that alcohol can have on people. I knew college freedom would only heighten the pressure to party, so I committed myself to balancing my social and academic life. I idolized older girls for their involvement and academic success while still having fun in moderation, and I surrounded myself with friends who wanted to do the same."

—Senior from the Northeast at a large public university

Campus prevention leaders genuinely want their drug and alcohol prevention efforts to have an impact with the students on campus; thus, quality evidence on the outcomes of their strategies and the processes used is essential. Evaluation documents actions taken; relays results; highlights areas of significant success, gaps, and resources; and drives future directions. Data collected will be most helpful for decision makers, stakeholders, and advisory groups and can shape strategic planning. Evaluation can also prove useful for sharing with other campuses, as they seek to implement quality approaches for their own needs.

Since many prevention efforts call for evidence-based approaches, central to that evidence is research. While research and evaluation often go hand-in-hand, the important focus for campus prevention efforts is upon program evaluation efforts. Research protocols and research findings can be illustrative and helpful for informing the program evaluation. In addition, research can help further substantiate the overall prevention efforts for the gatekeepers on campus.

Prevention specialists will benefit from a broad overview and basic understanding of evaluation. Regardless of the specific nature of the prevention specialists' skills—whether clinical, programming, planning, peer leadership, or training—attention to reasonable and appropriate evaluative approaches is essential. The blend of quantitative and qualitative methods, the examination of direct and indirect factors, and collaboration with specialists and other subject matter experts all help with implementing quality evaluations.

In this chapter, three contributors provide their insights and wisdom on evaluation. Case Study 9.1 addresses the importance of working collaboratively. Lessons From the Field 9.1 highlights specific considerations for evaluating a new initiative, with attention to a campaign. David Hanson, in Innovator 9.1, discusses broad and critical questions and offers down-to-earth perspectives.

MAKING A CASE FOR EVALUATION

Evaluation is a critical aspect of campus drug and alcohol misuse prevention efforts. Five overall perspectives are helpful in terms of evaluation activities. First, the societal context of health promotion efforts is important. Second, evaluation aids strategic planning and focus. Third, evaluation helps with documentation and justification. Fourth, evaluation supports program improvement, revision, and replication—both on campus as well as elsewhere. Finally, evaluation is essential for contributions to the field of drug and alcohol abuse studies.

First, with overall health promotion efforts in society, quality evaluation helps practitioners to determine the needs and optimal strategies to address identified health threats. Regardless of the prevention effort's focus—sexual decision making, interpersonal relationships, stress management, exercise—evaluation documents the results and the processes associated with that health-enhancing initiative.

The long-term context is critical. The fact that deaths due to impaired driving have been reduced shows that progress can be achieved; nonetheless, the problem remains. The fact that reductions are found with underage alcohol use and high-risk (binge) drinking among high school and college students demonstrates that progress can be made. But the persistence of such problems shows two things: first, that progress can be made; and second, that continued diligence is needed.

Human behavior, in individuals and in groups, is complex, so any expectations for change must be kept reasonable and appropriate. Even greater challenges surround drug and alcohol issues specifically: misinformation, many personal experiences, cultural overlays, and expectations about quick outcomes. Preventive work with drug and alcohol issues can be placed within the "hard sciences," which is typically associated with laboratory work. Any focus on hard science or laboratory research methods has a downside;.qualitative or descriptive data may be discounted or dismissed. An unintended consequence of a singular focus on quantitative, experimental research studies is a "one-size-fits-all" approach. Qualitative data allows for local variables to be considered alongside quantitative research methods.

The second point is that evaluation is essential for strategic planning efforts and should be incorporated actively in them (Anderson, 2008). Evaluation must be considered from the onset of a campus effort; all too often, however, evaluation is tacked on at the end of a project or is incorporated because the funder requires it. Having evaluation specialists at the table during the initial planning phases helps all stakeholders clarify desired results. Discussions help zero in on the outcomes and audiences with questions such as, "What is it that is desired, specifically, as a result of the planned efforts?" and "What would be most helpful to document that?" Thus, rather than having broad objectives such as "to reduce drug abuse," "to offer fun activities without alcohol," "to have a social norms campaign," or "to get more students involved with our efforts," program planners benefit from specificity and focus. Consider the following specific goals:

- to reduce the misinformation about marijuana among first-year students by 20% each year
- to increase the confidence of coaches talking with team members about drugs and alcohol, to a level of 75% following training, and sustained at 50% after 6 months, using a specified measure
- to increase awareness of helpful referral resources on campus by residence hall staff (to a 90% level), by student activities staff (to 75%), and by faculty (to 50%) by the end of a 3-year training series

The point of this list is to show how evaluation can help to focus planning. Being specific about the audience (e.g., first-year students, coaches, faculty), timing (e.g., annually, post-training and follow-up, and 3 years), and levels (e.g., 20%, 75/50%, and 90/75/50%) helps clarify what would be reasonable and appropriate for a campus at a specific point in time.

The third overall benefit of evaluation is the related documentation. Evaluation incorporates desired outcomes, a logic model, reasonable milestones, and appropriate measures to document campus prevention efforts. Worksheet 9.1: Logic Model Template helps with understanding the linkages between various elements typically included in the preparation of a logic model. Within the overall goals and strategies, and within the context of changing the campus culture, such documentation sheds light on moving the needle vis-à-vis drug/alcohol usage and related consequences. Although evaluation challenges often include how to measure what did not happen, the reality is that so much *can* be measured. Campus prevention efforts primarily aim to reduce negative outcomes; thus, lessening problems, increasing knowledge, enhancing skills, moderating attitudes, changing behaviors and patterns of use, and other variables are important elements to consider in terms of evaluation.

Appropriate documentation aids in not only systematic program improvement but also justification regarding the program and its components. Documentation will include descriptions of the efforts implemented as well as what helped and what hindered the strategy.

Understanding the achievement or lack of achievement of specified objectives is helpful. The intent of planning is to incorporate evidence-informed approaches and to have reasonable objectives. Just as a budget is a plan, objectives are also premeditated targets.

Fourth, information gathered via evaluation helps to improve programs and strategies. Because campus prevention personnel, campus decision makers, and stakeholders all want campus prevention efforts to be meaningful and appropriate, they will likely want to ensure good use of resources and time. For efforts that do not achieve the desired outcomes, rethinking and reorganization may be warranted; revisions are appropriate with the aim of improvement over time. Since affecting change with drug and alcohol abuse issues is challenging, attention to factors such as clearly defined objectives, a helpful logic model, and measures of proximate outcomes assist with modifications of programs as well as measures. Worksheet 9.2: Planning for Goals and Objectives helps with the differentiation of goals and objectives, and also includes scheduling and resources.

The final consideration regarding evaluation is more long term and idealistic and focuses on moving prevention science forward. The broader perspective is about drug and alcohol issues on campuses nationwide (and ultimately worldwide). Gaining insights about one campus' efforts and strategies that are working or not working as well will assist others. This shared knowledge and collective wisdom is essential for continuing to evolve and make progress, with the acknowledgment of a changing culture, updated student needs and learning styles, technological enhancements, the introduction of new drugs of abuse, and the complex interaction of human behavior. Gathering quality outcome and process evaluation, and sharing these results and insights through publications, presentations, blogs, media coverage, and a public presence will help move the field of prevention.

EVALUATION AND THEORY

Integrating theory with evaluation is critical. Strategic planning (see Chapter 10) takes advantage of the best science and evidence available and applies them to local needs and issues. Starting with the logic model, prevention specialists develop links between their desired outcomes and the strategies planned to achieve them. Prevention specialists incorporate evidence-informed approaches, including theoretical underpinnings. Prevention specialists will specify which theories will best guide the logic model toward the achievement of the desired outcomes (drawing from, as a starting point, many of the theories on health behavior, psychology, and sociology [see Chapter 3]). The insights, wisdom, and innovation of the planning group enhance such planning and inform the campus prevention strategies.

Several important points relate to this connection between theory and evaluation. First, as noted, theory undergirds the design of the campus efforts. Several theories are available for consideration, so the choice of relevant theory (or theories) is determined by local decision makers.

Second, much attention is paid to evidence-based strategies. Decades ago, many drug and alcohol abuse prevention efforts lacked this evidence foundation. At the same time, evaluation and documentation was emphasized; however, evaluation on its own does not necessarily translate into effective practices. Rigorous evaluation follows effective strategies. An emphasis on evidence-informed promotes campus efforts being planned with sound foundations, whether this evidence is from published professional literature, the application of theoretical constructs to a local situation, or another thoughtful and grounded approach. This evidence-informed process is in contrast to the "feel good" approach, the "we've done it this way for years" standard, or the "because that's what I want" directive. Evaluating feel-good strategies is difficult without sound theoretical foundations and the use of core components based on research and evaluation.

Third, the emphasis on theory blends well with innovation. If the only allowable approaches were based on existing evidence, then room for innovation becomes limited. New and creative approaches, when grounded, offer opportunity and hope for doing better—and achieving even greater progress toward specified aims. With innovation comes the chance to test theories and apply best practices in novel ways.

Fourth, locally developed strategic plans are vital, as they create greater local ownership, buy-in, and long-term viability. By drawing on theory to address local needs and local planners' aims, the best fit for the current circumstances can be designed.

Finally, the distinction between research and evaluation is useful. For campus prevention efforts, prevention specialists have their primary emphasis on strategies believed to have the greatest likelihood of making a difference locally. These strategies include policies, programs, training, campaigns, and other actions. Essential with these strategies is attention to documenting progress toward reaching the specified objectives, as well as assessing the processes used. Overall, this documentation is encompassed within program evaluation. Research efforts may also be conducted; research is important for moving forward the field of drug and alcohol misuse prevention. However, within the scheme of most campus prevention efforts, research per se is not the top priority. Research incorporates stricter standards, such as rigorous control group designs and levels of evidence and proof of effect. Prevention specialists can gather insights from research efforts, and seek to improve their own program evaluation activities with research-based foundations. Some research design features may help maximize the opportunity for new evidence and contribute to scientific discovery; faculty members with interest and relevant expertise are the likely leaders of these efforts. Case Study 9.1, prepared by Cynthia Wilson and Eric Gipson, emphasizes faculty member engagement and the critical role of collaboration.

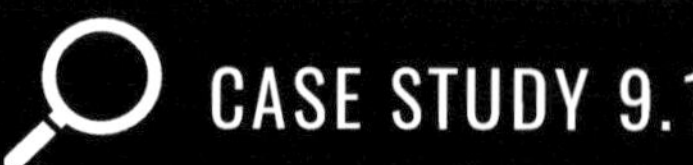

Working in Silos? That's NUTS!

Cynthia B. Wilson, PhD
Executive Director, Florida Center for Prevention
Florida State University

Eric Gipson, MA
Prevention Coordinator, Center for
Health Advocacy & Wellness
Florida State University

Collaboration is the key to campus success with drug and alcohol abuse prevention at Florida State University. The Center for Health Advocacy and Wellness (CHAW) provides all campus health education and prevention efforts and directly employs evidence-based interventions. By implementing strategies from *CollegeAIM* (National Institute on Alcohol Abuse and Alcoholism [NIAAA], 2019), CHAW uses intervention matrices built for individual and environmental levels. Individual-level interventions involve substance use classes for students required to attend due to infractions, and outreach efforts for specific populations (e.g., Greek-letter organization members, student-athletes, first-year and new students, students with disabilities, LGBTQIA+ students). Environmental-level interventions involve the routine and inclusive review of alcohol and tobacco policies to ensure their effectiveness and comprehensiveness.

Since 2002, the Florida Center for Prevention Research (FCPR) has implemented a social norms initiative called The Real Project (https://fsureal.com), which has demonstrated its ability to promote positive norms, reduce harmful misperceptions, and increase protective behaviors to reduce alcohol-related harm (Siebert et al., 2003; Wilke et al., 2005). The Real Project utilizes data collected from undergraduates in its yearly UCelebrate survey, which asks students to report on their perceived alcohol-related behaviors. Created in partnership with advertising students, print and social media are central to a campaign that corrects misperceptions and accurately reflects students' alcohol norms and seeks to reduce risk factors and promote protective ones. To help make the campaign engaging and relevant for students, a mascot (a cartoon squirrel named Micco) is seen as "just a squirrel who's nuts about telling FSU students the REAL facts about drinking habits on campus" (Micco the Squirrel, n.d.). Micco makes appearances around campus with promotional items such as water bottles, T-shirts, cell phone wallets, and blood alcohol concentration cards.

Collectively, the strategies by CHAW and FCPR promote a campus environment where students can be free from harm. Having both organizations work together strategically while sharing the same mission results in louder messages, resources more broadly shared, and a more positive campus culture.

THE MATTER OF EVIDENCE

With the various policies, programs, and other efforts undertaken with the universal, selective, and indicated strategies highlighted in the Institute of Medicine's framework (see Chapter 3), prevention specialists seek evidence about "what made a difference, and why." This evidence is precisely what the evaluation data and processes ultimately seek to provide, as it can help direct, shape, and reshape the campus effort.

With evidence-based strategies, the evidence may come from a compilation or a repository prepared by others, such as is found with

NIAAA's (2019) *CollegeAIM* or those cited in the Substance Abuse and Mental Health Services Administration's (2018) evidence-based practices book. The evidence may also come from theoretical grounding or other best practices compilations. The essential point is to specify what evidence is used to undergird campus decisions; however, two cautions emerge. One is that a strategy found to work elsewhere, and under certain conditions, is not guaranteed to work on another campus. The other is that just because a strategy is not included in a compilation does not mean that it will not work; it simply may not have met the specified criteria. In other words: Lack of proof of an effect is not proof of lack of effect. Campus leaders should be guided by the "best fit" approach (see Chapter 3).

A related concern is that a specific strategy identified as an evidence-based practice may be impractical to *implement locally with fidelity.* Consider, for example, the specific standards or conditions by which an evidence-based practice was selected; some of these particular criteria may not be appropriate, or not met, for a particular campus, thus making it understandable why the adoption of that strategy may not have the desired outcomes. If the design is compromised locally, the effectiveness may be reduced. Similarly, if an evidence-based approach is applied to a population not included in the original research, then it is not clear what results should be expected. Overall, although it is helpful to review and consider evidence-based practices, prevention specialists should not be constrained by their presence or absence. Campus prevention specialists are best served by understanding the theories that underlie evidence-informed practices.

Finally, attention to *types of evidence* helps provide some context for campus evaluation efforts. Because the primary purpose of campus-based strategies is to address specified areas of concern, and document relevant outcomes and processes, the main emphasis is on sound evaluation. Research approaches and the various types of evidence can help inform the quality of the campus evaluation.

Overall, researchers seek the highest level of evidence feasible. Because proof of effect at the most rigorous, scientific level does not always exist—or is too expensive or time-consuming to implement—researchers balance the ideal with the practical, based on the context of their needs. Typically, the higher scientific levels incorporate more rigorous methodology and thus provide more significant evidence of effectiveness. The following descriptions comprise a hierarchy of research design.

At the highest level are *systematic reviews and meta-analyses*. These are assimilations of others' research, based on established publication standards of multiple studies and acquired from searches of the professional literature and systematic methods of selection and review. Because systematic compilations take time, *primary studies* are a viable source of evidence. One approach is a randomized control trial, whereby participants are randomly assigned into experimental and control groups for the study, thus providing attribution to the treatment or intervention as the cause of differential outcomes.

Cohort studies, longitudinal in nature, track groups of people over time. These can be retrospective (historical) or prospective (moving forward) in nature. By recording characteristics such as protective factors and tracking exposure to treatment over time, the impact of exposure or treatment, based on personal characteristics, can be assessed. A *case-control study* is more retrospective in nature and seeks to identify factors that may have contributed to a current state of affairs; this compares those with a particular attribute with those who do not have that attribute (e.g., a control group) and looks for differential interventions or exposure (as a potential causal attribute).

Case series and case reports track individuals who have received a particular intervention or treatment and see what outcomes have been obtained. These forms of evidence are descriptive, with case series representing more than one individual. Finally, *editorials and expert opinions* represent the opinions or judgments provided by those with appropriate qualifications and experience.

Although campus planning efforts on drug and alcohol issues are not research projects per se, they may incorporate some more modest research activities and will want to integrate quality evaluation. Prevention specialists aspire to document their efforts as much as possible and thus seek for the evidence to be as sound as possible.

TYPES OF EVALUATION

The primary consideration with evaluation is that it is performed. Regardless of the size of the campus, available resources, or scope of effort, some type of evaluation at some level is essential. A second consideration is that whatever is done is useful to its audiences (the prevention specialists, the prevention leadership, the advisory group, and the decision makers). Third, based on the varied audiences, different elements of evaluation may be more or less helpful. Fourth, the evaluation should complement and be integral to the campus program and strategy; the results will help guide the effort. Fifth, no "one-size-fits-all" or "ideal" evaluation design exists; campus leaders are encouraged to be grounded with their evaluative strategies and operate within the context of local aims and resources. Finally, the evaluation, while important and essential, should not lead or control the campus effort—it should merely guide it. The data gathered should assist campus leaders as they plan strategies to address needs and gaps.

Three broad constructs help to examine various types of evaluation. One construct focuses on quantitative and qualitative approaches, a second focuses on outcomes and processes, and the third addresses direct and indirect attributes. Through blending these constructs, specific strategies, measures, and protocols can be developed and implemented. With any of them, attention to existing resources and instrumentation can help significantly with the planning efforts, such as the documentation done well with the Drug Enforcement Administration's (2020) prevention publication for colleges and universities.

The first construct of quantitative and qualitative measures stresses the use of both types in evaluation design; each helps inform the other. *Quantitative approaches* are numerical and statistical, including yes/no questions, Likert scales, percentages, prioritizations, dollars, or similar items. Gathered with such approaches as surveys, questionnaires, and pretests/posttests, quantitative approaches may also include archival data, environmental scans, policy reviews, and participation rates. Quantitative approaches are quite amenable to statistical analysis, which may consist of examining data results based on demographic factors (e.g., gender, age, race/ethnicity), group comparisons, and statistical analyses.

Qualitative evaluation is more open ended and observational. Examples include focus groups, key informant interviews, and discussions, and may involve observation, telephone polling, and narrative or open-ended responses. Qualitative evaluation methods are more labor intensive, in terms of information gathering, and the resulting data are challenging to code. That said, qualitative data can be coded, organized, and summarized in understandable ways and used to help interpret or illustrate other findings.

The second construct addresses outcomes and processes. *Outcome evaluation* focuses on goal achievement and specifically addresses the objectives. Objectives include clear and measurable criteria and typically emphasize shorter term results among participants, whether they are the ultimate audience (e.g., students) or intermediaries (e.g., staff, faculty, coaches, leaders). *Process evaluation* addresses the "how" factor, including approaches implemented, challenges faced, and what might have contributed to or hindered the achievement of specified outcomes. These measures describe what was done, so a greater understanding of the "why" regarding the results is obtained. With Worksheet 9.3: Planning Guide With Evaluation Measures, prevention specialists can discern ways in which outcome and process measures each have value with evaluating the campus effort.

The third construct addresses direct and indirect factors. The primary attention for prevention specialists is upon those *direct factors*, addressing drug and alcohol issues specifically. The evaluation will tackle such items as usage patterns and rates, attitudes about substances, intentions regarding use, skills associated with managing substance use and misuse (e.g., bystander training or conversational factors), and perceptions. Complementing these direct factors are the *indirect factors*, consistent with the prevention effort's theoretical grounding and logic model. These indirect factors may be protective and resiliency factors, such as assertiveness, decision-making, stress management, conflict resolution, communication, and relationship skills. They are labeled as indirect because of their causal linkage to drug or alcohol outcomes (e.g., stress management skills related to reduced substance misuse).

Prevention specialists benefit from attention to each of these three constructs. It is not sufficient to simply gather attendance or program satisfaction data with a post-event survey; consider each of these three, broadly constituted frameworks when developing the overall evaluation plan. It is also helpful to blend the various approaches; just as outcome data may inform the "what was achieved" question, process data may inform the "how" issue. Similarly, quantitative data may report the numbers and results, but the qualitative data may help "tell the story" and illustrate what occurred. Having multiple data points for pulling together the information represents triangulation, thus painting a complete picture of what is happening within the complexities of human behavior.

ASSESSING COMMUNICATIONS IMPACT

Specific attention with evaluation focuses on the communication efforts associated with the variety of campus strategies. That is, not only are the strategies important, but also important is how these strategies are seen or heard by the audience. Overall, the critical issue surrounding communication and messages is what, precisely, the audience heard—what is it that they infer from the policy, program, campaign, or other initiatives? The aim is to verify that what is heard is what the planners (i.e., the prevention specialists) intended.

If the intent is to make students aware of the importance of intervening with another person's misuse of substances, including but not limited to an overdose, it is important to ensure that the listener does not infer endorsement of a substance-using behavior. Similarly, harm reduction approaches, with the intent of getting individuals to achieve reductions of their heavy use of alcohol, is not designed as an endorsement of alcohol consumption that may still be illegal (for those under age 21).

Any communications assessment process benefits from using both quantitative and qualitative approaches. Quantitative strategies may incorporate questions in a campus survey, such as asking whether a campaign or messages were seen and, if so, what effect (if any) they had on the respondents' thinking, attitudes, behavior, behavioral intention, or other factors. Survey questions may ask whether the respondent found the communication credible, helpful, and accurate; survey questions may also ask whether the communication was clear with what it wanted the audience to do; examples include getting involved with a behavior that concerned them, making a referral, challenging a point of view, or correcting misinformation.

Qualitative strategies address many of the same questions, except that they provide the opportunity to tack on follow-up questions such as "why" and "how." With approaches such as focus groups, discussion groups, telephone polling, and one-on-one interviews, questions can be asked about the messages heard and their effects. These open-ended approaches could ask, "What messages do you hear from the campus (or from peers, or parents, or faculty) about alcohol (or high-risk drinking, or marijuana use, or illicit use of prescription drugs)?"

Observation is another qualitative approach; this may be in a large group, small group, or individual setting. Watching the audience when trying to inform or, ultimately, persuade them of a particular message can provide insight into their understanding, acceptance, tolerance, excitement, or other reaction. With opportunities for immediate modification with the message delivery, follow-on elaboration or clarification can be helpful.

These efforts of assessing and monitoring the impact of communications help prevention specialists identify ways of ensuring programmatic consistency and messaging effectiveness. Not only does this careful examination of communication strategies help with program and messaging improvement, but audience engagement can also help with moving the audience toward endorsement and, ultimately, embracing the campus effort. Some further details about ways of implementing quality evaluation is highlighted by William DeJong in Lessons From the Field 9.1.

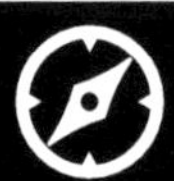

LESSONS FROM THE FIELD 9.1

How to Evaluate a New Campuswide Prevention Program

William DeJong, PhD

Professor (retired), Boston University School of Public Health

Adjunct Professor, Tufts University School of Medicine

Developing a research design to evaluate a new campuswide intervention presents a major challenge: How do college officials separate out what the program or policy may contribute above and beyond the college's other prevention initiatives? This is not an issue if a program reaches students individually or in small groups, when it is possible to conduct a randomized control trial—with half of the students (or small groups) randomly assigned to receive the intervention and the others assigned to a delayed-intervention control group. But what if the program reaches the entire student body, such as a campuswide social marketing campaign?

There are two research design options. A *time-series study* can reveal whether a data trend line shifts significantly after the campaign is implemented (Shadish et al., 2002). This is a strong design, especially when all the following conditions are met (Turner et al., 2008):

- Annual random-sample student surveys have been and will continue to be implemented for several years, or there are other official records or indicator data that align with the campaign's objectives.
- The campaign has a clear start date on which it is fully implemented, thus sharply defining the pre-intervention and intervention time periods.

- The campaign runs long enough to observe a significant shift in the trend line.
- No other policies or programs with the same outcome objectives are introduced simultaneously with the campaign.

Importantly, the evaluation team should track local, state, or national events that might influence students' behavior and thus obscure or exaggerate the campaign's true effect.

An *exposure study* requires a single post-intervention survey that asks questions (placed at the end) to ascertain which respondents the campaign reached. The data analysis examines whether students who have "unassisted message recall" are more likely to report behaviors that are consonant with the campaign (Surkan et al., 2003). Of note, this analysis can also be done each time a student survey is conducted in a time-series study. Positive findings may be a result of the campaign, but they could also mean that students who already endorsed the message paid greater attention to—and therefore more often recalled—the campaign. This weakness can be partly addressed by asking students to report whether their behavior had changed since the campaign's start date.

If neither research design is feasible, then focus groups or intercept interviews with a diverse and representative sample of students can also provide useful information, especially if each session begins with a short survey. This is a good fallback option, but this type of research can also be used in combination with a time-series or an exposure study.

These alternatives are less robust than a randomized control trial, but they are the best options available for evaluating a campuswide intervention and collecting the data needed to inform midcourse corrections and future intervention planning.

PRACTICAL GUIDANCE FOR PREVENTION SPECIALISTS

Building on the theoretical and evidence emphasis that grounds campus evaluation efforts, prevention specialists benefit from summary guidance. This provides overall direction for needs assessment and evaluation efforts. The specific design and "how-to" elements are locally determined, based on areas of interest, expertise, and resource availability. Seven major sections organize these guidelines: Overall, Planning Processes, Content, Organization, Implementation, Data Use, and Reporting.

Overall

1. Make sure evaluation is part of the overall campus strategic planning process. Discussions on evaluation approaches and context are essential as the goals, objectives, and strategies are determined. These evaluation deliberations can be most helpful in deciding the nature and scope of the campus initiatives.
2. Evaluation planning should always consider how the information gathered will be utilized and presented. With that endpoint, planners can assess whether the measures, questions, and protocols are helpful in achieving those aims.
3. Evaluation is important at the macro and micro levels. Systemically, evaluation can help answer whether and how the comprehensive campus strategies help address the needs of the campus. At the more focused level, evaluation can shed light on the extent to which specific learning or other outcomes are achieved, whether based on an event or overall strategy (e.g., policy, campaign, service).
4. Be clear and focused on what is desired from the evaluation. Be specific with what is necessary to know.
5. Make sure there is intent or commitment to use the data gathered. For example, do not ask questions if there will be constraints on using the results.

Planning Processes

6. Engage as many stakeholders as possible throughout the design, implementation, review, and distribution phases.
7. Leverage local technical expertise by engaging evaluation specialists on campus to help with instrumentation, sampling, implementation plans, data coding, analysis, and reporting. Participants will likely be faculty from various disciplines, including those with expertise regarding the target population.
8. Seek agreement from the campus prevention specialists regarding the nature, content, and use of evaluation processes and results. This includes documentation of the nature and value of the campus program.
9. Gain perspectives of campus decision makers regarding what, specifically, they would like to know, learn, or see as a result of the evaluation.
10. Include a focus on ways in which the campus effort links to and is supportive of the institutional and organizational/division mission statements.
11. Provide opportunities for student engagement, with professionals providing mentoring about the various phases of evaluation.

Content

12. Attend to measures that link directly to the campus efforts' aims. Direct measures are likely the most important, including behaviors, attitudes, beliefs, perceptions, knowledge, intention, and interests. Indirect measures about contributing factors (such as risk and protective factors) are important as they link to the campus' strategic plan and logic model.
13. Attend to both outcomes and processes. Overall, outcomes incorporate achievement of identified objectives, and processes address strategies used.
14. Evaluate as many strategies as feasible. They include programs, events, activities, training, policies, and campaigns.

15. Attend to challenging documentation on issues surrounding communication, such as credibility, messages heard, and impact.
16. Gain insight on each of the prevention strategies: universal, selective, and indicated.
17. Gather data from multiple sources. This includes self-report (e.g., student surveys), incident data (e.g., incident reports, policy violations, emergency transports, arrests or citations, property damage), stakeholder insights (e.g., staff, faculty, student leader reports), academic records, and environmental scans.
18. Include both quantitative and qualitative sources. Numerical data are meaningful, but narrative reports provide insights and help “tell the story” about what is or is not happening.
19. Blend data from multiple sources to triangulate results. This may include qualitative insights or examples that illustrate quantitative findings; it may also cite areas of overlap or inconsistency.
20. Prioritize evaluation needs and activities so that key questions and issues are addressed; acknowledge that every question and subquestion cannot be answered.
21. Maintain focus on multiple perspectives, including current (shorter and intermediate term) as well as longer term (ultimate outcomes).

Organization

22. Be systematic and organized with the needs assessment and evaluation activities.
23. When gathering information, attend to the credibility of the information collected and to be used.
24. Make sure the evaluation processes are manageable. Learn ways to conduct evaluation efficiently without compromising quality. This includes minimizing disruptions and maximizing response rates and honesty.

Implementation

25. To the extent possible, use instrumentation and tools that are valid, reliable, and culturally appropriate. These may include approaches previously developed and vetted; for new

approaches, develop high-quality evaluation methods, and objectively document outcomes.

26. Build in redundancies and cross-checks. This includes validating responses to ensure accuracy as well as securing storage in safe, duplicative settings.
27. Attend to details to maintain the integrity of the evaluation. These efforts are not like those used in a laboratory or a highly controlled environment; nevertheless, attention to professional standards and best practices will help assure quality outcomes.

Data Use

28. Monitor activity and progress throughout implementation of the campus effort. This helps frame evaluation beyond just the beginning and end of an initiative to include periodic assessments or "pulse checks."
29. Incorporate data and results in a timely way; adjust the instrumentation, protocols, or strategies as needed.
30. Be open to using results that may be challenging, such as those that document an initiative as not particularly useful or that raise questions about a strategy.
31. Maintain a commitment to gathering quality information and using that information. Acknowledge that detailed planning will be needed, but that the effort is both necessary and worthwhile.

Reporting

32. Present data clearly and accurately. Presentations should avoid confusion, ambiguity, exaggeration, and errors.
33. Make sure reporting is clear and understandable. The reports should be such that researchers and scientists appreciate them and that they are understandable by various audiences (e.g., administrators, staff, faculty, students).
34. Promote trust with reported findings. This incorporates sound, ethical, and approved protocols, data integrity, full reporting of

results, and confidential use and storage of data. It also includes an underlying aim of continuous improvement.

35. Report the data in ways that are helpful to the various audiences. This may involve different types of reporting, from summaries to more detailed analyses. Data for the campus prevention leadership group, general faculty, and campus decision makers will vary.
36. Share data, findings, conclusions, and recommendations to various constituencies in a planned and timely way.
37. With reporting, cite areas of confusion or contradiction. Include potential areas for further examination or consideration. Also include ways in which the evaluation design can be improved.
38. Consider how the media (campus or local) may use and report the findings. This helps provide awareness and support of the campus needs, issues, and opportunities.
39. Consider ways of sharing results beyond the campus. This may include professional journals as well as conference presentations.

These various practical suggestions make clear that no single approach exists—that is, there is not a single, specified evaluation design appropriate for all institutions. The method of the evaluation efforts can be viewed as a type of calculus, or even as a quilt, with different pieces coming together in an organized and systematic way. It is also an organic process, as approaches will be adjusted with changes in needs, personnel, expertise, and interests. The important factor is that evaluation must be included and done diligently throughout both the strategic planning and program implementation processes.

Building on these overall constructs and practical tips is a more global view of promoting culture change on the campus. David Hanson, a long-term educator, researcher, and innovator, offers valuable takeaways. In Innovator 9.1, he advocates for common sense approaches for addressing alcohol; these perspectives can aid prevention specialists as they connect with various constituencies.

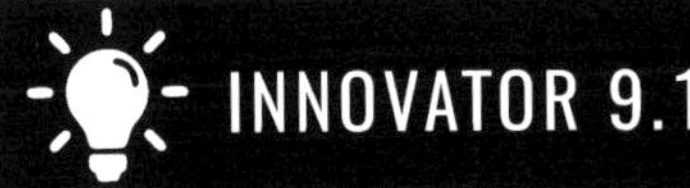

Promoting Change With How Drinking Is Viewed

David J. Hanson, PhD
Professor Emeritus
State University of New York at Potsdam

U.S. alcohol policy focuses on reducing consumption per capita—and for those under age 21, it promotes complete prohibition. But national Prohibition from 1920 to 1933 should have taught us that total prohibition leads to heavy episodic and other harmful drinking. So, I have long promoted harm reduction. U.S. society actually uses a harm reduction approach with many other issues, whether it be heroin dependence, safer sex, or homelessness.

Cross-cultural evidence indicates that light alcohol consumption isn't harmful to young people: It's the abuse of alcohol that's the problem—just as it is for those age 21 and older. This finding suggests moderation should be taught to young people. And this approach doesn't require them to drink. Consider that civics is taught in middle school long before students can vote, serve on juries, or hold public office. Similarly, geography is taught without taking students to Zimbabwe or Tibet. But harm reduction for those under age 21 is strongly opposed by both governmental agencies and many others.

In promoting harm reduction in my books, chapters, and scholarly papers, I reach relatively few people. Therefore, I decided to expand my audience. In 1997, I launched a nonprofit website, *Alcohol: Problems and Solutions* (https://www.alcoholproblemsandsolutions.org). It was and remains somewhat controversial. People have both praised and criticized it.

Largely as a result of the website, I have been invited to appear on national radio and TV. It has also provided a platform on national publications to promote harm reduction. There, for example, I can address common objections to parents serving their young people alcohol in the home, where the law permits doing so. And most states do allow this practice.

The vast majority of people will seriously consider logical evidence presented in a rational manner. Even when they remain unconvinced, they respect you. So don't fear offending people with rationality.

Here's an example. Our society fails to prepare young people to live in the United States—in which most people drink alcoholic beverages. That can reasonably be compared to how our society prepares them to live in a country in which most people drive vehicles. What if society prepared them to drive by the following approach?

- Start by telling young people that driving is dangerous and kills thousands of people annually.
- Say that driving requires knowing road rules (which are not taught to them to avoid sending them "mixed messages" about their ability to drive).
- Stress that good—and safe—driving requires guided practice (but which is not provided because they are too young to drive).
- Remind them that they lack the necessary emotional maturity to drive safely (but they will acquire this maturity on their 21st birthday). Then, on that magic day, they are handed the keys to the car.
- Remind them that using public transportation is much safer than driving their own vehicle. But if they insist on driving, warn them to be careful.

> What would the result be? Streets and highways would be unimaginably dangerous.
>
> My concern is that this same approach to driving is also used in preparing young people to consume alcohol if they choose to do so when they turn 21. And most youth will decide to drink before then. In fact, society's approach to driving is something called "graduated licensing." Perhaps we would do well to consider something similar for alcohol.
>
> People respond well to logic, but promoting change is a challenge. Humans have a natural inertia—we feel comfortable with the familiar. As a result, we often fear change. Evidence and logic can be powerful in persuading people.

CONCLUSION

Not only are comprehensive campus efforts based on data and theoretical constructs, but they also gather data of both a quantitative and qualitative nature. This evidence provides documentation on the efficacy of strategies and helps prevention specialists refine, remove, or enhance current efforts. As evidence-informed approaches are undertaken to develop innovative strategies that best meet the identified needs of students, data collected helps with decisions locally and more broadly (with the dissemination of findings). As an integral component of strategic planning efforts, evaluation encompasses both outcome and process measures and also addresses both direct and indirect factors related to drug and alcohol issues. Pay special attention to communications surrounding prevention strategies, as this is where meaningful messaging, receptivity, and engagement are found. When thoughtful planning takes place and content experts participate, substantive contributions for impact can be achieved locally and beyond.

REFERENCES

Anderson, D. S. (2008). *IMPACT evaluation resource.* National Collegiate Athletic Association. https://www.ncaa.org/sites/default/files/SSI_IMPACTEvaluationResource_20161109.pdf

Drug Enforcement Administration. (2020). *Prevention with purpose: A strategic planning guide to preventing drug misuse among college students.* http://www.campusdrugprevention.gov/preventionguide

Micco the Squirrel. (n.d.). *Bio* [Instagram profile]. Instagram. https://www.instagram.com/micco4fsu

National Institute on Alcohol Abuse and Alcoholism. (2019). *Planning alcohol interventions using NIAAA's CollegeAIM alcohol intervention matrix* (Publication No. 19-AA-8017). U.S. Department of Health and Human Services, National Institutes of Health. https://www.collegedrinkingprevention.gov/CollegeAIM/Resources/NIAAA_College_Matrix_Booklet.pdf

Shadish, W. R., Cook, T. D., & Campbell, D. T. (2002). *Experimental and quasi-experimental designs for generalized causal inference.* Houghton Mifflin.

Siebert, D. C., Wilke, D. J., Delva, J., Smith, M. P., & Howell, R. (2003). Differences in African American and white college students' drinking behaviors: Consequences, harm reduction strategies, and health information sources. *Journal of American College Health, 52*(3), 123–129.

Substance Abuse and Mental Health Services Administration. (2018). *Selecting best-fit programs and practices: Guidance for substance misuse prevention practitioners.* https://www.samhsa.gov/sites/default/files/ebp_prevention_guidance_document_241.pdf

Surkan, P. J., DeJong, W., Herr-Zaya, K. M., Rodriguez-Howard, M., & Fay, K. (2003). A paid radio advertising campaign to promote parent-child communication about alcohol. *Journal of Health Communication, 8*(5), 489–495.

Turner, J., Perkins, H. W., & Bauerle, J. (2008). Declining negative consequences related to alcohol misuse among students exposed to a social norms marketing intervention on a college campus. *Journal of American College Health, 57*(1), 85–94.

Wilke, D. J., Siebert, D. C., Delva, J., Smith, M. P., & Howell, R. L. (2005). Gender differences in predicting high-risk drinking among undergraduate students. *Journal of Drug Education, 35*(1), 79–94.

COLLABORATION: "The How"

Thoughtful planning processes to effect cultural change vis-à-vis drug and alcohol misuse is central to this section's three chapters. The focus of this section is upon the *how* of organizing strategies and personnel for implementing a comprehensive campus approach to drug and alcohol misuse prevention. Attention is provided to strategic planning; critical to effective and thoughtful planning is the nine-step planning model, which incorporates many of the foundations and key components provided in earlier chapters. Within the overall strategic planning process is the importance of working with various constituencies; prevention specialists have a vital role with orchestrating varied coalition efforts on campus, in the community, and in other settings. Finally, attention is provided to varied persuasion strategies for speaking out clearly and maximizing impact with varied audiences.

CHAPTER 10

Planning Processes
How to Mobilize Resources

"I was eager and ready to graduate high school and experience the independence that came with being a college student. Looking back, I was much more impressionable than I like to admit that I was, but through building relationships with older students whom I saw balance a healthy social life and academic life, I was able to find ways to make decisions I felt confident in."

—Senior from New England at a rural public university

By understanding the variety of concerns and opportunities surrounding drug and alcohol issues, reviewing current and desired norms, and knowing both theories and conceptual frameworks, prevention specialists have a firm foundation for moving forward. They must also perform a review of comprehensive campus efforts—with attention paid to policies, programs, education, training, support services, and evaluation—before starting to plan localized strategies. So, a planning guide for organizing, orchestrating, monitoring, and reviewing these efforts is helpful.

This chapter aids prevention specialists as they design, redesign, or reenergize their campus strategy. The entire campus-based effort revolves around "the campus culture," as described in Chapter 2.

A significant amount of commitment is required to achieve the strategy's desired results, and this dedication takes the form of personnel time—which means active support from institutional leadership.

The range of considerations and strategies documented in previous chapters are incorporated here. The thrust of this approach involves a nine-step model that is appropriate for all campus efforts. It applies to new or existing campus efforts and can be led by a seasoned or new professional.

Throughout this planning process are the dominant themes of "keeping it local" and "making it practical." Further, communicating the key elements of what is planned, to all relevant constituencies, is essential. Three contributions in this chapter drive home this point. Lessons From the Field 10.1 illustrates the importance of engaging campus police with the planning effort; similar arguments can be made for many other campus constituencies. Case Study 10.1 highlights a successful campaign with student participation. Innovator Dave Closson provides insights about the planning and implementation of a specific engagement strategy, sharing challenges and how they were overcome.

THE CONCEPT OF PLANNED CHANGE

The concept of *planned change* helps orient campus efforts regarding substance abuse issues. It represents a process whereby order and direction help guide the organization leaders toward some specified and desired results. Implicit within strategic planning, planned change incorporates various approaches such as a SWOT (strengths, weaknesses, opportunities, threats) analysis, the Eisenhower Matrix, Force Field Analysis, and prioritization efforts. Planned change is built around the process of being purposeful—as opposed to being reactive or piecemeal in approach.

Within this overarching concept of planned change, prevention specialists lead a process that moves the college campus toward the desired end (e.g., reduction of problems associated with drugs or alcohol). Planned change includes the creation, modification, or elimination of campus policies and procedures services and strategies, training and activities, and other initiatives. Intentional change assumes that some change is needed; with the issues surrounding drugs and alcohol, the specific issues to be addressed revolve around the nature of the problem for the campus (see Chapter 1) and also the various aspects of the current needs and desires regarding the campus culture (see Chapter 2). The basis of the need is dissatisfaction with the hundreds of thousands of alcohol-related injuries, more than 1,600 alcohol-related deaths, and many drug-related deaths—all annually, all college based, and virtually all preventable. Planned change uses organized efforts to modify this current state of affairs into a better one.

Essential within planned change efforts is an understanding of the variety of any potential obstacles and challenges faced. The construct of Force Field Analysis (Lewin, 1951) describes the movement from the current status to the desired outcomes being facilitated by "driving forces"; examples are policies, programs, and strategies. Worksheet 10.1: Force Field Analysis can be used to help define many of these factors with campus efforts.

It is helpful to seek the participation of multiple constituencies in this process of orchestrating change; the collective impact model (Turner et al., 2012) demonstrates how various entities can coalesce and collaborate toward a shared vision (see Chapter 11), rather than working in silos on campus. The reality is that many constraints or obstacles exist; these restraining forces include, among others, attitudes, incomplete or faulty knowledge, lack of funding, and vested interests. Further, many members of the campus community resist change, due to factors such as the uncertainty surrounding it, lack of trust with the planners, lack of preparedness or skills, or different visions or aims. One way to promote change and address the attendant challenges is by engaging key constituencies; in Lessons From the Field 10.1, Ryan Snow offers perspectives about collaboration for campus success.

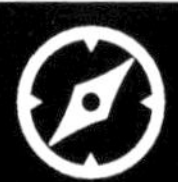

LESSONS FROM THE FIELD 10.1

Engaging Police in Campuswide Prevention Messages

Ryan Snow, MEd
Instructor
Preventionleaders.com

When I was asked to sit on a committee focusing on the university's alcohol and other drug vision and mission statement, I jumped at the opportunity. As a campus police officer, I saw firsthand the issues facing the campus and the student population. As I sat down for my first committee meeting, I looked around the room and became familiar with the faces: participants from counseling, Greek life, student discipline, housing, academics, and student events were all sitting around me. I immediately recognized that building a strong partnership with these individuals was important for the overall message the university was trying to send.

As I worked with these various units of the university, I realized they were using the police as a scare tactic to steer students away from underage drinking and illegal substance use. I immediately saw this approach needed to change, because the police department's aim (as a whole as well as with individual officers) is to be as helpful as possible. We are community partners, and focusing on the "trouble" factor wasn't our message at all. Previous messaging by the university showed hands in handcuffs or people behind bars to scare people away from using illegal substances. By pointing out our department's perspective, I was able to show committee members the damage that was being done by this earlier messaging.

I believe it is important for those in leadership positions—and on campus prevention committees—to remember who is being served; leaders should remain in alignment with the campus and department mission and vision statements when serving the campus community. Having various perspectives and points of view at the table helps to create and deliver clear, consistent, and positive messages. When messages about responsible choices are being conveyed, everyone involved must be aware of the unconscious biases they are projecting. Biases and stereotypes need to be recognized and changed to communicate effectively the true vision of where the community wants to go.

GROUNDING CAMPUS EFFORTS

Beyond planned change, decisions about the appropriate theories and frameworks (highlighted in Chapter 3) will further ground campus efforts. When folded into the planning model, these foundations keep strategies focused. Use of the step-by-step model, which is the emphasis of this chapter, is based in sound principles and theory; active use of this model as the planning framework helps keep all key personnel, stakeholders, and other interested parties focused and on task. Prevention specialists should also consider using Robert's Rules of Order for meetings; they allow for peaceful decision making and discussion, and without such rules, meetings would likely be disorderly and unproductive. Similarly, for planning campus efforts, an orderly framework and organized process ensure meaningful and effective strategies; in contrast, lack of planning and organization facilitates haphazard and spurious efforts with a limited opportunity for significant impact.

When orchestrating these efforts—with whatever framework, theories, and logic model selected—campus planners must make the strategy practical and local. National or state data document the initial need, but parallel local information validates the campus need and helps secure buy-in from stakeholders. Similarly, attention to evidence-based practices highlights the importance of grounding and identifying the best fit at the local level. Prevention specialists can then prepare to implement strategies deemed most helpful and appropriate for their campuses.

A final consideration for grounding the campus effort is to agree on the fundamental theories and framework. Prevention planners are encouraged not to belabor the specific process itself but to move forward with some organization and try it; revisions can be made based on local experiences and the addition of new personnel. Just as the entire campus effort will evolve, based on formative evaluation insights, the general planning process can also develop over time.

Although the details and logistics can be overwhelming, what is most important is that there be a quality planning process to organize the campus prevention effort. The process can be challenging, due to the personal nature of the issue and various obstacles, but honest discussions must take place if meaningful results are to be achieved. Taking stock of a campus's needs is risky; the results may not be popular or encouraging. However, it is through these efforts that opportunities for change—and positive outcomes with a healthier campus climate—await.

A STEP-BY-STEP PLANNING MODEL

Figure 10.1 illustrates a nine-step planning model that is prepared as a practical synthesis of a variety of elements: multiple theoretical constructs, different strategic planning approaches, overall experience, and local applicability. Central to this process is that each campus must determine its direction and approaches. It is incumbent upon leaders to determine the direction(s) based on the campus's unique needs, background, personnel, and resources.

These nine steps can be viewed as a sequence, which is most appropriate for a campus beginning its drug/alcohol abuse prevention efforts; however, the process is likewise valuable for those institutions undertaking a review of campus efforts. The steps can be viewed as a framework for reviewing and renewing the campus effort either as a whole or with regard to specific aspects. Some elements here draw upon more focused explanations detailed elsewhere in this volume.

Figure 10.1
Planning Model

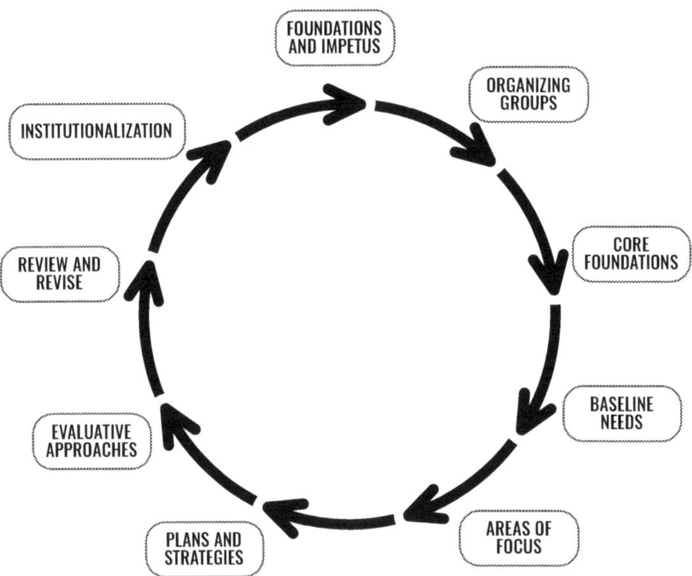

Step 1: Validate Foundations and Impetus

This initial step seeks to generally clarify and affirm why some organized effort is even needed to address campus drug and alcohol issues. Campus leaders or instigators of this process may be motivated because of a recent death or overdose on campus or nearby. The motivation may be based on a sense that "things" are out of control; perhaps the local data continue to demonstrate usage patterns or perceptions that are no longer deemed acceptable. The foundation may be to revamp campus approaches by taking a fresh look; or, it may be based on the biennial review specified by the federal government. This process may be based on the desire to have a campus strategy that is planned, organized, and grounded on sound conceptual foundations, perhaps in contrast to more reactionary or haphazard, although heartfelt, approaches of the past. The grounding of the effort may be to identify ways of better preventing problems and promoting increased resiliency. It may be as simple as identifying ways to create new opportunities to distinguish the institution from peer institutions. The impetus may be a mandate from the campus's governing board and/or president/chancellor, such as with a blue ribbon committee.

This first step can be a "fuzzy" or "soft" start. Essentially, it addresses the fundamental question: "Why are we embarking on these efforts regarding drugs and alcohol?" This foundation can serve as a constant reminder for the organizers and members of the planning group of their aim or mission, as it provides the overall shape and direction for the planning and specified efforts.

Step 2: Convene Organizing Groups

Central to an organized planning process is having several clearly designated groups that will guide the campus effort (see Figure 10.2). The detailed discussion in Chapter 11 on coalitions highlights the importance of having key constituencies involved in each of these groups; additional detail about engaging various constituencies is found in the last section of this chapter. The diverse interests of different organizations, and the varied areas of expertise, are all critical for inclusion when developing or revising the campus strategies.

The primary group for organizing the campus effort is labeled here as the leadership group. The leadership group should have broad and substantive representation from multiple offices on campus and perhaps in the community. Representatives should include a wide range of individuals with vested interests, areas of concern, and potential reach. The caution is that it not be weighted too much in any one sector of campus; instead, ensuring broad representation from health and counseling, resident life, fraternity/sorority life, athletics, the faculty, student activities, student government, academic advising, and media relations is a priority. This group may have 15 to 20 individuals included and should meet regularly (e.g., monthly).

Within that leadership group should be a much more limited assemblage—a steering committee—of four to five people who can be nimbler and meet more regularly to ensure that the direction and activities remain on track. Its role would primarily be oversight, monitoring, and problem solving, with most attention paid to ensuring an appropriate and engaged process.

Beyond the leadership group may be a much broader constituency, such as an advisory body. It could incorporate the wide range of interests and perspectives throughout the college community; this larger group could meet less often, perhaps two or three times a year. Its primary purpose would be to keep its members informed and engaged. It may serve as a sounding board for the leadership group's activities, whether planned or current. This advisory body can further anchor campus effort in meaningful ways, as it can help the campus prevention effort extend its reach, identify related issues, support access to resources, and communicate its messages; each of these roles assists with the ultimate aim of institutionalization of the prevention effort (see Chapter 3).

Figure 10.2
Organizing Groups

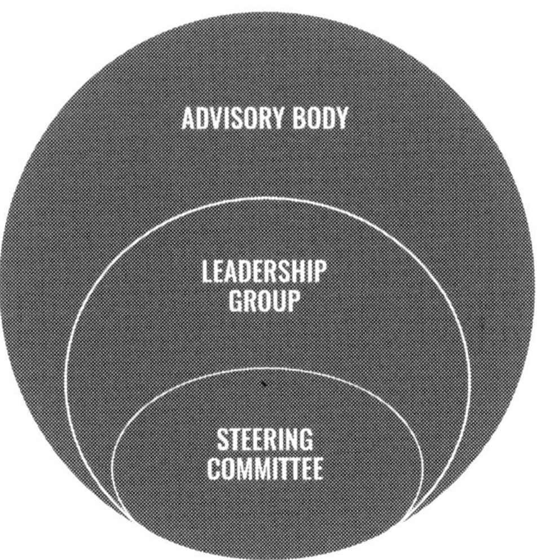

The leadership group's overall responsibility is managing the entire process of defining and refining the campus strategy. As the various activities and duties unfold, different individuals or groups may take responsibility for specific tasks. One way of configuring this delineation is to have subcommittees of the leadership group address particular items (e.g., policy, training, evaluation, public awareness, funding). These subcommittees may engage others beyond the leadership group for their expertise; these individuals could be from the advisory body or other offices or individuals (e.g., faculty expertise to aid in evaluation efforts, or a public affairs office to help prepare awareness campaigns). Highlighted at the end of this section is Case Study 10.1 by Delynne Wilcox; she illustrates ways in which active student involvement helped with both the results achieved by and the longevity of the efforts.

Also critical for the leadership group is having meaningful, substantive—not "token"— engagement. It is vital that individuals' and groups' expertise and long-term tenure in the institution be respected. Consider, especially, the role of faculty members; their position is important, as they are typically the longest serving members of the institution and have varied fields of study and expertise that can help meaningfully ground and implement plans. Further, their involvement can result in cost-effective and student-engagement approaches through research projects, classroom activities, field experiences, and internships. A complementary benefit is that involved faculty members gain a greater understanding of the importance and nature of prevention efforts and thus can serve as advocates for the campus effort.

A related question addresses where the leadership should be based. In Chapter 3, attention focused on the appropriate placement of the prevention specialists themselves, including their organizing office. A similar question arises here with the administration of the leadership group. It may be determined that the campus's coordinator of drug/alcohol issues is the most appropriate person to spearhead this effort; alternatively, it may be determined that the leadership of the planning would best come from a separate office, division, faculty member, or administrator, as such expertise would provide the appropriate institutional influence and prestige. This local decision should be based on the needs and aims of the institution itself and what best serves the campus prevention effort.

Step 3: Develop Core Foundations

The primary task of the leadership group is to specify the direction and focus of the campus effort. Within this step are four distinct yet overlapping actions. First, develop the overall general vision for the campus vis-à-vis drug and alcohol issues. Much of the specific vision will be based on what was identified in Step 1, which determined the general foundations and impetus behind the campus effort. This vision may include what campus leaders want to see for the campus regarding drug and alcohol use behavior. It may also be based on the current and desired status of student and staff attitudes, ways in which drug or alcohol situations are handled from a policy or support services perspective, and the nature of conversations among students or between students and staff or faculty. With each of these (as well as other items), an understanding of the current state of affairs helps with determining if change is desired and, if so, what the desired results would be.

Second, the leadership group should answer two questions: (1) What do you want to prevent? and (2) What do you want to promote? The responses clarify the focus of the effort. Each thrust—"prevent" and "promote"—has an important role, similar to those outlined in Chapter 2 on campus culture and in Chapter 3 with frameworks. When the answers get operationalized with service delivery, both aspects—what is wanted for someone not to do (the "prevent" question) and what is wanted for them to do (the "promote" question)—are addressed.

Third, the group should determine guiding principles. Specifically, campus organizers should agree upon specific elements that will underlie their efforts, as these aspects will help steer the planning and the actions. These elements should be agreed to at the onset, reviewed periodically, and revised as needed. Examples may include membership, meaningful involvement, nurturing engagement, timing, reporting, audiences, monitoring, quantitative and qualitative documentation, visibility, implementation, follow-through, and funding. These guiding principles may include needs-based approaches, decision making, defining the effort, administrative support, comprehensiveness, and long-term perspectives. See Worksheet 10.2: Guiding Principles for help with determining appropriate foundations for the campus effort; this worksheet encompasses elements appropriate for individual participants as well as for groups or the coalition as a whole.

Finally, the leadership group should specify the desired outcomes and processes, thus making concrete the approaches appropriate for the campus. With clearly defined outcomes, prevention specialists can build objectives with solid measures. By focusing on a specific behavior (e.g., impaired driving, marijuana use, support of recovering students, bystander engagement, use of drugs to help with studying, alcohol-fueled violence), prevention specialists can develop appropriate strategies to address those issues. Processes may also evolve directly from the guiding principles, so consider meaningful involvement of students, active engagement of multiple faculty members, or close collaboration with coaches. Specific processes may address decision making (e.g., voting vs. seeking consensus) and engagement (e.g., ensuring that discussions actively involve all parties and are not unduly influenced by a particular office).

Step 4: Document Baseline Needs

Prevention specialists benefit from having detailed information on the specific needs and areas for interventions. Although some documentation may have helped inform Step 1, this effort substantiates the issues and opportunities facing the leadership group. Also, quality needs assessment can be blended with evaluation efforts, including both quantitative and qualitative approaches (Step 7). The needs assessment focuses on specific desired outcomes; here it may be determined that a particular issue is more prevalent with a certain audience (e.g., marijuana use among first-year students, or high-risk drinking among student-athletes or a specific athletic team). The assessment process helps prevention specialists focus on and identify strategies within the framework of universal, selected, and indicated approaches; it also helps allocate the campus's limited resources to those areas with the greatest documented need.

Step 5: Use Constructs to Determine Areas of Focus

This step blends the results of the needs assessment efforts with the detailed foundations from this book's first section on context (Chapters 1, 2, and 3). The needs assessment results help point prevention specialists toward the audiences and issues worthy of attention. The incorporation of evidence-informed foundations, including theoretical constructs, take place at Step 5. In short, the universal, selected, and indicated approaches are blended with the stages of change model, other theoretical models, and prevention specialists' knowledge of the campus culture, to ascertain what might work. With this mix, prevention specialists then create the logic models that would be appropriate for each of the specified outcomes. Some logic models will overlap from one specified outcome to another. The important part is to make clear what the leaders believe would be appropriate and then pursue those concerns more deliberately.

Step 6: Prepare Plans and Strategies

This step focuses on the specific actions deemed by prevention specialists to be most appropriate to meet the needs of their audience; these actions are consistent with the logic models. All too often, campus program implementers turn initially to this step—without first establishing the necessary grounding. They may do this because they are comfortable with certain strategies, get directives from supervisors, are uncertain of change, or have a sense of urgency to act; however, it's a type of "ready, fire, aim" approach. As this preparation is being conducted, Worksheet 10.3: Menu of Strategies provides a general framework within which specific approaches may be considered.

As cited in Chapter 3, the appropriate tactic is to look for the best fit. Strategies that work elsewhere may or may not be suitable for another campus. When considering theoretical and evidence-based foundations, prevention specialists should draw upon but not be limited to established approaches. Excellent resources and approaches abound in the National Institute on Alcohol Abuse and Alcoholism's (2019) *CollegeAIM* publication; this resource can serve as a useful starting point for strategic planning, particularly with regard to environmental and individual perspectives. As part of the planning process, prevention specialists must assess ways in which individual approaches cited in *CollegeAIM* are reasonable and appropriate for the campus; this will be based, in large part, upon the identified needs, desired outcomes and logic models used with the campus planning efforts. In addition, it is important to note that *CollegeAIM* approaches are focused on alcohol and based on published literature only.

Similar concerns are relevant regarding other evidence-based strategies. Many campus efforts have a reliance on evidence-based practices (EBPs), which promote strategies with a proven track record. While this is a helpful starting point, it is important to note that not all strategies work as planned on every campus. Leaders must be comfortable with discontinuing any EBPs that do not meet the intended outcomes. Modifying EBPs for the campus risks compromising the model integrity of the intervention. Thus, creating a mix of local theory-based interventions or interventions based on core components of EBPs may be a viable alternative to address what to do when EBPs are less effective in the specific local campus and community setting. Overall, what is important is that campus decision makers implement evidence-informed efforts, with that evidence coming from published literature, theoretical grounding, local needs, specified outcomes, localized logic models, and the insights of the campus leaders. This evidence-informed approach allows for innovation and creativity, with this construct of being evidence-informed.

Once specific actions are selected, classic planning approaches are relevant: having goals, objectives, strategies, and measures. The various strategies can be couched within measurable objectives. For each strategy, identify areas of responsibility for implementation; timelines; and resources needed and available. Planners may include a type of Gantt or PERT (program evaluation review technique) chart that shows the various subtasks for implementing the strategy with relevant timelines. Details and their associated milestones can help prevention specialists with oversight and monitoring; as challenges arise, they can problem-solve to address these concerns promptly.

The matter of innovation and creativity warrants further illustration here, as novel efforts will best connect with students. Prevention specialists, in conjunction with the leadership group, have pertinent knowledge about the campus. By working together, these groups can harness their creativity and innovation, which will aid in selecting and locally implementing specific strategies.

Step 7: Implement Substantive Evaluative Approaches

As detailed in Chapter 9, evaluation design is an essential aspect of any drug and alcohol abuse prevention effort. Evaluation and measures should be part of any initial discussion about the overall strategic plan for the campus and then also considered when specific objectives are crafted. Evaluative efforts must be both quantitative and qualitative; quantitative approaches are helpful with data, and qualitative methods help with understanding the data as well as "telling the story."

Objectives should be reasonable and appropriate. For example, the expectation that "binge drinking should be eliminated" or "illicit drug use should be zero" is neither reasonable nor achievable. The standard should be what prevention specialists, in consultation with overall campus leaders, deem appropriate. Then, stakeholders can establish tactics to achieve these outcomes. Essentially, standards allow for the allocation of necessary resources.

Also significant is that attention is given to both the outcomes and the processes. The outcome evaluation addresses what results are sought, and the process evaluation focuses on what was done and what might be improved. When developing the logic model, attention must be paid to how its various elements will be assessed; the results obtained will help with the later review of relevance and appropriateness of each of these elements. Messaging—including what messages are heard and what impact can be attributed to them—is also crucial. Effective messaging is a result of sound assessment strategies.

Campus faculty can be a helpful resource with implementing evaluation efforts. Prevention specialists should identify different faculty members with a range of subject matter expertise, to ensure that sound theoretical practices will be followed. Linkage with academic departments may result in collaborative efforts such as class projects, internships, affiliations with resource centers and institutes, dissertations and theses, and published research. Because campuses are institutions of higher education, collaboration with researchers and scholars on evaluation as well as on overall strategic guidance is both logical and appropriate. Ideally, top academic administrators (e.g., vice president for student affairs, provost, president) will promote collaboration between student affairs and faculty departments. Faculty certainly benefit from these opportunities for research, publication, service, and cross-campus collaboration.

Step 8: Review and Revise

After the campus strategies have been implemented and various types of evaluation conducted, a regular review of results and processes is appropriate. This review of evaluative data provides insights regarding the campus efforts, especially from an overall perspective of the entire campus effort. The review needs to ask, from both a holistic and a focused perspective, how well things worked toward achieving the specified outcomes; the holistic aspect focuses on the entire campus and the campus culture, and the focused perspective addresses specific components (e.g., training, campaigns, policies). If the intent was to address marijuana use, and if the implemented strategies were consistent with the logic model, how well did this approach work? If the plan was to promote understanding and support for students in recovery from a substance use disorder, what was the impact on recovering students, and what results were achieved with other students as well as faculty and staff? The results of a review process will help prevention specialists understand not only the extent to which the objectives were achieved but also what contributed to those results and what might have limited their attainment. Evaluation data shed light on what may need to be changed. The assumptions made, the logic model, the theoretical grounding, the strategies chosen, or the implementation may warrant adjustment.

The review process should be undertaken regularly. Some reviews may be finite (such as the immediate and follow-on results obtained after training key intermediaries or peer educators, for example); they can be conducted periodically over the academic year. Others, such as an overall review of the campus effort, are appropriate to do on an annual, biennial, or 5-year basis. Much more detail about reporting is found in Chapter 13. Useful with this review process is having clear documentation regarding what was intended with the strategy, and what the results were. Worksheet 10.4: Prevention/Outreach Checklist and After Action Report provides a helpful document for each strategy. Not only does this link clearly with the Institute of Medicine framework with universal, selective and indicted approaches, but it also highlights risk and protective factors as well as results and observations.

Prevention specialists should keep in mind that the context of planning, implementing, and reviewing the campus effort evolves. Student needs and issues continue to change. Further, the challenge of changing human behavior is a massive task—and one that can be overwhelming. When people talk about the "hard sciences," they are typically referring to those fields undertaken in a laboratory with controlled conditions; however, it may be more appropriate to refer to this type of human-focused work, particularly with drug and alcohol issues, as the "hard sciences," as it is genuinely challenging.

Finally, the leadership group should share findings regularly, such as the evaluation results, the review of the nature and appropriateness of the campus efforts, and the desired evolution of the campus strategies. This sharing of findings and directions should also be done with the advisory body as well as other key stakeholders on campus and in the community; their perspectives and insights can further clarify the content as well as the breadth of messaging locally. Not only does this sharing of findings keep the overall campus leadership and decision makers apprised of the campus needs and efforts, but it also can garner their continued interest and support.

Step 9: Promote Institutionalization

Through the entire process of implementing these planning steps, prevention specialists' aim is global: The campus drug and alcohol prevention effort is viewed not as a compilation of discrete events or things, but as an integrated whole seeking to address a range of issues and needs. The identified strategies seek to address a range of students' needs based on their current, past, and intended behaviors; these include students not using substances at all, those doing experimentation, those needing modification to reduce patterns or quantity of use, and those involved with treatment and recovery services. With such a diverse behavioral pattern, a variety of supportive and educational messages are critical, all done within a consistent overall campus strategy. These aims are accomplished through numerous specific strategies within the framework of universal, selected, and indicated approaches (see Chapters 5, 6, and 7).

Finally, the aims of addressing drug and alcohol issues are not short lived; these are long-term strategies designed to offer long-term solutions. Continued attention and diligence are required for progress with moving the needle for the campus. Neither a problem nor a series of problems to be solved within a finite period, these issues are enduring and evolving.

CASE STUDY 10.1

Experiential Education: The LessThanUThink Campaign

Delynne Wilcox, PhD, MPH, CHES

Assistant Director, Department of Health Promotion and Wellness

University of Alabama

A decade after it started, a student-run campaign designed to engage students in reducing heavy episodic drinking is still going strong. The LessThanUThink (LTUT) campaign originated in 2009 as a result of a national Ad Team competition sponsored annually by the Ad Council for college students majoring in advertising and public relations (APR). The cosponsor that year was The Century Council (now The Foundation for Advancing Alcohol Responsibility). A collaboration between students in APR and a university representative from the campus health promotion department brought about this award-winning campaign. But placing second in the Ad Team competition was just the beginning of the accolades for the LTUT campaign. Included among its numerous awards is the Silver Anvil Award, in which a student-run PR firm competed against nationally recognized corporate PR organizations. Even more important, the campaign continues to demonstrate a positive impact on recalibrating students' alcohol expectancies that predict heavy episodic drinking; it seeks to lower their desires to consume large quantities of alcohol quickly, by promoting the social desirability of less intoxication.

The LTUT campaign (https://www.ltut.org) is much more than a catchy slogan and flashy graphic design. LTUT is a student-run, student-generated campaign that uses humor to emphasize the negative and physical consequences of heavy episodic drinking. A campaign example is, "U think you won't Text your Ex. And you wouldn't. Three drinks ago. It takes LessThanUThink.org." The design incorporates campaign-specific color schemes, fonts, and graphics that fit the LTUT brand. While the slogan and graphics may be what attracts students initially, the campaign is actually grounded in the principles of health communication and health promotion. To achieve the results that were scientifically based on and consequential for student behavior, the campaign involved careful planning.

LTUT is the result of true multidisciplinary collaboration, innovation, and a willingness to embrace students as valuable stakeholders. Flexibility is also a key, as both the messaging and processes of campaign development have evolved over time and remained relevant for over a decade and with multiple cohorts of students. This is due, in part, to the intensive grounding in the principles and practices of advertising, public relations, and public health. Students are drawn to the LTUT campaign because the messaging is developed by students for students. Noteworthy is that students working on the campaign quickly realize that there is another degree of difficulty working with a "product" that is a complex social issue, such as alcohol consumption, and especially among their peer age group. The students are continually challenged to stretch beyond common alcohol prevention messages (e.g., "drink responsibly," "don't drink and drive") and critically contemplate the personal and societal values encapsulated around alcohol consumption. In addition, they are challenged to utilize the knowledge and skills they are gaining in the classroom as aspiring APR professionals. Similarly, administrators working with the campaign are challenged to embrace new ideas toward alcohol prevention through the innovation provided by the students. The result is a model of true experiential education.

ENGAGING VARIOUS CONSTITUENCIES

Having multiple individuals, groups, and organizations involved in planning the campus drug and alcohol abuse prevention effort is essential for various reasons. As highlighted in Step 2 of the planning model, this diversity gives a broad perspective; it incorporates myriad points of view as a result of participants' organizational affiliation, past experiences, professional codes of behavior, and personal attitudes. The blending of these factors makes the campus effort stronger. This broad-based participation helps with garnering campuswide support for the effort. When challenges arise about the nature or content of policies or strategies, such broad-based support is helpful, as the justification for the approaches selected will be grounded with multiple perspectives (e.g., health and safety and legal and educational), rather than one single approach (e.g., legal). Broad support from a variety of perspectives and backgrounds can also assist with program growth and institutionalization.

For the overall planning of the campus prevention effort, prevention specialists will benefit from considering traditional as well as nontraditional groups; traditional ones may include, among others, counseling, judicial, housing, law enforcement, and wellness offices. Nontraditional partners may consist of student government, alumni, public affairs, and marketing classes.

Essential questions for determining partners—individual, group, and organization—include the following:

- Who should be at the table, and for what purpose(s)?
- Who is essential for success?
- Who might be a roadblock or a challenge to implementation?
- What skills and perspectives are critical for inclusion?
- What perspectives or interests seem to be lacking?
- Whose needs can be met by participating?
- Who would be upset if they were not involved?
- Who wants to see a certain kind of change or no change at all?
- In what ways can students be involved at a meaningful level?
- Whose voice is essential for reaching specific audiences?

When approaching an individual or group, prevention specialists benefit from stressing the win–win nature of such participation. For example, involvement of faculty members may aid with their research agendas; contributing students get hands-on experience with research, marketing, training, or other initiatives of the comprehensive campus effort.

On a related note, prevention specialists should identify things that potential contributors could accomplish—or better accomplish—by partnering with the campus prevention effort. For example, a potential partner may have a question it wants answered, and this query could get answered by being included in a survey prepared by the campus prevention effort. A potential partner could get staff members trained on a challenging topic, or a faculty member may benefit from having a specialized lecture or class engagement by a prevention specialist (this class session could even be offered during a time when the faculty member is absent, thus providing class coverage).

Partnership efforts are designed to get the overall campuswide prevention effort more infused and integrated into other campus offices and initiatives. Whether it is students undertaking field research, classes developing public service announcements, volunteer artists creating advertisements or marketing, offices placing questions into campus surveys, or departments offering service hours for substance-related judicial infractions, the opportunities are many.

When building these partnerships, prevention specialists should consider individuals from unconventional or innovative settings. One example may be a faculty member who has a personal connection to the important work of drug and alcohol abuse prevention; another may be a high-level key decision maker who wants to be involved and supportive but also wants the leadership group to pursue its interests more independently. Members of an institution's governing board or campus alumni may have an interest in prevention efforts; these individuals may have personal reasons for wanting to help. The important thing is for prevention specialists to be attentive, creative, visible, and welcoming.

The overall aim is to ground the campus effort with diverse perspectives, varied talent, and a range of power settings. Through collaborations, dialog, and creative problem solving, these partnerships can guide the prevention effort and set an example of effective interconnectedness.

The Innovator 10.1 segment describes hands-on experience, illustrating the importance of perseverance and, ultimately, grit. Dave Closson, with his long-term innovative spirit of bringing ideas to action, tells how he managed to take the grounded approach of motivational interviewing (see Chapter 7) and engage others with it. The lessons in this segment help prevention specialists and other campus leaders as they seek to promote change and a positive campus culture.

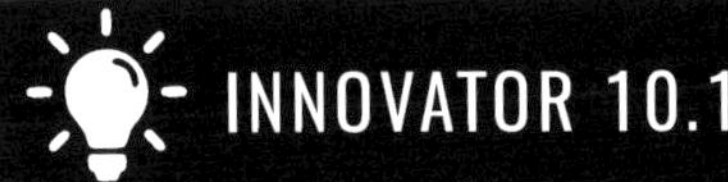

Motivational Interviewing for Campus Police

Dave Closson, MS
Owner, DJC Solutions, LLC

While working as a campus police officer, I saw how students' substance misuse affected our responsibilities and how we did our jobs. Over a typical weekend, call topics would range from an intoxicated/incapacitated individual, to a fight, to an odor of cannabis in the residence halls, or to a possible intoxicated driver. Students' substance misuse kept us busy, and the solution seemed obvious: substance misuse prevention. I asked myself, "What else can we, as police officers, do to help?"

To help answer that question, I observed fellow officers have what I call "do-better" talks with students. Typically, after resolving the initial reason for the interaction, officers would talk to the student about staying out of trouble. Every officer had a different style: Some would lecture, while others tried scare tactics. Regardless of approach, these "do-better" talks could be the first step in helping a student change his or her life. Frankly, I thought these discussions could be handled better; I thought how officers talked to students about their alcohol use, drug use, and behavior could be improved.

I already knew about motivational interviewing (MI), and I thought that an MI conversation could be effective for officers' "do-better" talks. The current skill set of police officers makes for the perfect foundation for MI: Officers are trained in expressing empathy, building rapport, and spotting ambivalence. They are exceptionally good at asking questions. Refocusing these skills in "do-better" talks could mean changing student outcomes. As offenders enter the student conduct process that follows a campus police citation or referral, they have already started the change process.

I started using my MI skills on patrol, and my fellow officers saw me doing things a little differently and didn't seem to understand it. They told me I was being too soft, wasting my time, and not doing "real cop stuff." Some even felt I might let them down in a violent situation since I was "too nice."

I faced a lack of support from both my fellow officers and my command, and I felt unrelenting pressure to "get back out there" on patrol. I felt discouraged; nevertheless, I thought it was essential to take an extra 15 minutes to have an MI conversation with a student. Other campus leaders saw how students were engaging in these conversations, and I felt encouraged to stay the course using MI.

Through all of this, I had to believe in myself and remember that what mattered most was the powerful conversations with students. As I walked patrol across campus, students eagerly came up to share how they were doing in making positive changes in their lives. Those students helped me persevere, and I owe them a big thank-you!

As my own experiences with MI continued and I saw other officers using it, I was inspired to write my book, *Motivational Interviewing for Campus Police*. I am now blessed with the opportunity to train police officers in MI so they can help change even more lives. This journey from a new idea to a national training program was filled with challenges, struggles, and grit.

CONCLUSION

A step-by-step process guides the design or redesign of campus prevention strategies. Nine steps help organize prevention specialists and campus leaders in ways that are grounded, evidence-informed, thorough, and visionary. The planning model is based on engaging various constituencies so the ultimate strategies are meaningful and appropriate. Three types of organizing groups—steering committee, leadership group, and advisory body—help anchor the effort for participatory decision making and ownership. Locally appropriate "best fit" strategies are likely to emerge when plans are grounded by universal, selective, and indicated approaches and a theoretical model.

REFERENCES

Lewin, K. (1951). *Force field analysis*. MIT Institute for Social Research.

National Institute on Alcohol Abuse and Alcoholism. (2019). *Planning alcohol interventions using NIAAA's CollegeAIM alcohol intervention matrix* (Publication No. 19-AA-8017). U.S. Department of Health and Human Services, National Institutes of Health. https://www.collegedrinkingprevention.gov/CollegeAIM/Resources/NIAAA_College_Matrix_Booklet.pdf

Turner, S., Merchant, K., Kania, J., & Martin, E. (2012). Understanding the value of backbone organizations in collective impact: Part 1. *Stanford Social Innovation Review*. https://ssir.org/articles/entry/understanding_the_value_of_backbone_organizations_in_collective_impact_1#

CHAPTER 11

Coalition Building

Engaging Partners in Prevention

"My first few semesters in college, my friendships revolved around going out and drinking. I felt like there was something wrong with me if I stayed in on a Friday night. I realized that I needed to surround myself with people who share the same balance of having fun and doing well academically. Getting involved with organizations on campus really allowed me to foster healthy friendships."

—Junior from California at a large university

The engagement of a variety of partners is critical for successful and sustained campus prevention initiatives. Having the assistance and support of others—whether through advisory groups, expert panels, review bodies, task forces, or other entities—ensures quality, depth, breadth, and impact. Whether the campus is large, midsize, or small—and regardless of the number of prevention personnel—broad support through formal and informal coalitions is crucial for success.

The point of coalitions is to extend the perspectives, expertise, and advocacy beyond the core prevention personnel. Different types of coalitions help prevention specialists better achieve their goals. The primary aim centers on the campus's comprehensive effort; a secondary one addresses campus and community relationships; and a third goal is directed toward efforts at the state or regional level. Coalitions and partnerships exist with various entities both on and off campus.

This chapter examines the "what" and "how" regarding these various opportunities for collaboration, and the concepts and strategies highlighted are relevant to each of the different coalition settings. These structures and tips dovetail nicely with the topics of several chapters in this book, most notably those of Chapters 10 and 13. Having an engaged coalition is key for grounding, for success, and for the institutionalization of the campus effort. Further, coalitions help to sustain the commitment of prevention specialists as they navigate the challenges and barriers associated with their actions.

Diverse perspectives prepared by various practitioners and policy makers shed light on how partnerships and coalition efforts can be implemented. This chapter boasts six contributions, culminating with the Innovator segment prepared by Eric Davidson, who discusses the vital role of a statewide coalition for its members, its institutions, and state policy makers. The Lessons From the Field highlights the important roles for law enforcement as part of a campus coalition. Four case studies are also included; two elaborate on elements of success for two statewide coalitions, and two highlight the role of the alcohol beverage industry as a partner at the local and state levels.

THE CONTEXT OF CHANGE MANAGEMENT

The use of coalitions is grounded in collective wisdom and influence; their purpose is intentional and strategic, with the ultimate aim of helping campus prevention efforts thrive. With the complexity of campus prevention efforts, the inherent obstacles and barriers, and the limitations with staffing typically found, a more extensive support network is essential for achieving positive outcomes. Change management strategies help campus prevention efforts, community partnerships, other campus efforts, and state or regional coalitions.

Within the overall context of "planned change" (see Chapter 10), change management encompasses comprehensive *campus-focused strategies* for orchestrating, in an organized way, efforts toward the desired healthy campus culture; these efforts depend on the engagement of others—the coalition. For the campus coalition, consider three general stages of functioning: startup, ongoing efforts, and review.

1. The *startup of the campus prevention effort* may take the form of convening a blue-ribbon committee, a task force, an expert panel, or a planning committee. By their nature, these groups would be task oriented and time limited, and their focus would be specified based on institutional considerations, including current and emerging needs, crisis response, necessary services, alignment with mission statements, resource availability, and future project outcomes. Worksheet 11.1: Planning for Collaboration can help with identifying potential individuals or organizations that can be part of this oversight and leadership group.
2. For *ongoing efforts*, an example would be the ongoing advisory or committee that serves the prevention specialists. Ongoing efforts may incorporate a core leadership group, the coalition as a whole, and an extended group of advisors or stakeholders. As outlined in Chapter 10, there may be different functions within each of these overlapping groups, as well as supplemental ad hoc groups (e.g., a committee focused on topics such as communications, evaluation, or volunteers).
3. A *review group* may be constituted to aid with the biennial review mandate as well as the other recommended program review processes (see Chapter 4). This can be a group that is designed and perceived as neutral, so honest appraisals of the prevention effort's accomplishments, needs, and opportunities can be performed.

The specific composition of these various coalitions will vary based on individuals' interests, expertise, and availability.

Community-oriented coalitions are the second way of employing strategic and beneficial change management approaches. Overall, community coalitions remind campus stakeholders of "the campus IN the community," acknowledging the critical role that campus leaders can play as "good citizens" and "good neighbors." Some colleges represent the lifeblood of the community, with much activity revolving around the institution. Other colleges are in rural settings with limited community involvement, while institutions in urban settings have very different dynamics. Regardless of the nature of the community, opportunities exist for coalition engagement. Consider four potential scenarios with community-based coalitions:

1. Campus leaders may believe that a campus–community partnership for drug and alcohol issues is appropriate. This joint partnership would focus specifically on substance misuse issues and identify independent and shared strategies.
2. Parallel to the focused partnership on substance misuse is a joint initiative on a related issue or on various issues, to which drug and alcohol issues are added.
3. Campus leaders may invite community representatives to participate with the campus coalition. Participation could include community representation with a campus advisory group or a campus coalition committee.
4. The community may have an existing coalition, whether on drug and alcohol issues, or on related matters; the prevention specialists may seek involvement with this group.

Regardless of the nature of the relationship, the focus is on collaboration. The aim is to achieve mutual benefit, with both campus and the community leaders identifying opportunities to work together to address and, ideally, prevent substance-related problems in the community. Varied issues may require attention, such as alcohol beverage licenses, alcohol sales hours and advertising, sponsorship of events, noise, public urination, traffic, impaired driving, trash, property damage, and overall quality of life. These concerns may be addressed through formal approaches (e.g., laws and ordinances, policies, and procedures) as well as informal approaches (e.g., dialog, collaboration, communication). The aim is to be proactive and collaborative for a win–win scenario. When constructing community-based coalitions, it is critical to consider who would be appropriate partners. Karen Moses highlights a collaborative and productive approach in Case Study 11.1.

Third, campus prevention specialists can help with change management by becoming *involved with related initiatives*, such as sexual assault, violence, quality of life, academic success, health promotion and wellness, student support, and professional achievement. Although many of these initiatives may be present on campus, the role of campus prevention specialists may not be prominent. Thus, such specialists will benefit from exploring how the voice of prevention can be incorporated with these other issues. Data are clear about the extent to which drugs and alcohol permeate other problems on campus and community issues; what is important is that prevention specialists find ways to collaborate in other coalitions and topic areas. Insight into emerging trends can help infuse substance misuse prevention messages and strategies into other initiatives, as well as identify collaborative partners for campus prevention efforts.

The final consideration concerns a *statewide or regional coalition*. Regional partnerships allow for prevention professionals from campuses throughout the state or region to gather regularly. These individuals may include those with direct involvement with drug/alcohol issues (e.g., campus prevention specialist, counselor) and those with indirect involvement (e.g., faculty member, researcher, clinician, health promotion specialist, law enforcement personnel, judicial affairs, someone in student leadership, other student affairs role). Coalition members can share respective institutional strategies, emerging issues, best practices, research, and resources; they can engage in collaborative problem solving while networking and offering personal support. Further, the coalition can identify ways to advocate for needed resources, policies, and leadership; strategies may include open discussions, conferences, training, annual retreats, drive-in workshops, webinars, website resources, listservs, policy statements, and resource development. In Case Study 11.2, Joan Masters and Margo Leitschuh go into rich detail regarding a productive and engaging statewide coalition.

Change management draws on campus and community collaboration. Coalition work relies on subject matter experts and other stakeholders engaged in advocating for healthy communities. This group approach provides allies and spokespersons from various parts of the campus and community to share vision and energy for collective impact.

CASE STUDY 11.1

A Partnership for Prevention: Wholesalers Advocating Moderation

Karen S. Moses, PhD
Director of Wellness and Health Promotion
Arizona State University

Wholesalers Advocating Moderation (WAM) was a 16-year collaboration between Arizona State University (ASU) Wellness and Health Promotion and the three largest beer wholesale distributors in the Phoenix area: Budweiser, Miller, and Coors. WAM members adhered to a set of jointly developed and self-directed guidelines regarding campus-based promotions. These guidelines included restrictions on beer ads on campus, restrictions on marketing to groups whose members were primarily students under the age of 21, use of the WAM logo and/or the company's moderation message instead of distributor or beer logos, and a focus on moderate and responsible use of alcohol, should students choose to drink.

Each WAM distributor contributed $700 a year to ASU for alcohol education. The WAM Designated Driver Program, hosted at bars and other drinking establishments surrounding campus, was founded through WAM connections with the managers and owners. WAM sponsored the ASU drinking norms campaign for several years, with the campus staff having the freedom to control the messages and graphics in the ads. WAM funded many educational programs, including Training for Intervention Procedures training for the Greek life community at ASU. WAM representatives were an active part of the ASU alcohol education team and attended conferences with prevention staff members. Owing to changes in corporate leadership, funding once provided to ASU is now used for other educational efforts to reduce underage and high-risk drinking in the community. Although annual funding is no longer available, the many positive contributions made through this collaboration continue to have a presence among other ASU prevention efforts.

Through WAM, campus prevention and health leaders were able to build trust, discuss evidence-informed strategies for prevention and risk reduction, and generate opportunities to partner toward common goals: reducing underage and high-risk drinking.

CASE STUDY 11.2

Using Connectedness to Fuel Prevention

Joan Masters, MEd
Senior Coordinator of Partners in Prevention
University of Missouri

Margo Leitschuh, BS
Communications Coordinator
Missouri Partners in Prevention

As coalition leaders of Missouri Partners in Prevention, we are often asked about the most effective ways to create change on campus. We believe that when we build the capacity of our colleagues and our campus coalition, positive outcomes follow. We also believe that campus leaders can never go wrong investing time and effort into developing their campus coalition, assessing readiness, and listening to colleagues.

Assessing readiness is vital in engaging partners in prevention. It provides a solid foundation and gives initial strength to the prevention efforts. Start with the following question: Is there readiness to make change? Coalition members must also be ready to put in the time and effort necessary to do alcohol and other drug prevention. Implement a formal readiness assessment (Plested et al., 2006) or determine a set of key questions to ask. You might ask new coalition members about their knowledge gaps or areas where they may have limited confidence or experience; inquire about what they think their participation might mean, what they might bring to the table, how much work it might be, what opportunities exist, and how important prevention is.

Be intentional and authentic in your approach. Connection is, quite simply, the fuel for prevention efforts. Get to know your colleagues on both a personal and a professional level. On many campuses, coalition membership includes student affairs professionals, law enforcement, faculty, or community business owners who may lack knowledge of public health strategies or the strategic prevention framework (Drug Enforcement Administration, 2020; Substance Abuse and Mental Health Services Administration, 2019). You can provide online or in-person training to help them understand the context of and specifics about the prevention work.

Building connectedness in your coalition involves developing win–win situations for your colleagues. For example, talk with Greek life staff or athletics department staff about engaging with the coalition, noting that you can train their employees as well as student leaders in evidence-based strategies while they gain a voice on the coalition. Remember: Don't just gain initial engagement—sustain it with regularly scheduled, positive, and productive meetings.

STEPS FOR ACHIEVING A COLLECTIVE IMPACT

Coalitions gather together individuals to address a shared vision and common goals. Whether these individuals are likeminded at the onset, are included in the coalition by virtue of their position, or are "assigned" to participate, their purpose is to help implement a shared agenda. The coalition involves individuals from different parts of the campus, and potentially the community, to achieve "collective impact" regarding drug and alcohol issues. The specific outcomes for each campus—while varied and based on factors such as current and anticipated needs, local context and priorities, and values of decision makers—benefit from an understanding of collective impact (Hanleybrown et al., 2012; Kania & Kramer, 2011, 2013).

The focus of collective impact is promoting and sustaining innovation. Comprehensive drug and alcohol prevention efforts rely on institutionalization of best practices. Innovation, vision, and leadership require being open to change. Collective impact emphasizes cooperative efforts—through coalitions. Participants engage in thoughtful and grounded planning and decision making; they have shared aims and, ultimately, specified outcomes. The five steps of collective impact can be incorporated in campus-only coalitions, campus–community coalitions, prevention specialists' engagement with other campus or community efforts, or statewide or regional coalitions.

Step 1: Create a Common Agenda

The first step of collective impact is creating a *common agenda*. Participants agree on the overall vision. They develop a shared understanding of the issues to be addressed, acknowledging that many individuals arrive with different perspectives and backgrounds. For example, the campus coalition will likely include health services, law enforcement, resident life, judicial affairs, and academic support staff, each coming together with varied experiences with students as well as with how drugs and/or alcohol have affected students' lives. Each person has a professional code of ethics and standards—and will likely have different strategies for addressing the issue. Through discussion and negotiation, the coalition aims to determine what its members can agree on, learn the nature and scope of the problem for their setting (campus and/or community), and outline parameters appropriate for this setting. Given their backgrounds, history, culture, context, resources, and vision, coalition members will define the nature and scope of appropriate action steps.

Step 2: Specify a Shared Measurement System

Second, the coalition must specify a *shared measurement system*. The group will identify what constitutes "success"—that is, members will articulate indicators or metrics that demonstrate the extent to which their efforts are achieving the desired outcomes. A logic model is the basis for creating measurable goals and objectives. Objectives that are Specific, Measurable, Achievable, Realistic and Time-Bound (SMART) may be included in a shared measurement system (see also Chapter 9). For example, coalition leaders may specify measurable goals (e.g., 90% proficiency) or a rate of change (e.g., a 2% increase each year). They may also determine specific aims for different audiences (e.g., first-year students, student-athletes, staff members, faculty), and they may have targets specified for the short term (e.g., 1 year) and over a longer term (e.g., 5 years). Some indicators may already exist, and others may need to be developed. The important point is that the coalition, at the onset, must have consensus about the desired outcomes and indicators of success. Ongoing development includes monitoring, review, and strategic modifications to the original aims.

Step 3: Develop Mutually Reinforcing Activities

The third step of collective impact activities emphasizes *mutually reinforcing activities*. Collaborative efforts negate the risk of a "silo approach," in which different organizations and agencies have independent, unconnected efforts under the umbrella of a comprehensive campus plan. These mutually reinforcing activities involve coalition members determining who and which sectors of the coalition are best suited to implement specific strategies. One radical approach is for everything associated with drug and alcohol issues to be handled by one office—and potentially, for small campuses, one person. Another radical approach is to divide up responsibilities with no overlap; for example, all enforcement is performed by police and security, professional psychologists or counselors do all counseling and advising, all instruction is carried out by faculty, student affairs professionals handle all programming, and trained methodologists do all the evaluation.

The collective impact approach is embedded within the philosophy of shared responsibilities. With the Task Force Planner (Anderson & Milgram, 1998), specific strategies are identified in a matrix; multiple campus individuals or groups (e.g., campus leadership, counseling, faculty, resident life, student government) have roles and responsibilities within the matrix of campus effort (e.g., policy, training, evaluation, curriculum). This approach demonstrates how each group can be meaningfully involved. While specific areas of expertise are indeed valid and to be honored, significant overlap in the type of effort is reasonable and appropriate. The collective impact approach helps to identify and coordinate these responsibilities and opportunities.

Step 4: Promote Continuous Communication

Continuous communication is essential for active coalition development. This ongoing dialog between and among the key stakeholders ensures an organized and strategic approach, and this enduring community within and between participating organizations encompasses negotiation, clarification, adaptation, and refinement. The communication must be clear, honest, and timely, as these aspects help to develop and nurture trust. With the overall aim of change within the campus culture, and with the individual and organizational challenges facing any change, communication is key for managing this change process. Approaches such as shared agendas, collaborative leadership, timely minutes, periodic reminders, and positive accolades likewise help.

Step 5: Have A Backbone Organization

The last step of the collective impact model is having a *backbone organization*. Although a coalition brings together multiple constituencies for a shared vision, having professional and support staff is essential for following through on the coalition's plans and activities. Some or all of these staff members may be active in the coalition; the important point is that the coalition is not left without the necessary professional support to sustain its efforts. This backbone organization typically covers six roles (Turner et al., 2012):

1. **Guide the vision and strategy.** This involves helping facilitate the planning processes through meeting design, group facilitation, documentation, and follow-through.
2. **Support aligned activity.** Facilitate continuous communication among members of the coalition. Look for opportunities to create opportunities for enhanced collaboration.
3. **Establish shared measurement practices.** Appropriate metrics, processes, timelines, implementation logistics, and reporting are essential to organize the coalition's vital efforts.
4. **Build public will.** This dovetails with the vital role of ongoing and effective communication, both within the coalition and with other stakeholders and decision makers on campus. The context of the coalition's work, particularly as it is new and unfolding, will require ongoing public relations efforts with a variety of constituencies.
5. **Advance policy.** Professional and support staff must work within the institutional structure to advance the coalition's decisions. Staff may take on resource allocation, staffing assignments, revised responsibilities, procedural changes, and structural realignments.
6. **Mobilize funding**. Mobilize and align resources to realize the goals of the initiative. Leverage institutional and community support to mobilize necessary funding. Working in concert with the coalition members, the backbone staff work to keep the initiative moving forward.

Overall, collective impact approaches transform how the campus prevention effort is planned and implemented. Through sound and thoughtful processes and the continuous reminder about the shared visions being sought, campus leaders can aspire to, document, and make progress toward campus culture changes. Also worthy of consideration is that campus prevention specialists do not need to think about doing this alone; a range of allies and stakeholders exist, one of which is highlighted by Steve Schmidt in Case Study 11.3.

CASE STUDY 11.3

Alcohol Control Agencies as Allies

Steve Schmidt, MS

Senior Vice President of Public Policy and Communications

National Alcohol Beverage Control Association

In the 1990s, as higher education and community leaders across the country increased efforts to address high-risk drinking by students, an unexpected ally emerged in several states to help take on this challenge: alcohol control agencies. Two examples, Pennsylvania Liquor Control Board and Virginia Alcoholic Beverage Control, provided resources and leadership for statewide initiatives to prevent high-risk college drinking. The components of these decades-long initiatives included a state leadership group; regional coalitions; training and consultation by national and state experts; statewide conferences; and grant funding for implementation and evaluation of local actions.

Today, these and several similar agencies are still active in their states and communities. Some may ask why an alcohol control agency would be an important ally or lead in addressing high-risk college drinking, but a close look at the mission and objectives of these agencies shows they are responsible for balancing the protection of public health/safety with the legal distribution and sale of alcohol within their borders. In other words, these agencies play a key role in access to alcohol and control of alcohol in local communities, including on college campuses.

In many states, campus and community leaders may not have considered alcohol control and regulatory agencies as possible allies and resources. These agencies differ from state to state, primarily as a result of the 21st Amendment (Repeal of Alcohol Prohibition) that established alcohol regulation as a state responsibility. Campus leaders should reach out to their state alcohol regulatory agencies; further, these state agencies can serve as a liaison to other state bureaus, such as education, health, public safety, and human services. These efforts can help the school achieve its mission, and the agency may benefit by achieving its own mission. The National Alcohol Beverage Control Association can provide assistance and serve as a resource for identifying possible contacts, resources, and next steps to engage alcohol control and regulatory agencies with efforts for impactful prevention.

NAVIGATING INSTITUTIONAL AND COMMUNITY POLITICS

Although the concept of a coalition is worthy, and the collaboration achieved through the collective impact approach is essential, the reality can often be troublesome. The processes of change, the achievement of outcomes, and the cooperation of all constituencies are rarely achieved perfectly. This is not to suggest that coalition use should be minimized; on the contrary, it is to highlight the importance of political factors facing coalitions.

At the onset, the coalition's role and scope of responsibility must be specified. Generally, a coalition is an ongoing, long-serving group of individuals; it stands in contrast to a focused task force or committee.

What needs to be made clear is whether the coalition is an active, engaged group, or more of a superficial, "rubber stamp" body. It is also helpful to create an expectation that coalition members advocate for the shared mission with their respective groups and constituencies—and even beyond campus.

Another factor to be specified is the relationship between the coalition and the professional staff working on drug and alcohol abuse prevention issues. Are some or all of these personnel members of the coalition itself? Is the coalition a board of directors to whom staff members report, or is it more of an advisory and consultative group? It's important to decide this role at the outset because coalition membership will be based on it. Ideally, the coalition will include the range of constituencies served by the campus prevention effort. Also, ideally, the membership will consist of individuals with expertise in the various core functions of the prevention services (e.g., education, health promotion, marketing, personal support, policy, enforcement, evaluation).

As the coalition and staff work together to achieve their aims, they must view their responsibilities and opportunities from a strategic perspective. As described in Chapters 10 and 13, participants must acknowledge the obstacles and intentionally incorporate them into strategic plans; this work is critical for achieving the desired outcomes.

This strategic approach is particularly appropriate for issues surrounding drugs and alcohol. People have direct or indirect personal experience; this background, coupled with emotions and knowledge (often outdated, inaccurate, and incomplete), results in many individuals in leadership and decision-making positions believing that they have the requisite expertise to address this complex issue. How the coalition acknowledges this belief and proceeds with its efforts is critical for its success and ultimate impact.

To deal with this political reality, coalition leaders benefit from their use of both hard power and soft power. This power emphasis complements the distinctions between instrumental leadership and expressive leadership (see Chapter 2). The hard power approach is consistent with a coalition that has clearly outlined decision-making authority, such as over the direction, philosophy, strategies, and resource allocations for the campus effort. It is more likely, however, that the coalition will have to rely on soft power (Nye, 2004); in this case, the use of appeal, credibility, shared values, and influence are emphasized. Lessons From the Field 11.1, by Dave Closson, shares some helpful insights about soft power and the important role of law enforcement in coalition efforts.

Ultimately, the campus prevention effort will be well served with collaborative and thoughtful planning that engages coalition partners. Some of this planning involves personal and group commitments as well as negotiation with others. Worksheet 11.2: Coalition Leadership Action Steps helps leaders specify what they are willing to commit themselves to, and where they envision other groups having responsibilities; each of these action steps can be viewed with a short-term and a longer-term perspective. By clearly defining the roles, engaging appropriate constituencies, and advocating openly, prevention specialists will increase the likelihood of sustained impact. Although many campus personnel do not want to—or like to—think and act politically, they must do so if they want to achieve their aims. A political orientation does not need to be overwhelming, nor does it need to compromise ethical standards: Thinking in terms of a win–win scenario, at the highest levels of the institution as well as at the more local levels, is helpful. By employing a variety of communication and advocacy strategies (see Chapter 12), and incorporating the collective impact approach, prevention specialists can find navigating campus and community politics more feasible. Insights provided by Lindsey Hanlon in Case Study 11.4 are helpful here.

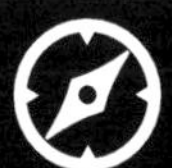 LESSONS FROM THE FIELD 11.1

Engaging Law Enforcement: Building a Foundation of Trust

Dave Closson, MS
Owner, DJC Solutions, LLC

Two of the most common questions I get about campus alcohol and other drug prevention are: "How do we engage law enforcement?" and "How do we partner with the police?"

The simple answer is to build a relationship before coming with an "ask."

When I served as the campus crime prevention officer, I built lasting relationships with the goal of changing the previous not-so-popular reputation of the police department. My hope was to put a face and a name to the department so people would feel comfortable and confident about our department. This approach succeeded in building relationships across campus and strengthening the department's reputation. Those relationships generated opportunities to collaborate and support prevention efforts—first me supporting theirs, and, later, them supporting mine.

So, I challenge all prevention leaders to examine what's at the core of quality relationships. Trust is at the very center; a relationship built without trust is simply a group of people who work together, and that engagement is mostly transactional. Trust is a feeling and cannot be taught; it must be earned through actions. When people trust you, they are more comfortable stepping outside their comfort zone and are willing to try new things.

When you seek to engage campus law enforcement in prevention strategies, realize that you are asking them to step outside their comfort zone. Environmental and individual strategies, prevention science, assessment, and evaluation are not taught at the police academy. If you want them to join you on the prevention journey, seek to build a foundation of trust.

Using my experience and taking from some key resources (Carnegie, 1998; Sinek, 2019), the following are a few tips to build trust with your campus police:

1. Express empathy.
2. Emphasize trust first.
3. Show genuine interest.
4. Be a good listener.
5. Talk in terms of the other person's interest.

No magic formula exists, but the outcome of any journey is enhanced when it is based on a foundation of trust.

CASE STUDY 11.4

Making a Coalition Thrive

Lindsey Hanlon, MS, CPH
Network Prevention Manager
Division of Behavioral Health
Nebraska Department of Health and Human Services

Nebraska has a number of community and campus coalitions with a variety of backgrounds and settings. While each group has its own missions, goals, and objectives, these coalitions serve a variety of local needs, including youth substance use, suicide prevention, prescription drug misuse, mental health promotion, or a combination of community health topics. From my statewide perspective, I see the range of shared strengths and challenges faced by these prevention professionals. My outside viewpoint allows me to identify what makes a coalition thrive and what gets in the way. Six key takeaways can help any coalition, regardless of whether it is new or more established.

I found that, first, it helps to have a dedicated evaluator to assist in guiding and shaping the plan; a rich background in working with many coalitions helps. Second, having a coalition capacity survey is useful for identifying local issues for attention, as well as common themes (needs, gaps, and barriers). Third, building local capacity is vital; it is accomplished by bringing together a network of experienced professionals and having peers share successes and barriers to implementation, educational opportunities, and tools.

Fourth, it is important to connect people to others with shared interests and have these individuals reach out to nontraditional stakeholders. Prevention can sometimes feel like a lonely pursuit, and these connections can be the link as well as the support that someone needs to make an impact within their community. Fifth, scanning the landscape of current prevention strategies and resources—and connecting them to local and statewide gaps and needs—helps with leveraging and coordinating funding streams. Finally, nurturing the broad perspective is helpful; this includes capitalizing on a workforce with so much history grounded in prevention science and integrating with a community of professionals willing to influence how prevention is viewed as a state.

Collectively, these six items can help coalitions truly thrive in order to make a difference—both locally and statewide.

TIPS FOR COALITION ENGAGEMENT WITH COMPREHENSIVE PREVENTION

Effective coalition engagement is vital for shifting the campus culture. Not only is expressive leadership essential for deepening stakeholders' definition and understanding of meaningful change, but affiliations with various departments and groups help expand the breadth and reach of campus prevention strategies. Through collective impact processes and strategic negotiation and implementation, coalition activities can be consequential and instrumental.

Beyond broad-based considerations, many practical suggestions and tips can aid campus prevention specialists as they engage coalition members individually and collectively. This advice can help "bring to life" the various concepts and constructs previously described.

Be very clear about the coalition's defined roles and responsibilities. This includes the specification and limitations of various group roles, decision-making processes, advocacy, and expectations about implementation timelines for selected initiatives.

Establish guiding principles. These should complement the overall guiding principles for the campus prevention effort as a whole. With these guiding principles, the focus may address the coalition roles, sources of information, outreach activities, how the coalition's reports and recommendations are to be handled, additional responsibilities, and philosophical frameworks.

Develop operational standards for the coalition's functioning. In conjunction with the guiding principles, specify standards of conduct for the coalition, such as how meetings will be conducted and their frequency; determine at the outset the decision-making processes and how members will interact (because many different backgrounds and professionals will be represented). Maximize group interaction, and facilitate ways of respecting diverse perspectives and methods for demonstrating continued respect for the broader mission of the coalition. Last, attend—with grace—to coalition members who are inactive or unengaged, overactive, domineering, or disruptive.

Ground the coalition's work in sound and current needs assessments. For the coalition's work to be meaningful and respected, it must operate with sound data. Where feasible, local data of a quantitative and qualitative nature should be gathered to complement state and national data.

Maintain a positive, proactive, and strategic orientation. Help the coalition look for opportunities to enhance its influence and impact. Although the primary emphasis is on reducing problems, additional attention to finding solutions and being constructive helps with engagement.

Focus on the overall campus environment while attending to individual needs. Both the campus environment (inclusive of the overall campus culture) and the needs of individuals (including respect, cultural appropriateness, and attention to developmental stages) are essential to the coalition's work. An appropriate balance between each factor will help with the campus effort.

Maintain a comprehensive focus that includes universal, selective, and indicated prevention strategies. The Institute of Medicine (IOM) prevention framework ensures a multi-faceted comprehensive campus prevention effort (Springer, & Phillips, 2007). The IOM framework provides clarity for those who strive to provide grounded and cost-effective prevention programming.

Create a supportive and productive environment that fosters members' engagement. Review coalition membership to ensure a sense of value and appreciation. Coalition membership is typically a volunteer, add-on responsibility for members, so attention to elements of coalition membership, meetings, and ongoing engagement is essential. Offer professional development opportunities to coalition members to foster a supportive and productive environment.

Continue to monitor coalition membership. Identify potential additions to the coalition based on an assessment of institutional needs and service gaps. Coalition leaders should seek to identify ways in which underrepresented groups can be identified and engaged in supporting the coalition's work.

Respect and use the expertise of coalition members. Coalition members are included for a strategic reason. Their skill sets and philosophies are strengths that warrant being tapped and nurtured.

Periodically take stock of the coalition's status, engagement, roles, and impact. It is helpful to review the various aspects of a coalition's activities, including membership, functioning, efforts, and efficiencies. Timely and relevant coalition efforts support member engagement in the collective impact process.

Reward coalition engagement. The coalition, as a group and as individual members, warrants periodic rewards. This positive response to members and their crucial roles helps maintain individual commitment and promote group sustainability. As detailed in Chapter 14, this reward helps with long-term institutionalization.

A functional and positive-oriented coalition has a significant impact on the quality and outcomes associated with the campus prevention effort. Though day-to-day responsibilities rest with the professional staff, graduate interns, peer educators, and other support personnel, the coalition helps ground prevention efforts within various academic disciplines and specialty areas, and its presence with support and advocacy provides crucial political power.

The perspectives of Eric Davidson are helpful and illustrate his innovative leadership at the campus, state, and national levels. In Innovator 11.1., he offers ways in which a statewide coalition can be helpful for campus efforts as well as for many of the policy decisions at the state level.

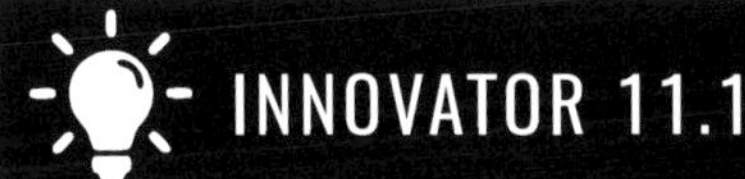

One of Illinois's Best Kept Secrets: Ready for Replication

Eric Davidson, PhD, MCHES
Interim Director, Health and Counseling Services
Eastern Illinois University

The Illinois Higher Education Center for Alcohol, Other Drug and Violence Prevention (IHEC) is one of the oldest collegiate substance abuse statewide initiatives. Founded in 1991 to serve rural community colleges, IHEC began serving all Illinois institutions of higher education in 1996. Since its creation, IHEC has played an important role for institutions and the state. Participating schools have benefited from training, resources, guides, consultation, networking, and data collection, allowing them to expand their capacity to deliver more cost-effective and impactful substance use prevention services, through policy development, education, student assistance, enforcement, assessment, campus/community collaboration, and social-ecological interventions. The state has also benefited from strengthening the statewide prevention system through increased collaboration between local and higher education prevention systems, keeping students healthy and enrolled (tuition dollars), and sharing data reporting, resources, and technical expertise.

Higher education faces multiple challenges and needs. Whereas, in the past, substance use prevention may have been granted preferential status, legislatures and college administrators have now given other issues higher priority. As a result of the defunding of higher education, the 2016–2017 Illinois budget impasse, and lower enrollments, resources once allocated to reducing substance use are often redistributed to other concerns. Maintaining substance use prevention as both relevant and a priority is a need at the local and statewide levels. Through persistence, data collection, and networking with leaders within and outside of higher education, IHEC staff have helped keep the flame of prevention alive during these dark times.

IHEC continues to serve as a voice and advocate for the needed substance use prevention services in Illinois higher education. With assessment essential to such advocacy, IHEC administers a biennial statewide substance abuse student survey to establish incidence and prevalence of collegiate substance use and other important metrics. A statewide aggregate is reported, and institutions that participate are provided with their campus data. Institutions also participate in a State of Prevention survey, which provides insights on institutional substance use prevention commitment, funding, staffing, policy, and programming efforts. Individuals served by IHEC are encouraged to complete a professional development survey highlighting any prevention competencies they believe they need. All programs and services are assessed for satisfaction and, when applicable, learning outcomes. The results of these three assessment strategies are used to articulate the prevention needs at both the state and local levels, as well as to demonstrate program success and impact.

Attracting and engaging key constituents is also required. IHEC focuses on developing advocates, who testify to the benefits and rewards of IHEC involvement. Strong advocates are often selected to become IHEC advisory board members, to help share the impact of IHEC within their professional circles and associations. Their testimonies allow IHEC staff to broaden networking and mobilization opportunities of key target audiences and organizations from inside and outside of higher education.

Regrettably, IHEC seems to be one of the best-kept secrets in Illinois. When possible, IHEC staff attend professional events to be visible and accessible to constituents. To expand its network and to enhance communication among the many disciplines within higher education, IHEC staff have developed databases of key roles (e.g., health educator, Clery compliance officer, vice president for student affairs). Use of social media, listservs, and direct mail promote involvement opportunities to these individuals.

Substance use remains a relevant and vital concern among colleges and universities. A statewide initiative such as IHEC helps support and propel efforts that are scientifically grounded, relevant, and current; collectively, they address needs at statewide and local levels. Developing and sustaining a statewide initiative requires significant resources, but the returns greatly exceed the investment.

CONCLUSION

The critical role of multiple collaborators with campus prevention efforts is grounded within the overall context of change management. Whether the coalition is campus focused/campus only, campus–community, or otherwise participatory, the efforts must be grounded in strategy. By incorporating the necessary steps to achieve collective impact, coalition members lay a foundation for long-term rewards. Prevention specialists can be forward-thinking and innovative as they help campus leaders navigate campus and community politics. By paying attention to practical considerations, engaging, functional, and determined coalitions can help propel campus strategies forward.

REFERENCES

Anderson, D. S., & Milgram, G. G. (1998). *Task force planner and task force planner guide promising practices: Campus alcohol strategies.* George Mason University. https://caph.gmu.edu/resources/college/create

Carnegie, D. (1998). *How to win friends & influence people: The only book you need to lead you to success.* Simon & Schuster.

Drug Enforcement Administration. (2020). *Prevention with purpose: A strategic planning guide for preventing drug misuse among college students.* t.ly/HTLn

Hanleybrown, F., Kania, J., & Kramer, M. (2012, January 26). Channeling change: Making collective impact work. *Stanford Social Innovation Review.* https://ssir.org/articles/entry/channeling_change_making_collective_impact_work

Kania, J., & Kramer, M. (2011, Winter). Collective impact. *Stanford Social Innovation Review.* http://www.ssireview.org/articles/entry/collective_impact

Kania, J., & Kramer, M. (2013, January 21). Embracing emergence: How collective impact addresses complexity. *Stanford Social Innovation Review.* http://www.ssireview.org/blog/entry/embracing_emergence_how_collective_impact_addresses_complexity

Nye, J. S. (2004). *Soft power: The means to success in world politics.* PublicAffairs, Perseus Books Group.

Plested, B. A., Edwards, R. W., & Jumper-Thurman, P. (2006). *Community readiness: A handbook for successful change.* Tri-Ethnic Center for Prevention Research.

Sinek, S. (2019). *The infinite game.* Portfolio/Penguin.

Springer, J. R., & Phillips, J. (2007). *The Institute of Medicine framework and its implication for the advancement of prevention policy, programs and practice* (SMA-4205). U.S. Department of Health and Human Services. http://ca-sdfsc.org/docs/resources/SDFSC_IOM_Policy.pdf

Substance Abuse and Mental Health Services Administration. (2019). *A guide to SAMHSA's strategic prevention framework.* https://www.samhsa.gov/sites/default/files/20190620-samhsa-strategic-prevention-framework-guide.pdf

Turner, S., Merchant, K., Kania, J., & Martin, E. (2012). Understanding the value of backbone organizations in collective impact: Part 1. *Stanford Social Innovation Review.* https://ssir.org/articles/entry/understanding_the_value_of_backbone_organizations_in_collective_impact_2#

CHAPTER 12

Promotion and Advocacy

"When I was 13, my mother passed away from alcoholism. As I grew older, I knew I had to be conscious of my experience with alcohol especially in a college environment. The impact the loss of my mother had on me has exceptionally influenced my awareness of the effects of overconsumption and has inspired me to share my story with others."

—Junior from the West Coast at a public university

Prevention specialists lead comprehensive efforts to address drug and alcohol issues on college and university campuses. Managing this sizable effort requires knowledge and skills; however, much more is needed to truly integrate the prevention effort into the campus life and decision-making structure. Promotional and advocacy efforts, for example, are essential to bring others along toward a shared understanding of, and support for, prevention efforts. These communication strategies are necessary for "sharing the word" and "growing the support," typically in conjunction with coalition efforts. Since most audiences and decision makers do not have professional backgrounds in or expertise with prevention strategies, strong advocacy and promotion efforts are needed to move beyond a simply logic-based approach (i.e., "here are the facts"). Promotion and advocacy work are essential for moving the needle.

Communication skills and strategies, and the confidence to use them, serve campus professionals well as they make their case with others about the importance of prevention work. Many of the approaches and insights can be embedded within the marketing efforts used with campus programming strategies, and the audience for these communication efforts includes stakeholders, intermediaries, decision makers, group leaders, and policy makers.

The need for these communication skills is compounded by the societal context of substance misuse issues: Found all too often are minimization, denial, and lack of understanding, whether about the extent of the problem, the role of prevention, or the opportunity for impact. Based on these and other challenges, campus prevention specialists must continuously "sell" prevention concepts and strategies to various gatekeepers. Further, prevention specialists have an essential mission to stress these gatekeepers' roles as a critical part of the campus effort; the shared responsibility of various constituencies is necessary for the campus's comprehensive prevention approach.

The four contributions in this chapter can help prevention specialists with advocacy issues. The initial Lessons From the Field segment emphasizes strategies for becoming a "prevention influencer," a phrase introduced in Chapter 2. The other Lessons From the Field highlights some suggestions, and topics to avoid, when working with Generation Z students. The Case Study is particularly relevant during these times because it provides helpful perspectives about the essential nature of leadership. The Innovator segment is provided by long-term educator and clinician Robert Chapman, who offers his insights about perspective and innovation, both of which are most helpful for the work of prevention today and tomorrow.

SPECIFYING THE AUDIENCES

For promotion and advocacy efforts to be effective, the messages need to be crafted to address each audience's needs and issues and to incorporate their frame of reference and perspectives. By addressing "What's in it for them?" the message contents and style can be targeted appropriately while maintaining overall consistency with overriding prevention strategies and messages.

The first step is to *segment the audience*, as is done with selective prevention and indicated prevention strategies (see Chapters 6 and 7). This segmentation may be based on group affiliation or individual role. While making plans for promotion and advocacy, the drug/alcohol specialist should consider these two broad groupings:

- **Intermediaries:** These are essential connectors with the ultimate audience: the students. As the "frontline" workers, these individuals enhance prevention efforts by understanding, supporting, and implementing the desired approaches. They can aid by espousing helpful messages (and, at a minimum, not espousing contradictory messages). Intermediaries include residence hall staff, student affairs specialists, student organization advisors, counseling and health professionals, faculty members, counselors, athletic trainers, and law enforcement personnel as well as student leaders, who can be student organization officers, student-athlete team captains, paraprofessional residence hall staff, orientation leaders, and peer educators.
- **Decision makers:** These individuals and offices are the power brokers on campus who control budgets, allocate resources, and make policy decisions. It is vital that they understand, appreciate, and support the overall campus effort and its varied elements. These people may include the chief student affairs officer, the chief financial officer, the president/provost/chancellor, and the student government. Others who may have real or unrealized power include the faculty senate, the staff senate, as well as various individuals (consider influential faculty members, the chief of police, the directors of health and counseling services, distinguished alumni, and vital community leaders). Further, the institution's board of trustees can serve an important role for support and leadership.

The second step with planning these efforts is to *gain an understanding of the audience's world.* To the extent possible, learn what is important to them in their role and what their respective constituencies find important. Where feasible, it is helpful to identify some personal connection, whether about areas of interest, hobbies, recreation, culture, or family. In planning the communication, prevention specialists should identify what these intermediaries and decision makers need to know as well as what they might want to know. The aim is to establish some connection.

The prevention specialist's planning or advisory group can be instrumental in identifying the audiences, specifying strategies, and crafting messages. Some group members may also be an intermediary or decision maker and thus can share insights about outreach to other individuals or groups. These planning or advisory group members can help the prevention specialist with understanding other individuals' and groups' perspectives and issues; they can also specify ways to promote a greater understanding of the problems at hand and gain the support of the ultimate constituents (i.e., students). Carlton Hall's strategies for becoming a prevention influencer, found in Lessons From the Field 12.1, are helpful for the prevention specialist, as well as for many of those reached, who in turn can themselves become influential in this role.

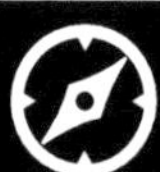

LESSONS FROM THE FIELD 12.1

Becoming a Campus-Based Prevention Influencer

Carlton Hall, MHS
President and CEO
Carlton Hall Consulting

In many important ways, influencers are encouraging mass engagement with substantive issues, leading to a rise in youth activism in recent years. Think about, among many others, Malala Yousafzai, an activist for female education, and

Greta Thunberg, an environmental activist. The same type of influencer role is valid and appropriate for preventing substance use and misuse on college campuses.

Campus-based prevention influencers can be defined as professionals or students who take positions on and influence alcohol, tobacco, and other drug prevention policies, programs, services, and messages. These individuals seek to improve the lives of students on campus by influencing others to prevent drug and other substance use.

Becoming a prevention influencer is a three-step process that builds on the aim of addressing—effectively—specific campus issues that need to change.

1. Identify the issue to address. The first step is to become knowledgeable—even an expert—on

- the issue (as specifically and narrowly focused as possible);
- potential strategies to address the issue; and
- potential partners with whom to work.

2. Take a position and determine your message. Prevention influencers create position papers and talking points critical to engaging others, communicating, and taking action. This step creates specific messages that target specific audiences to enable them, in turn, to address the issue:

- Formally state ideas on the issue.
- Provide a "defensible" position.
- Create "compelling talking points."

3. Move to action! Identify specific ways to use the power to influence others to take action:

- Build "consensus" and "unity."
- Create a basis for taking action.

> Campus-based prevention influencers tap into others' passion, gather supporters, and develop thoughtful plans for change. These steps help an influencer work with others to provide a clear and consistent description of the issue, strategies, and reasons why people should become involved.

REFINING THE MESSAGES

Messages to the intermediaries and decision makers are crafted in timely and appropriate ways. The focused planning begins with overarching themes of audience relevance, clarity, consistency, and action orientation.

The first step is to clarify the outcome or outcomes sought. Because different audiences will desire different results, prevention specialists must be specific about what they want the audience to know, feel, and/or do. Once this goal is clear, prevention specialists can take steps to clarify the aims desired with the identified audience, and then specify ways to accomplish this communication. The messages need to be relevant to the audience and address their needs, issues, and overall context.

Prevention specialists benefit from considering a variety of items that can be addressed with their various audiences. As the prevention specialist prepares to engage with an audience, they should consider each of the following items and select those deemed most appropriate for the audience. When making this determination, the prevention specialist should think about what is needed for and what will resonate with audience members.

- **Importance:** Since drugs and alcohol cause so many campus problems, prevention strategies help reduce these issues. Individual and group involvement in the prevention effort is vital for helping the campus, overall, achieve its mission and goals.

- **Problems:** Issues associated with drugs and alcohol affect much of campus life, including academic productivity, student preparedness for life after college, and faculty and staff engagement. Prevention efforts help reduce troubles in these areas, and thus affect the quality of life with audience members.
- **Reputation:** Prevention strategies can make a difference in keeping the institution as well as groups and organizations out of the "bad news" headlines. The campus, as well as groups and organizations, can also gain positive attention for achievements and progress that demonstrate how local prevention efforts address a societal problem.
- **Positioning:** By speaking up, the organization can show its leadership and unique place with addressing drug and alcohol misuse.
- **Accurate knowledge:** When prevention specialists know about the incidence and prevalence of drug and alcohol issues on campus and nationally, they can use this information to motivate individuals and groups to action. These facts may include typical student substance use, including their heavy and frequent substance use; incidents and problems associated with student substance use; students' perceptions of other students' use of drugs and alcohol; students' attitudes and personal knowledge; opportunities for individual and group engagement; and what messages are heard by students. Prevention specialists can compare campus data with national and state data, as well as longitudinal perspectives, to motivate others to action.
- **Drug/alcohol facts:** With prevention specialists having current knowledge about drugs and alcohol, including what is known and not known about their short- and long-term effects, they can better inform audiences with the latest information; ideally, prevention specialists can then be seen as resources for future inquiries. This includes understanding substance use disorders as well as brain health development. Countering misperceptions and inaccurate information is vital. Quality information is available from national sources, such as the Substance Abuse

and Mental Health Services Administration, the National Institute on Alcohol Abuse and Alcoholism, the National Institute on Drug Abuse, the Drug Enforcement Administration, and the Centers for Disease Control and Prevention.

- **Misperceptions:** Since many people have incorrect perceptions of others' drug or alcohol use patterns, it is appropriate for prevention specialists to challenge these inaccurate views. Many people overstate high-risk behaviors such as illicit drug use and heavy alcohol use. More about correcting misperceptions can found in Innovator 6.1 (see Chapter 6).
- **Denial:** Attitudes such as denial and minimization of problems serve as roadblocks to engagement by individuals and groups, and thus warrant special attention by the prevention specialist. Many students see the misuse of substances as "no big deal"; many faculty members, administrators, and parents see substance misuse as a "rite of passage" similar to what occurred during their own young adulthood. Some of these audiences appear satisfied with the status quo of existing problems among individuals or organizations by saying "we're no worse than our peers"; this laissez faire attitude can be addressed by the prevention specialist.
- **Prevention:** The critical role of prevention is worth emphasizing and promoting by the prevention specialist. Individuals and groups can be encouraged to engage in quality prevention efforts; while not a guarantee of eliminating problems, these efforts can help reduce the harm caused by substance misuse.
- **Goals:** Prevention specialists can provide the perspective about the overall context of the campus, group and individual prevention efforts. They benefit from stressing that any goals must be reasonable, and cite that although drug and alcohol problems will never be eliminated, they can be better managed.
- **Comprehensive approach:** Another contextual focus for prevention specialists is that having a comprehensive approach overall is essential for affecting the campus culture as well as the culture within individual groups. This comprehensive approach

involves a shared responsibility by numerous individuals, groups, and offices; it also involves using a variety of methods, including policies, programs, training, education, support services, and evaluation. The prevention specialist can highlight ways in which individuals and groups can have a meaningful role within this context.

- **Stigma:** Prevention specialists can help audiences understand stigma, and ways in which individuals and groups can help reduce it. Attention can be provided to not stigmatizing those with a substance use disorder or those engaged in healthy decision making.
- **Language:** It is helpful for prevention specialists to emphasize the message that "language matters" and "words matter." They can stress this message, as well as the use of current science and current knowledge, with their audiences. Appropriate language includes "alcohol and other drugs"; "drunk and impaired driving"; "recovering alcoholic"; "substance use disorder"; "low-risk choices"; and "responsible decision making."
- **Honoring success:** Prevention specialists can make a difference by empowering individuals and groups to become engaged with prevention efforts. This can be done by promoting the positive, and citing the small and large steps that have been made locally. Prevention specialists might cite evaluation results, stories that illustrate helpful impact, and positive comments that celebrate the "brand" or "norm" of low-risk drinking.

Using these potential communication anchors, specific examples and illustrations relevant to the audience can build meaningful connections. For example, when working with a group such as a fraternity, sorority, or an athletic team, group-appropriate language emphasizes the relevance of the message. Similarly, with decision makers, identifying relevant examples creates linkages to their frames of reference. With a focus on reaching Generation Z students, prevention specialists benefit from specific insights regarding approaches that are most helpful, and what might not be appropriate, with this audience.

Carolyn Capern and Greg Trujillo highlight these insights in Lessons From the Field 12.2.

Finally, whatever examples or messages are used, the prevention specialist must identify specific, actionable behaviors. By first clarifying what the audience should "know and feel," prevention specialists can then articulate specifically what the audience should "do." That action step may be to make references in a talk or conversation, to take a specific stance on a policy, to review a proposed action, to allocate resources, and so on. Worksheet 12.1: Communication Foundations provides a template for organizing appropriate strategies for various audiences (within the Institute of Medicine's universal, selective, and indicated framework). This worksheet helps with specifying key messages for different audiences, with attention to the aim of changing, reinforcing, or introducing some behavior, attitude, or other attribute.

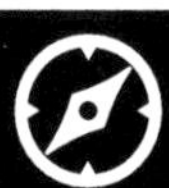

LESSONS FROM THE FIELD 12.2

Talking to Generation Z About Substance Misuse

Carolyn Capern
CTS Agency

Greg Trujillo
CTS Agency

To communicate effectively with someone, you need to think how they think and feel how they feel. The Pew Research Center studied millennial trends for more than a decade as the generation grew up and entered the workplace (Dimock, 2019).

Now, here comes Generation Z.

Millennials grew up in the comparatively peaceful 1990s. Generation Z—comprising individuals born between 1996 and the early 2010s—grew up in the shadow of the War on Terror, school shootings, the Great Recession, and a global pandemic (Parker & Igielnik, 2020). For this generation, 9/11 is a historical event comparable to their parents' experience with the Kennedy assassinations (McBride, 2020).

Developing effective prevention messages for Generation Z requires a different approach than was used for past generations. Consider the following guidelines for this new group of young adults:

- DO focus on mental health. Generation Z is more likely to misuse substances as self-medication because they are trying to escape anxiety than because of social pressure (Taylor, 2018).
- DO showcase diversity. Generation Z is the most diverse generation in U.S. history—and they celebrate that fact. Your images and messages should embrace people from a variety of races, ethnicities, genders, sexual orientations, and lifestyles (Parker & Igielnik, 2020).
- DO communicate in images. This is the generation of GIFs, emojis, and streaming video. They live online, and they can absorb information at a rapid pace. Communicate frequently and in short bursts that get to the point (Williams, 2015).
- DON'T use questionable data. Generation Z was born into the era of smartphones and tablets. They are adept at finding answers via Google and YouTube. Assume they are capable of fact-checking everything you say.
- DON'T use gateway analogies. Avoid slippery slope logic with Generation Z. Rather than lumping "all drugs" into a bucket, campaigns and outreach should emphasize realistic levels of harm caused by individual *substances* and addictive *behaviors*.

- DON'T leave them out of the conversation. Social media has given Generation Z a political voice since before they could vote. They are entrepreneurial and motivated, so help them get involved! Give your online audience the opportunity to be an active part of the conversation.

Staying relevant is about taking your audience seriously and tapping into the things that make them (and you) unique. Look for opportunities to bring them to the table. Generation Z's tech savvy and creativity alongside your subject matter expertise could be a powerful combination behind your next great campaign.

A MENU OF COMMUNICATION APPROACHES

As the prevention specialist prepares to communicate with specified audiences, available are a wide variety of tools and resources. These can be viewed as a type of "menu" from which to select those most appropriate for meeting the desired outcomes with each audience. With the planning efforts for a specific audience or setting, all of these approaches will not be used. The prevention specialist will benefit from considering which ones would be most likely to resonate with, and thus influence, audience members. When selecting approaches, it is appropriate to blend them; this may be done by illustrating data with examples, or linking desired outcomes with the campus mission statement.

It is also helpful for the prevention specialist to consider which emphasis, or coupling of emphases, would be influential with the audience. Aristotle is known for his three forms of proof: logos, pathos, and ethos (Daniels et al., 2007). With logos, attention is provided to logic, and the communicator focuses on the intellect of audience members and what might appeal to their rational nature. With pathos, the emphasis is upon emotions, and what might influence the passion or feelings of audience members. Ethos focuses on ethics and character; the prevention specialist will look at factors of credibility, and may include the appeal of knowledgeable sources as well as celebrities.

In making a calculated judgment about which elements within this menu are most helpful, the prevention specialist can select from the following 12 approaches for preparing the communication strategy. These approaches, a blend of these, and others identified by the prevention specialist can be helpful:

1. **Data** include prevalence and incidence and may consist of national, state, and local information. Data may also include comparisons among demographic groups, trends over time, projections, and analyses. (Robert Wood Johnson Foundation & the University of Michigan Center for Health Communications Research, 2020).
2. **Facts and scientific knowledge** incorporate authoritative statements, such as definitions (e.g., substance use disorder, harm reduction), facts (e.g., how drugs work in the body, effects of current and new substances), higher risk populations, and documented strategies.
3. **Expert statements** from relevant fields of study offer insights, interpretations, conclusions, and recommendations on topics such as prevention science, data, strategic approaches, and the importance of collaborative efforts.
4. **Testimonials** may emanate from students, faculty, staff, or others who have a positive or negative experience related to drugs or alcohol. Their stories may directly relate to current strategies or situations; they may also have stories that relate to strategies under consideration.
5. **Case studies** involve situations that illustrate the nature of concern from different perspectives as well as how the application of various approaches might play out.
6. **Visuals and videos** may provide a quick snapshot of key points, such as a sample promotional piece, or an illustration of an area

of concern (e.g., a photo of property damage or a video of disruptive behavior).

7. **Social norms marketing** is an approach designed to challenge and correct the misperceptions many people have about others' behavior; the use of local and current data highlights the desired behavior by documenting what the majority of students are doing.
8. **Creative epidemiology** is an innovative approach that converts often-confusing data into brief, impactful, and memorable examples. This approach highlights the scope of the issue with parallel images by saying "This rate or number is as if . . . " and links it with cost equivalents, time comparisons, or similarities with demographics.
9. **Positioning** is used to help prioritize the prevention specialist's message with the audience. Since many messages compete for audience members' attention, positioning helps identify how the proposed consideration is unique or different. For example, the prevention specialist may suggest that the desired behavior or attitude is better than, newer, more innovative, more cost-effective, or more attractive in some way other than what is currently being done or considered by the audience.
10. **Self-efficacy** provides confidence regarding one's potential influence. It includes tips, motivational statements, and reflections on how others view the issue. Self-efficacy may also include talking points that can help guide the audience's engagement and background reading for further clarification.
11. **Linking and pairing** identify ways of "attaching" the approach to a current event or feature. Affiliation may occur with a national, state, or local celebratory month, week, or day; associations or comparisons can be made with something historical or seasonal. This relationship with an existing offering can also orient an initiative as a repeat or renewal, a contrast, or an occasion to celebrate.
12. **Visualization** reviews what might be incorporated with the campus effort as well as what might be accomplished. It includes

"what if" or "imagine this" scenarios, both of a problematic situation and the overall desired outcomes.

By incorporating some of these approaches strategically and seeking the "best fit" with the audience, prevention specialists can communicate clearly and effectively. Blending quantitative and qualitative methods enhances the opportunity for the audience to hear and "get" the messages. Clear communication helps the audience understand the messages and to know specifically what is desired of them.

PERSUASION STRATEGIES

The issue of persuasion is best thought of as an ongoing process. While many efforts are finite and focused in nature (such as with an "elevator speech"), it is more likely that persuasion will be a slow, formative process. The aim is to get the specified audience support and ideally "own" the campus prevention efforts. Persuasive approaches are based on an orchestrated, engaged process that guides decisions and initiatives for audiences, messages, timing, and strategies. They are also based on the importance of maintaining perspective throughout this journey, especially during particularly challenging times, as highlighted by Dolores Cimini in Case Study 12.1.

Persuasion is best accomplished when the prevention specialist has a regular presence in various settings. This presence can enhance the investment of others in the campus prevention effort. Specific steps that the prevention specialist can take include the following:

- Include individuals and organizations on the prevention advisory body.
- Identify ways campus specialists and experts can assist; consider needs assessments, evaluation, planning communication campaigns, and marketing.
- Reach out to faculty for their engagement for specific areas; offer opportunities for research, grants, projects, publishing, and service.

- Suggest student experiential engagement as class projects, internships, and research for a thesis or dissertation; consider students in public health, community health, marketing, public administration, health promotion, and education.
- Identify how student organizations can undertake an initiative by sponsorship or partnership with a prevention strategy.
- Offer expertise to campus offices and departments to help them address an identified or unidentified need.
- Volunteer to participate on campus committees, whether an advisory group or a staff/faculty search committee.
- Conduct a presentation at a campus, state, or national conference.
- Participate in the campus or community speakers bureau, sharing expertise and awareness of the campus prevention effort.
- Encourage campus public relations and external media coverage of prevention activities and strategies as well as staff presentations and publications.

The important feature of having a regular presence throughout the campus community helps prevention specialists to become known as knowledgeable and dedicated personnel. Ultimately, these various integrations into the fabric of the institution are designed so the prevention specialists and their strategies will be viewed as essential for the institution.

With increased engagement and interweaving within the institutional fabric, the aim of respect for and incorporation of prevention specialists and their expertise is more likely to be achieved. This engagement with various faculty and staff provides opportunities to engage and negotiate toward shared understandings and mutually beneficial outcomes.

This process should be viewed as a journey toward collaboration and engagement. Prevention specialists should prepare to engage in various opportunities for persuasion by having talking points ready for use. This type of "elevator speech" approach takes advantage of planned and unplanned opportunities, such as with committee work, before or after events, during a commute, or more spontaneously on or off campus. Figure 12.1 provides a nine-step model for persuasion planning.

Figure 12.1
Steps for Persuasion Planning

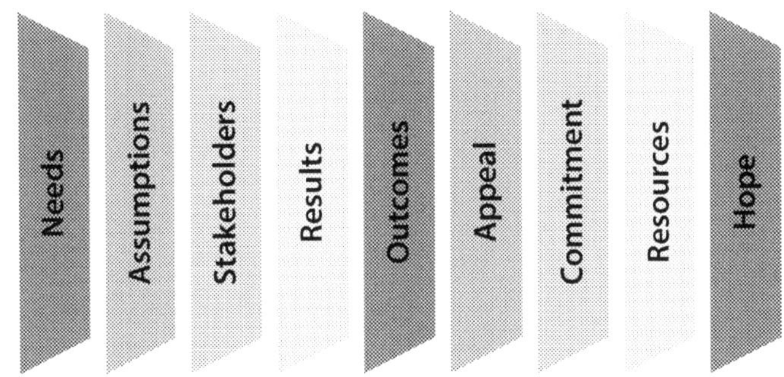

1. **Needs:** Understand clearly the needs to be met. Be grounded and up to date, acknowledging current and factual information, and identify knowledge gaps.
2. **Assumptions:** Clarify what might make a difference. Address theoretical underpinnings for the campus effort, including the logic model and guiding principles.
3. **Stakeholders:** Understand stakeholders' needs and issues. Identify ways of being personally relevant to decision makers. Frame the problem within the institutional context, and engage assets and resources.
4. **Results:** Define desired results from proposed initiatives. Keep goals reasonable and consistent with campus needs and visions; include measurable milestones to monitor progress.
5. **Outcomes:** Specify outcomes sought by stakeholder(s), including areas of interest to other constituencies. Specify strategies to help address their needs and concerns. Identify specific ways stakeholders can be helpful and supportive.
6. **Appeal:** Utilize varied approaches to appeal to intellect and emotions by incorporating logic, passion, and ethics. Be attention getting and maintain credibility.

7. **Commitment:** Demonstrate personal engagement with short- and long-term strategies and periodic reviews. Equip stakeholders with directions, tools, and speaking points.
8. **Resources:** Incorporate references and resources from reputable sources. Be supportive of those engaged with the process.
9. **Hope:** Remain aspirational and hopeful. Incorporate idealism, dreams, and optimism throughout the process, and maintain the courage to speak up and speak out regularly.

To persuade individuals and groups to support and embrace the prevention message for the campus, paying attention to multiple strategies in a planful way is essential. At a minimum, these various stakeholders and decision makers should not be counterproductive, whether by design or unintentionally. Worksheet 12.2: Persuasion Worksheet provides a template for summarizing many key elements for planning persuasive communication initiatives.

CASE STUDY 12.1

Leadership in Turbulent Times: Reflections on What Really Matters

M. Dolores Cimini, PhD
Psychologist and Director
University at Albany

Recently, when I met virtually with the alumni board of our university's peer education program to share the news of the cancellation of our 50th reunion due to the COVID-19 global pandemic, the founder of the program shared some recollections. He cited campus disruption and the shutdown of academics and other operations on campus during the spring semester 50 years ago when he was a student. At that time, students struggled with national concerns such as racial tension, the consequences of the Vietnam War, and increases in alcohol and other drug misuse among college students. Violence during that era was at a peak, with campus buildings destroyed and protests taking place on both campus and in the community. Alcohol and drug misuse across colleges and universities nationally, and on our own campus, were prominent. Further, no prevention strategies as we know them today were available on campuses in the United States.

This discussion made me reflect on leadership during times of turbulence on our campus: the Vietnam War, concerns related to equity and inclusion, a shooting on our campus in 1994, alcohol- and drug-related student deaths, and the coronavirus global pandemic. While campus issues have varied over time, the critical importance of steady and visible leadership from senior administrators has remained most constant and critical. Over the years, we have not been defined by the challenges we faced but by how we learned from these tragedies as we shaped our future.

In the end, it is not necessarily how challenges present themselves at any point in time but how campus leaders find a ray of optimism in the midst of tragedy and model the courage to move forward in the face of challenges that really matters. We must lead with a spirit of optimism in the face of uncertainty and tragedy, be transparent in our approach and messaging, and proceed with a spirit of inclusion and respect for all members of campuses and communities.

Incorporating persuasion strategies into campus prevention efforts helps prevention specialists to obtain the support of intermediaries and decision makers. Ongoing engagement with various constituencies and audiences provides multiple opportunities to ask audiences about any questions they may have, as well as about their suggestions for improvement. Answers to those questions and modifications can help move the audience toward endorsing and, ultimately, embracing the campus effort. The other question emanating from this engagement is more pointed, and yet is the ultimate aim of this engagement: "What are you willing to commit yourself to doing?" While that question may not be explicitly asked, it can serve as an anchor toward which the prevention specialist moves the conversation. A clear answer and a clear commitment are what is ultimately being sought.

Finally, as prevention specialists strive to orchestrate campus efforts that will move the needle and engage many stakeholders through their persuasive engagement efforts, the important role of innovation remains. Robert Chapman, a long-time and innovative educator and clinician, cites how both innovation and perspective are essential in moving forward with changes to the campus culture. Innovator 12.1 provides helpful views about "inventing" the desired future.

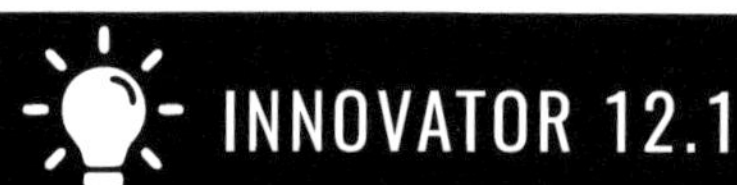

Innovation: The Father of Invention

Robert J. Chapman, PhD
Associate Clinical Professor (retired)
Drexel University

In his book, *A Whole New Mind,* Daniel Pink (2006) argued that innovators arise from that group of individuals who are willing to cross boundaries—intellectual, academic, and professional boundaries. The innovator is the individual who *thinks outside the box* and therefore is inspired by the inherent potential in another's idea to address current problems. For this to happen, however, innovators often need to experience a change in perspective that opens the mind to the possibilities that exist beyond perceived boundaries.

I used to ask my counseling students, "Is 2 minutes a short or long time?" Almost immediately I would hear, "Short!" I'd turn to that student and with a smile on my face say, "Okay; hold your breath for 2 minutes." The class would chuckle and we'd then discuss the importance of a practitioner's perspective when trying to engage a client in a conversation about change. The same is true for prevention specialists; it is important to consider one's perspective before attempting to change student drinking or other drug behaviors.

So how do we stimulate those responsible for addressing collegiate drug/alcohol use to attend to these student perceptions rather than simply relying on their own understanding of collegiate drinking or just looking at the data? How about metaphor as a catalyst for innovation?

Imagine you are standing in the aisle of a moving train, bouncing a ball. The ball leaves your hand at point A, drops to the floor and bounces straight back into your hand, which to all in the passenger car is in the same place as when the ball was released. Meanwhile, outside, standing on a station platform as the train passes through, an observer views you bouncing the ball. The observer sees the ball leave your hand at point A, drop to the floor and bounce back at point B several feet in front of where you dropped the ball. The experience of the observer and the observed differ significantly.

Now, consider the observed passenger on the train represents our collegiate drinker, and the observer on the platform our prevention specialist. It may be clear from the prevention specialist's perspective that the student's drinking is high risk if not problematic, but not from the student's perspective.

Problematic behavior will itself register as such *only when it causes a perceived problem*. If the results of a behavior appear untoward to the prevention specialist yet present no concern to a student, why would that student be motivated to consider changing—especially if that behavior presents a solution to a real problem, say, social shyness or anxiety? To the practitioner, the student drinking is an issue because it is underage drinking, results in missed classes, or causes problematic behavior. To the student, the drinking accomplished social engagement and interpersonal confidence, with any accompanying results (e.g., missed classes) acceptable consequences.

If necessity is the mother of invention, then innovation is its father—and perspective the matchmaker that brings these two together.

CONCLUSION

Effective communication skills are vital for prevention specialists, particularly as they seek to garner support from campus and community leaders and decision makers. By using varied evidence-informed strategies, such as those highlighted with the menu of communication approaches, messages can be crafted based on specific interests and needs of identified audiences. Nine specific steps for persuasion planning are identified to enhance the likelihood of garnering support for locally appropriate strategies.

REFERENCES

Daniels, M., Bowen, H., & Adgani, P. (2007). Aristotle's forms of proof: The keys to teaching recreation marketing. *SCHOLE, 22*(1), 103–106. https://www.nrpa.org/globalassets/journals/schole/2007/schole-volume-22-pp-103-106.pdf

Dimock, M. (2019, January 17). *Defining generations: Where millennials end and Generation Z begins.* Pew Research Center. https://www.pewresearch.org/fact-tank/2019/01/17/where-millennials-end-and-generation-z-begins

McBride, T. (2020, February 12). *The Marist college mindset list, class of 2023.* https://www.marist.edu/mindset-list#2024

Parker, K., & Igielnik, R. (2020, May 15). *On the cusp of adulthood and facing an uncertain future: What we know about Gen Z so far.* Pew Research Center. https://www.pewsocialtrends.org/essay/on-the-cusp-of-adulthood-and-facing-an-uncertain-future-what-we-know-about-gen-z-so-far

Pink, D. (2006). *A whole new mind: Why right brainers will rule the future.* River Head Books.

Robert Wood Johnson Foundation & the University of Michigan Center for Health Communications Research. (2020). *Visualizing health.* http://www.vizhealth.org/gallery

Taylor, K. (2018, February 21). Millennials are dragging down beer sales—but Gen Z marks a "turning point" that will cause an even bigger problem for the industry. *Business Insider.* https://www.businessinsider.com/millennials-gen-z-drag-down-beer-sales-2018-2?r=UK

Williams, A. (2015, September 18). Move over, millennials, here comes Generation Z. *The New York Times.* https://www.nytimes.com/2015/09/20/fashion/move-over-millennials-here-comes-generation-z.html

CHOICES: "So What"

The book's final two chapters encompassed in this last section address the choices made by campus leaders regarding whether and how to become involved with campus drug and alcohol misuse prevention efforts. These chapters offer a broad perspective about the important work being undertaken by prevention specialists with the engagement and support of campus leaders. While significant attention has been made in previous chapters about having strategies that are evidence based and thoughtful, a priority that remains is to actively review and report on the efforts; this includes the biennial review as well as more detailed review processes. Periodic self-monitoring is essential for maintaining locally appropriate strategies to meaningfully engage with varied constituencies and audiences. The book concludes with discussion on taking the time to step back and reflect on the importance of having campus efforts address drug and alcohol misuse, and the value and contributions of the campus strategies with this aim. This assessment incorporates celebration of the progress of individual and collective efforts, as well as an identification of potential next steps and new directions. Collectively, the efforts and processes result in impact and culture change that illustrate the *so what* for the campus strategies as a whole.

CHAPTER 13

Reporting Results and Processes

"When I was a freshman, I made the choice not to drink and have upheld that decision to this day. The decision unfortunately influenced who would be friends with me and how separated I would be from some of my collegiate peers. Regardless, this has not stopped me from seeing the effects of over-consumption and how it has completely altered the path and futures of college students."

—Junior from the Mountain states at a large public university

The job of effecting change with campus prevention efforts is large, but meaningful and appropriate strategies exist and results large and small are achievable. Still, with the value placed upon grounded strategies and attention to cost-effective approaches, prevention specialists must stop periodically and review the status of their work. Whether for short-term strategies (e.g., specific events, training), broader approaches (e.g., policies, campaigns), or systemic reviews (e.g., assumptions, theoretical grounding, logic model, outcomes, processes), meaningful assessments are essential to maximizing results on students' well-being, productivity, and success.

This chapter's perspectives and strategies equip campus leaders to implement appropriate and necessary monitoring and review activities. Attention to specific local data, national guidance, and challenges is provided to help prevention specialists revitalize and renew, as well as reorient and adjust, the campus strategies.

Three different contributing segments offer practical insights on the reporting of campus strategies and results. The Lessons From the Field segment describes the biennial review and how sharing its results can aid with the promotion of the campus prevention effort. The Case Study offers some suggestions regarding evaluation and highlights the importance of qualitative approaches. The Innovator piece is prepared by long-term scholar, educator, and advocate William DeJong; he addresses some challenges faced when promoting environmental management, thus offering inspiration and insights helpful for prevention specialists as they provide leadership and advocacy.

IMPORTANCE OF REVIEW AND REPORTING

Consistent with the role of institutions of higher education as repositories of knowledge, settings for human development, foundations of critical thinking, and centers of excellence, the campus prevention specialists must periodically review their work to ensure they are on the right track and make necessary adjustments as needed. Investments of time and resources are essential for impact and progress. Complementing the evaluation details and strategies (see Chapter 9) are systematic review and reporting processes.

Overall, program monitoring is designed primarily to ensure that specified outcomes are being achieved. A related purpose is to review the strategies and processes used to assess areas for improvement, greater efficiency, lessons learned, potential inconsistencies, and unintended consequences. The review process examines the return on investment for the campus effort. Review processes, conducted on a regular basis, keep those involved with the campus prevention effort up-to-date and engaged with policies, programs, procedures, and strategies. With personnel turnover, these review processes help significantly with maintaining the momentum of the campus effort and, as such, support the overall institutionalization of the campus prevention effort.

Individual campus strategies warrant similar review processes. In the case of staff training, media campaigns, or policy implementation, for example, the examination of outcomes as well as procedures is warranted. From data gathered to testimonials shared, the insights help to reaffirm the approaches used as well as to rethink these efforts for improvement.

Beyond program improvement, outcome and process results aid those planning and implementing prevention efforts. For prevention specialists, results that demonstrate how efforts have paid off are affirming; further, identifying areas for improvement helps motivate leaders to attain a constructive impact. Less-than-desired results can serve to inspire campus leaders to rethink and redesign the effort.

Periodic reviews of campus prevention efforts are also essential because of changes among the student body. New students, with varied backgrounds, arrive on campus several times a year; some are recent high school graduates, some are transfer students, some are veterans, and some are adult learners. Further, students' learning and interaction styles, interests, and priorities change continuously. These differences in backgrounds and learning styles are further compounded with continual evolutions in technology, including social media; the impact of technology upon factors such as learning styles, the nature of interactions, self-esteem, and critical thinking may be consequential, to be examined with further research. Of specific interest in this regard is the large group of new students arriving from high school: Generation Z students (see Chapter 12 for more details). The best ways to reach and interact with Generation Z students is different than for millennials as well as for older students such as Baby Boomers and Generation X. Further changes among any students being reached by campus efforts may include the substances used, including marijuana and its increasing potency, other illicit drugs, and prescription drug use for nonmedical purposes. Coupling these issues with increased societal stress and uncertainty, limited coping skills, and compromised relationship and communication skills results in continued needs to modify the campus prevention effort to keep it relevant.

A final contextual role with review processes concerns the larger community. Monitoring efforts demonstrate that prevention specialists are sincere in their efforts to address campus challenges as well as larger societal issues. Review processes demonstrate a commitment to the campus mission and the campus's efforts to serve as a leader for society as a whole. Conducting the review, and sharing the results, shows a commitment toward continual improvement and, ultimately, for positive impact. The contextual view of seeking to better manage (rather than solve) drug and alcohol issues serves as a model for acknowledging challenges as well as opportunities. These outward-oriented roles promote trust and credibility with campus leadership, thus setting the stage for future support. See Worksheet 13.1: Synthesis and Review for help organizing this review and reflective effort with regard to campus strategies.

THE BIENNIAL REVIEW

A review of campus prevention efforts is specified by federal law and applies to institutions of higher education that receive federal funds or financial assistance. The "biennial review," as it is commonly called, is required every 2 years—the even-numbered years. The U.S. Department of Education standards are specified in the Education Department General Administrative Regulations (EDGAR Part 86) and emanate from the Higher Education Act of 1965 and the 1989 amendments to the Drug-Free Schools and Communities Act (also known as the Drug-Free Schools and Campuses Act).

The biennial review mandates that colleges and universities take drug and alcohol misuse seriously on their campuses. Designed to promote accountability, the law underscores the importance of having campus prevention efforts, since drug and alcohol misuse is contrary to the mission of institutions of higher education. While the law allows flexibility for local authorities to determine their own actions and documentation, it does require compliance with the implementation of a prevention program and a biennial review of it.

Institutions of higher education are expected to have efforts designed "to prevent the unlawful possession, use, or distribution of illicit drugs and alcohol by students and employees" (U.S. Department of Education, 1997, p. 3). Further, the program "must include annual notification of the following: standards of conduct; a description of sanctions for violating federal, state, and local law and campus policy; a description of health risks associated with alcohol and other drug (AOD) use; a description of treatment options; and a biennial review of the program's effectiveness and the consistency of the enforcement of sanctions" (U.S. Department of Education, 1997, p. 3).

For the review process itself, two objectives are specified:

- "To determine the effectiveness of, and to implement any needed changes to, the AOD prevention program
- To ensure that campuses enforce the disciplinary sanctions for violating standards of conduct consistently" (U.S. Department of Education, 1997, p. 13).

The institution must certify that it has adopted and implemented an AOD program, as quoted above. This regulation requires three things:

1. The institution must notify each employee and student of the standards of conduct, legal sanctions, health risks, and treatment programs; this must be done on an annual basis.
2. The institution must prepare a sound process for distributing this annual notification information.
3. The institution must prepare a report on the effectiveness of its AOD programs as well as the consistency of its sanction enforcement; this must be done on a biennial basis.

To address the legal requirements, prevention specialists benefit from preparing a summary of policies for students and staff as well as their distribution channels. Also critical is a summary of prevention, intervention, and recovery services initiatives. A review of programmatic goals and objectives, their accomplishment, and strengths and weaknesses will help identify future directions, recommendations, and revisions.

The documentation of this biennial review should be maintained and readily available, since periodic monitoring may require this review to be shared. Some federal assistance applications require higher education institutions to certify that they have these programs. The requirements also call for all records to be maintained for 3 years. Beyond the legal requirements, the biennial review offers other opportunities for solidifying the campus prevention effort; Eric Davidson illustrates several approaches with Lessons From the Field 13.1.

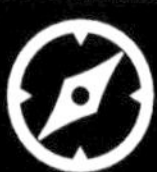

LESSONS FROM THE FIELD 13.1

Sharing the Biennial Review Is Important

Eric Davidson, PhD, MCHES

Interim Director, Health and Counseling Services

Eastern Illinois University

The biennial review process, mandated by the U.S. Department of Education's Drug-Free Schools and Campuses Regulations (EDGAR Part 86), ensures that campuses are engaging in quality prevention (The Drug-Free Schools and Communities Act Amendments of 1989). The intent of the law was to ensure that each institution of higher education addresses policies and services and also reviews the effectiveness of its prevention efforts. This biennial review serves as a strategic planning process and also as an assessment and evaluative process that captures large amounts of data (U.S. Department of Education, 1997).

Sharing results with key stakeholders is one of the less widely implemented actions of the biennial review process. Sharing results may be enacted through a variety of strategies, including formal presentations to an institution of higher education's various governing bodies, Substance Abuse and Mental Health Services Administration Town Hall Meetings, brief highlights documents shared to stakeholders, and infographics. Often, data collected can assist with an analysis of overall strengths, weaknesses, opportunities, and threats. The strategic planning aspect of the biennial review should also be shared. Findings of the biennial review are intended to drive improvement and success. Sharing results, as well as recommended strategies and initiatives planned to strengthen an institution's prevention program, demonstrates institutional commitment to addressing substance use while also making others more likely to want to join the effort.

Within this trove of biennial review information, there is bound to be something of interest to almost any audience invested in higher education, including administrators, faculty, community members, student leaders, alumni, and government leaders. Biennial review results and findings can be used with these audiences to increase interest in (and ideally support of) prevention through illustrating student substance use behaviors and attitudes, evident problems, and the need for increased prevention focus and resources, as well as program successes. To garner further buy-in, these audiences may identify specific interests they would like to see reviewed during the subsequent biennial review process, thus further enhancing local relevance.

Transparency of key results and conclusions is important. When possible, the biennial review report should be openly shared. Since the report may contain lots of data, it may be important to simplify results or develop different summaries for particular audiences. Knowing and understanding the wants and needs of specific audiences and providing the desired data will help attract stakeholders and allies to the cause.

As an assessment action, it is important to close the assessment loop. As the strategic planning portion moves to implementation, it is essential to continue collecting data; reviewing programs, services, and strategies; and informing stakeholders and allies about the progress the institution is making in addressing substance use issues. As progress is made, be sure to celebrate the wins with the various allies and stakeholders.

THE DETAILED REVIEW PROCESS

Just as campus academic programs are reviewed regularly, such as for certification, accreditation, or programmatic renewal, the campus prevention effort merits similar regular scrutiny. Systematic and detailed programmatic examination can help with the development of grounded strategies designed to reduce current harms associated with substance misuse, to promote the desired campus culture, and to be as cost-effective as possible. This more extensive, full-scale, periodic review is recommended every 6 to 10 years, thus incorporating the biennial review processes.

Five steps are recommended for conducting this review. While these steps complement the planning processes for developing the campus effort overall, they are distinguished here for the purpose of programmatic study.

Step 1: Establish a Review Committee

A broad-based committee, with comprehensive campus representation, should oversee the review process. It may help to choose a committee chair who is independent of the campus prevention office; this person may be a faculty member with interest and appropriate expertise and who may be provided an incentive (e.g., course release) for undertaking this responsibility. The committee should be provided a specific charge of nature, scope, and desired outcomes for its effort. Considerations include a review of the previously established vision, mission goals and objectives, the grounding and logic model, the strategies used, and the results obtained. The committee should also specify any return on investment elements and make recommendations for improvement and future initiatives.

Step 2: Examine Documentation and Generate Insights

With an established set of timelines and review processes, the committee should examine findings from various sources, such as annual reports, biennial reviews, and localized data (e.g., campus surveys, environmental scans, event summaries). Attention to some of the more detailed descriptions, such as those from training events or campaigns conducted, will be necessary.

The review committee will also benefit from focused discussions, key informant interviews, and focus groups with stakeholders and varied groups. The decisionmakers' and key leaders' insights about the strengths and challenges of campus prevention efforts are essential. Appropriate sources include health and counseling services, residence halls, student activities, judicial affairs, athletics, police and security, and community relations. Special consideration should be given to the groups and organizations involved with the selective approaches (e.g., first-year students, fraternities and sororities, student-athletes) since these and other groups have professional staff members and offices providing services specifically for their audiences. And because many of these organizations have elected student leaders, specific outreach regarding their experiences and insights is important.

Step 3: Reflect on Progress

The review group should examine the achievement, or lack thereof, of programmatic objectives. Productive discussions include what helped and what hindered the campus effort, both broadly and specifically. Assessment of the logic model, supporting theories, and strategies will help determine the validity and appropriateness of the logic model and its contents. With evolving student needs, interests, and learning styles, the appropriateness and value-added of the campus strategies, and how they contribute to the achievement of desired outcomes, benefit from the review. A review of new resources and updated evidence-informed strategies will prepare the foundations for the future. Illustrative for this purpose, and other evaluative purposes, are the insights provided by James Lange in Case Study 13.1; he emphasizes instrumentation as well as qualitative strategies.

Step 4: Prepare Recommendations

Action steps include any needed redesign of the logic model, infusion of new strategies, refinements of the current strategy, reassessment of personnel and resource needs, and specifications of potential new evaluation and measurement processes (including those helpful for future reviews). Recommendations must clearly identify the resources and personnel needed to accomplish the specified aims. The recommendations may also include ways of increasing cost efficiencies as well as identifying new partners and potential changes in programs, policies, and services.

As recommendations are being developed, the review committee has the opportunity to clearly articulate the case for the future. The recommendations should include ways in which the prevention specialists envision how the campus may address needs and issues on the horizon (e.g., student body changes, emerging drugs, changes in usage patterns, new or anticipated legislation). These factors become opportunities for the campus prevention effort to be proactive, and demonstrate a commitment to a healthy and safe campus. Being attentive to such new factors anchors the prevention initiatives in current affairs, thereby remaining relevant to the issues and needs of the primary audience of students.

Step 5: Finalize and Distribute Report of Findings

The report of the review group's findings should include an executive summary, extensive detail, illustrative narrative, and appendices with more detailed documentation. The information is vital for further institutionalizing and refining the campus prevention effort.

When writing the report, include some narrative that frames the content in ways that resonate well with the report's audience. Reports are often organized around content areas such as goals, objectives, activities, staffing, evaluative measures, and recommendations; these and other areas are helpful and appropriate. However, prevention specialists should also consider using trigger points that engage the audience; the following should be considered to accomplish this purpose:

- "This is what our students need, drawn from local documentation."
- "This is what the science says about what we should do."
- "This is what we did and what we achieved."
- "This is what we have learned."
- "This is what we aspire to for the future."

Dissemination of the report and its findings is vital. Key findings are helpful for public dissemination, and public relations efforts can help engage and further grow various stakeholders and constituencies.

Overall, this thorough and systematic review process provides campus leaders, as well as those supporting the prevention effort, with the confidence that the strategies and approaches are well grounded. The detailed review process can demonstrate that the campus prevention effort has strong foundations. The review can specify clearly the theoretical and practical grounding for the initiatives, including limitations based on budget, staffing, approval processes, challenges faced, and changing needs. When documentation of processes used and outcomes achieved are specified, and when the metrics are in place and illustrate what results are achieved, a clear picture is provided to campus leadership and other constituencies about the nature and scope of services and strategies. Further, actively engaging in this process demonstrates to leaders and supportive audiences the level of commitment held by prevention specialists to the prevention effort and its continued successes.

CASE STUDY 13.1

Mind the Measurement Gaps

James E. Lange, PhD
Coordinator of Alcohol and Other Drug Initiatives, San Diego State University
Executive Director, Higher Education Center for Alcohol and Drug Misuse Prevention and Recovery

Using data to identify new problems or trends is integral to the work of prevention. However, I've found that sometimes the data are limited. Perhaps most frustrating is when a single data point is available with little context. Knowing that 23% of the population is doing X-risky-thing does not always provide enough context for action. Knowing instead that over the past 4 years, the population has gone from 13% to 23% of that behavior, or that all the surrounding communities are at 13%, while ours is at 23%, provides the clue that something is different in the environment that is facilitating that risky behavior. This knowledge can both provide direction and galvanize action toward meaningful change.

Another serious limitation is the measurement instrument itself. Often, those of us trying to create interventions are working with large, standardized questionnaire-based surveys. But for such surveys, the specific items define the universe of possible understanding. In my experience, listening to community members (often either medical professionals or just people in the know) has led me and my colleagues toward uncovering emerging drug use that was being missed by preexisting surveys: Consider the use of Ritalin/Adderall (McCabe et al.,

2005; Schulenberg et al., 2020; Shillington et al., 2006) and *Salvia divinorum* (Lange et al., 2008) as examples of researchers adding new items to a survey, thus resulting in the identification of significant novel substance use missed by previous standardized surveys. Additionally, standard surveys often provide little information about the context (both physical and social) for substance use behavior. Systematic observational studies—for instance, of bars and parties (Clapp et al., 2007), or even of social media posts (Lange et al., 2010)—can lead to far better understanding of motivators and drivers for the behaviors than an item on a population survey.

In other words, get out of your office and away from your computer, and talk with people. Do your best to understand the context, motivations, and breadth of their behaviors. Only then can the data provided from standardized measures be understood and used appropriately to create change.

CONSIDERATIONS FOR THE DETAILED REVIEW

Numerous resources and documents are valuable for inclusion in the detailed review, depending on the specifics of the campus review group's charge. With the aim of keeping the final report meaningful and helpful, consideration should be given to a range of broad and narrow issues.

General Review

Questions appropriate for the large-scale review would include the following:

- Is the mission for the campus prevention effort clear, focused, and reasonable?
- Is this mission consistent with the institution's overall mission, as well as that of the division hosting prevention efforts?

- What are the goals and affiliated measurable objectives?
- In what ways does theory undergird campus efforts and inform the logic models?
- To what extent are prevention efforts informed by the Institute of Medicine (IOM) model of universal, selective, and indicated strategies? (See Chapter 3 for an overview of the IOM model, and Chapters 5, 6, and 7 for more details on each of these strategies.)
- How strong are the connections between goals, objectives, and strategies?
- Are the specified strategies reasonable, appropriate, and contributing to meeting the objectives?
- How is current, local data used to monitor progress and students' needs and issues?
- In what ways are the program design and strategies updated based on the changes with the student body?

Data Elements

Current, localized data are essential for reviewing and monitoring campus efforts. Data should be gathered based on locally appropriate needs, emanating from the goals, objectives, and logic model of the prevention efforts. The needs identified and the logic model will go hand-in hand, with identified needs being considered for inclusion in the logic model, and items in the logic model needing local data to help provide documentation. In addition, the specific data collected can help with initiatives undertaken by other campus offices (e.g., counseling and psychological services, campus health services, sexual assault services). Further, the data to be collected may be defined by what is needed and appropriate for the detailed campus review. The data can be generally organized within three areas: (a) drug/alcohol consequences (see Table 13.1), (b) overall student issues (see Table 13.2), and (c) intermediaries (see Table 13.3). Note that the data identified in these three tables are illustrative and not intended as exhaustive; the specific data to be collected will be based on what prevention specialists and campus leaders determine is necessary and most useful, as well as what can be gathered in a reasonably efficient manner.

Table 13.1
Drug/Alcohol Consequences

Death	Hospital transports	Suicide attempts
Property damage	Impaired driving arrests	Arrests
Personal injury	Injury to others	Sexual assault
Public intoxication	Public disturbance	Interpersonal violence
Violent behavior	Health center contacts	Counseling center contacts
Alcohol poisoning	Underage alcohol use	Possession of substance
Alcohol use	Marijuana use	Other illicit drug use
Nonmedical use of prescription drugs		

Table 13.2
Overall Student Issues

Knowledge of alcohol or drug effects	Attitudes about drug/ alcohol use	Perceptions of others' use of alcohol/drugs
Awareness of campus AOD resources/strategies	Attitudes about campus AOD resources/strategies	Satisfaction with campus resources
Assessment of the campus climate overall	Attitudes about recovery and those in recovery	Understanding of bystander roles
Understanding of amnesty and Good Samaritan policies	Engagement and connection with the campus overall	Resiliency skills (e.g., stress management, time management)
Understanding of campus policy	Awareness of rationale and respect for policy elements	Attendance at specific events (AOD and general)
Skills for communication and interpersonal relationships	Overall self-esteem	Overall confidence

Table 13.3
Intermediaries

Staff knowledge of drugs, alcohol, substance use disorder	Staff knowledge of campus AOD resources/strategies	Staff skills with problem identification and referral
Staff support of campus AOD strategies	Staff understanding of the intersectionality of mental health, wellness, and alcohol/drug issues	Staff confidence with discussing AOD issues with students
Faculty knowledge of campus AOD resources/ strategies	Faculty awareness and skills on responding to problematic behaviors	Faculty infusion of AOD issues in their courses
Staff and faculty belief in the importance of their role with student AOD issues	Staff and faculty understanding of their role in shaping the campus culture overall	

The data can be examined for the campus overall as well as for groups and individuals specified for more focused interventions (per the IOM model, highlighted in Chapter 3). For example, a specific group of individuals (e.g., first-year students, student-athletes) may have divergent results and focused needs, thus warranting focused efforts.

Process Elements

Focused attention on the planning and implementation of the range of strategies and processes used is essential for the campus review. This helps with understanding what contributed to the success of these efforts, as well as what could be strengthened and what is worthy of replication.

Central to this review is the clarification of the success criteria. Is success based on attendance, as well as repeat attendance by individuals? Is it based on participants' satisfaction or acknowledgement of the strategy being helpful or meaningful? Is success based on demonstrated changes in participants' knowledge or personal attitudes, or is it based on changes in their perceptions of others' knowledge and attitudes? Or, is success based on changes in participants' reported behavioral intentions, their confidence, or their commitment to trying to reduce drug and alcohol problems? Whatever the choices are, the important factor is for campus leaders to be clear with the criteria for success. With that determination, assessments can be made regarding specific programmatic components, thus aiding with decisions about sustaining and adjusting these strategies for the future. Specifically, those strategies that do not meet the specified criteria for success may be modified or eliminated, and replaced with other strategies deemed more appropriate.

While many of these elements are gathered with the event evaluations and follow-up assessments, a "big picture" compilation is appropriate. These quantitative and qualitative data help decision makers understand the role of specific strategies and programmatic elements within the context of the comprehensive campus effort. For example, it is important to know the results that can be attributed to specific training events, as these results can be used to assess the "value-added" of each event to the overall achievement of the campus prevention efforts. Examples of specific training topics include handling a medical emergency, making a caring confrontation (a gentle intervention), making responsible decisions, and avoiding shame surrounding substance use disorders.

Valuable in this process are staff members' perspectives, key informant interviews, participant insights, and observational data. When combined with focused reports about individual programmatic and policy elements, these views provide a large-scale understanding.

A Holistic Perspective

When conducting the detailed review process, a crucial consideration is the interconnectedness between the overall campus experience and the prevention strategies. While the review process examines elements of the prevention effort, it also assesses ways in which these prevention strategies are interwoven into the overall fabric of the campus and its culture. This assessment includes identifying how drug and alcohol prevention efforts contribute to or detract from the range of initiatives, strategies, and programs undertaken on campus. Specifically, it is useful to review how the prevention strategies fit within the overall context of the entire campus and the campus culture. Generally, the students' college experience emphasizes a balanced and well-rounded approach for their intellectual, cultural, social, and physical development, focusing on their college years as well as preparing them to thrive for the rest of their lives.

Having this holistic perspective helps with articulating the intersection between wellness and drug/alcohol abuse. This intersection includes the coping mechanisms (often substance misuse) used by students to address challenges such as poor academic performance, heightened stress, distress, or problems with relationships. Similarly, celebratory strategies—whether with academics, social life, or other personal considerations—warrant attention for emphasis with drug and alcohol misuse prevention, as these celebrations often include the use of substances and could be reframed to be substance-free. Finally, as part of the review from a holistic perspective, prevention specialists should consider factors related to drug and alcohol misuse (from a causal or correlational perspective). These factors emphasize wellness, resiliency, protective factors and root causes (see Chapter 1); these factors can also promote a strong sense of values, healthy life skills, good relationship skills, problem-solving abilities, connectedness to the institution, and a sense of purpose. This examination incorporates the theoretical constructs for the prevention effort, with attention to the positive youth behavior model, positive psychology, and well-being issues (Bowers et al., 2010; Seligman, 2002; Seligman & Csikszentmihalyi, 2000; Seligman et al., 2005).

Obstacles and Challenges

Embedded in the review process is an examination of challenges and obstacles facing the successful implementation of the campus prevention effort. Whether anticipated or not, some issues will be event-specific (e.g., weather, competing campus events, broader societal considerations) and others will be systemic (e.g., resistance to recovery approaches, unrealistic expectations of "solving" concerns with underage drinking or marijuana use). Through the use of techniques such as a campus survey, focus groups, organizational self-assessments, or discussion groups, the review team can gather greater insight.

Four broad clusters of challenges are relevant:

1. **Individual and personal issues,** such as coping skills, mental health concerns, societal and cultural norms, beliefs and attitudes, resistance to help seeking, and limited healthy opportunities
2. **Professional issues,** including job responsibilities, time restrictions, burnout and compassion fatigue, lack of resources, and limited professional development
3. **Institutional issues,** such as limited staff, lack of funding, alcohol availability, competing priorities, inconsistent enforcement, campus traditions, risk avoidance, lack of knowledge, low interest, weak collaboration, denial, and limited data
4. **Community issues,** including alcohol availability, marketing and promotion efforts by bars, limited police enforcement, high-density housing, limitations with regulations and monitoring, competing priorities, lack of understanding by local decision makers, lack of resources, and local cannabis access

Prevention specialists should have a broad understanding of the world within which they, as professionals, work. The first three clusters of challenges identified focus primarily on professionals themselves, as these factors can constrain or negatively influence the impact of the planned strategies. Similarly, with the last item of community issues, it is important to understand the world within which students live. That is, college students are typically not isolated on campus; they visit, experience, participate with, and are engaged in the local community. Thus, pinpointing challenges and obstacles helps with identifying circumstances surrounding campus-based efforts. When couched within the broader context of such challenges, this review can help identify ways in which the campus leadership can better support and promote the prevention effort. By addressing many of the challenges identified, greater progress and documented outcomes can be obtained.

Communications

A central element of the review process focuses on communication, including the intended messages versus what was heard by targeted audiences. With the aim of having these two aspects of communication match, messages should be heard, understood, believed, and ultimately have the desired effect.

The review process benefits from first ascertaining what prevention specialists intended, and then assessing audience reactions. Potential messages may include some of the following, acknowledging that specific wording will be more refined:

- The use of drugs or alcohol is a personal choice.
- Many students overestimate others' use of substances.
- Heavy drinking (binge drinking) is dangerous.
- Underage drinking laws are in place for a reason.
- The campus has a zero-tolerance policy.
- Regular marijuana use can cause problems with attention and memory.
- There are many ways to have fun without alcohol.
- Have the confidence to ask for water or juice.
- Be an active bystander; be courageous and step up.
- Social media emphasizes the "highlights" of others' use of substances.
- It is important to know the dangers of high-risk drinking behaviors.
- It is OK not to drink or use drugs.
- Look after friends, roommates, and teammates should you choose to drink.
- Celebrate recovery.

Regarding what the audience hears, consideration focuses first on whether the message was even heard. For messages seen, potential queries include the following:

- What was the message?
- Was the message believable?

- Was it clear?
- Did it point to the next step?
- Was it consistent with other messages heard?
- Was it clear who the sponsoring organization was?
- Did it identify where additional information or resources could be obtained?
- Did it provoke personal thinking?
- Did it promote considerations of taking action or doing something different?
- Did it result in doing anything different?

An ongoing review of these questions is relevant for a focused campaign, social norms marketing campaign, or awareness initiative. Whether through specific assessments or by embedding queries in the ongoing campus survey process, taking stock of the impact and potential value of this aspect of the campus effort is essential.

An Organizational Self-Assessment

Another strategy for the detailed campus review is an organizational self-assessment, an approach that can be done in several different ways. One way is to have the prevention specialist review all components of the campus effort, such as policies, support services, training, educational efforts, and evaluation. The specialist can rate the extent to which each element is included and the quality of the action. Parallel to this is having various entities on campus complete the same assessment; this may be include a sampling of staff members, faculty, students, and student leaders. Comparing results between the specialist and others, and among campus groups, provides insight about the understanding of the campus efforts and areas for future attention. Including reflections about various scores and differences further informs the campus review.

Final Considerations

Although conducting the detailed review is a large undertaking, the work is vital for guiding prevention specialists and informing campus leaders about the current status and future opportunities for the prevention effort. Incorporating multiple data points and sources serves to orient and triangulate campus strategies. When strategies are oriented toward being current and relevant, and continually improving, this review process guides informed choices. The aim of the prevention strategies overall is to maximize the impact of whatever campus efforts are undertaken toward the ultimate goal of helping students make healthy choices regarding drugs and alcohol; having a thorough review process keeps the campus prevention strategies meaningful, appropriate, and ultimately effective.

The detailed review is important for "taking stock" of current efforts; more critical, this review provides opportunities for reshaping and redirecting the overall campus strategy. As William DeJong highlights in Innovator 13.1, the movement toward environmental management was, in its earliest days, an innovation for higher education's drug and alcohol abuse prevention efforts; since then, it has been widely validated and adopted. Similarly, prevention specialists can shape the discussion and strategies appropriate at the local level for current and anticipated campus needs and issues.

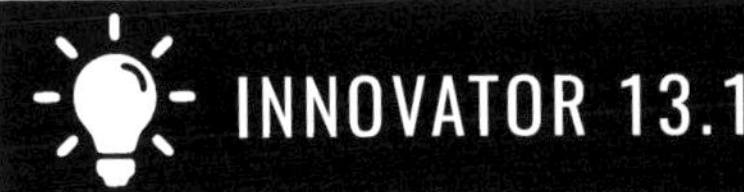

Taking the Leap Into Environmental Management

William DeJong, PhD
Professor (retired), Boston University School of Public Health
Adjunct Professor, Tufts University School of Medicine

My work for the U.S. Department of Education's Higher Education Center for Alcohol and Other Drug Prevention (HEC) began when the center was launched in late 1993. One of my first assignments was to write a guidebook on campus policy options for addressing substance use problems on campus (DeJong & Langenbahn, 1996).

During the 1960s, the courts put aside the legal doctrine of *in loco parentis*, ruling that colleges do not have a duty to control student conduct. In the 1980s, however, judges had begun to assert that colleges must take reasonable protective measures to guard against foreseeable hazards and risks in the school environment, just as any other property owner or manager must do (Bickel & Lake, 1999; Gehring & Geraci, 1989).

This emerging doctrine provided a legal basis for adopting the public health approach I wanted to propose: *establishing and maintaining an academic, legal, economic, and social environment that would guide and motivate students to make safer and healthier decisions*. Yes, college officials must hold students accountable, but they also need to take on the job of remaking and managing the campus environment and working collaboratively with community stakeholders. I called this approach *environmental management* (DeJong & Langford, 2002;

DeJong et al., 1998; National Institute on Alcohol Abuse and Alcoholism, 2020; Zimmerman & DeJong, 2003).

A key aspect of environmental management is revising and enforcing campus policies, but the approach is much broader than that. For example, I urged colleges to create a more rigorous academic environment by having more early morning and Friday classes, raising academic standards, boosting faculty–student contact, and improving student mentoring. Other examples include offering and promoting substance-free social, recreational, extracurricular, and public service options; restricting alcohol advertising and promotions; and implementing a responsible beverage service program. The list of potential strategies was long then and is even longer now.

When the HEC began, campus officials had been focusing on a mix of individual-level strategies, in particular awareness education, harm-reduction programs (e.g., safe rides), and disciplining and counseling students with substance use–related infractions. This work, while vitally important, does little to change the campus and community environment and thus leaves intact the conditions that enable the problem and virtually ensures its continuation. Student affairs staff were invested in this work, so it was unsurprising that environmental management initially received a mixed reception. Some critics dismissed the approach as the "flavor of the month," and one even denounced it as "fascism." Astonishingly, a Department of Education official said the HEC had no business encouraging prevention efforts in the local community.

More commonly, people questioned whether the "social engineering" I was calling for would actually work. Environmental-level strategies had been successful in reducing cigarette smoking, increasing seat belt use, and fighting drunk driving, but did I have evidence to support this approach to address student substance use? No. I had taken a leap of faith—an informed leap, but a leap nonetheless—because at the time there were very few published studies on college alcohol and other drug prevention. That soon changed, and now the National Institute on Alcohol Abuse and Alcoholism's (2020) updated review of college drinking prevention research, *CollegeAIM* (Alcohol Intervention Matrix), has two major sections: individual-level strategies and environmental-level strategies.

My contribution was modest. Other public health experts were trying to move the field in the same direction, but becoming the HEC director in 1995 gave me a singular platform to present the argument for environmental-level strategies. Most importantly, I had the privilege of working alongside a talented and dedicated staff of professionals who were willing to take that leap of faith with me—and to do the lion's share of the hard work required to realize our shared vision.

CONCLUSION

Ongoing monitoring and periodic reviews of campus strategies help ensure their cost effectiveness and relevance. While a biennial review is specified by federal law, less regular yet much more detailed assessments are critical, as these assessments can examine the soundness of the theories and the logic model undergirding campus strategies. While all assessments, whether event or strategy specific, will help monitor outcomes and processes, holistic reviews and reporting allow for adjustment of campus interventions. Particularly with the implementation of innovative approaches, monitoring and reporting promotes accountability. Numerous considerations for the detailed review process help prevention specialists organize and orchestrate information-gathering systems that inform sound decision making.

REFERENCES

Bickel, R. D., & Lake, P. F. (1999). *The rights and responsibilities of the modern university: Who assumes the risks of college life?* Carolina Academic Press.

Bowers, E., Li, Y., Kiely, M., Brittian, A., Lerner, J., & Lerner, R. (2010). The five Cs model of positive youth development: a longitudinal analysis of confirmatory factor structure and measurement invariance. *Journal of Youth and Adolescence, 39,* 720–735. https://doi.org/10.1007/s10964-010-9530-9

Clapp, J. D., Holmes, M. R., Reed, M. B., Shillington, A. M., Freisthler, B., & Lange, J. E. (2007). Measuring college students' alcohol consumption in natural drinking environments: Field methodologies for bars and parties. *Evaluation Review, 31*(5), 469–489. https://doi.org/10.1177/0193841X07303582

DeJong, W., & Langenbahn, S. (1996). *Setting and improving policies for reducing alcohol and other drug problems on campus: A guide for administrators.* U.S. Department of Education, Higher Education Center for Alcohol and Other Drug Prevention.

DeJong, W., & Langford, L. M. (2002). A typology for campus-based alcohol prevention: Moving toward environmental management strategies. *Journal of Studies on Alcohol, S14,* 140–147. https://doi.org/10.15288/jsas.2002.s14.140

DeJong, W., Vince-Whitman, C., Colthurst, T., Cretella, M., Gilbreath, M., Rosati, M., & Zweig, K. (1998). *Environmental management: A comprehensive strategy for reducing alcohol and other drug use on college campuses.* U.S. Department of Education, Higher Education Center for Alcohol and Other Drug Prevention.

The Drug-Free Schools and Communities Act Amendments of 1989, Pub. L. No. 101-226, 103 Stat. 1928 (1989). https://bluetigerportal.lincolnu.edu/c/document_library/get_file?p_l_id=142227&folderId=1695938&name=DLFE-18424.pdf

Gehring, D. D., & Geraci, C. P. (1989). *Alcohol on campus: A compendium of the law and a guide to campus policy.* College Administration Publications.

Lange, J. E., Reed, M. B., Croff, J. M. K., & Clapp, J. D. (2008). College student use of *Salvia divinorum. Drug and Alcohol Dependence, 94*(1–3), 263–266. https://doi.org/10.1016/j.drugalcdep.2007.10.018

Lange, J. E., Daniel, J., Homer, K., Reed, M. B., & Clapp, J. D. (2010). *Salvia divinorum:* Effects and use among YouTube users. *Drug and Alcohol Dependence, 108*(1–2), 138–140. https://doi.org/10.1016/j.drugalcdep.2009.11.010

McCabe, S. E., Knight, J. R., Teter, C. J., & Wechsler, H. (2005). Non-medical use of prescription stimulants among U.S. college students: Prevalence and correlates from a national survey. *Addiction (Abingdon, England), 100*(1), 96–106. https://doi.org/10.1111/j.1360-0443.2005.00944.x

National Institute on Alcohol Abuse and Alcoholism. (2020). *CollegeAIM (Alcohol Intervention Matrix).* NIAAA. https://www.collegedrinkingprevention.gov/CollegeAIM

Schulenberg, J. E., Johnston, L. D., O'Malley, P. M., Bachman, J. G., Miech, R. A., & Patrick, M. E. (2020). *Monitoring the future national survey results on drug use, 1975–2019: Volume II, college students and adults ages 19–60.* Institute for Social Research, The University of Michigan.

Seligman, M. (2002). *Authentic happiness: Using the new positive psychology to realize your potential for lasting fulfillment.* Free Press.

Seligman, M., & Csikszentmihalyi, M. (2000). Positive psychology: An introduction. *American Psychologist, 55*(1), 5–14. https://doi.org/10.1037/0003-066X.55.1.5

Seligman, M., Steen, T., Park, N., & Peterson, C. (2005). Positive psychology progress: Empirical validation of interventions. *American Psychologist, 60*(5), 410–421. https://doi.org/10.1037/0003-066X.60.5.410

Shillington, A. M., Reed, M. B., Lange, J. E., Henry, S., & Clapp, J. D. (2006). College undergraduate Ritalin abusers in southwestern California: Protective and risk factors. *Journal of Drug Issues, 36*(4), 999–1014. https://doi.org/10.1177/002204260603600411

U.S. Department of Education, Office of Safe and Drug-Free Schools, Higher Education Center for Alcohol and Other Drug Abuse and Violence Prevention. (1997). *Complying with the Drug-Free Schools and Campuses Regulations [EDGAR Part 86]: A guide for university and college administrators.* https://safesupportivelearning.ed.gov/sites/default/files/hec/product/dfscr.pdf

Zimmerman, R., & DeJong, W. (2003). *Safe lanes on campus: A guide for preventing impaired driving and underage drinking.* U.S. Department of Education, Higher Education Center for Alcohol and Other Drug Prevention. https://safesupportivelearning.ed.gov/sites/default/files/hec/product/safelanes.pdf

CHAPTER 14

Identifying and Celebrating Progress

"Before college, I had never been one to party or drink, nor had I been exposed to it. Coming into my freshman year, I was exposed to binge drinking and consistent partying for the first time and found that I did not enjoy the culture that surrounded it. Because I prioritized my grades, extracurricular involvement, and aspired for career success, I found that binge drinking did not fit into the aspirations and visions that I held for myself, thus leading me to develop friendships that positively impacted my goals and my concept of healthy alcohol consumption."

—Sophomore from the Midwest at a public research university

As institutions of higher education, colleges and universities abound with idealism and experimentation, critical thinking and scientific expertise, and tradition and innovation. As such, the challenges of implementing and sustaining positive cultural change regarding drug and alcohol issues, although numerous, are both appropriate and manageable. That is, these institutions of learning are founded upon the growth and development of students. Therefore, it is incumbent upon institutions to address problems as widespread as drug and alcohol misuse, so that the larger goal of student success can be achieved. Further, higher education institutions have—within their faculty, staff, and alumni ranks—specialists and experts in various fields of study;

these individuals have many of the requisite skills for planning and orchestrating comprehensive campus strategies. Prevention specialists have knowledge and experience in the content area of drug and alcohol misuse prevention; they will benefit from drawing upon other campus personnel with varied areas of expertise. However, without grounded and comprehensive prevention efforts to address current and anticipated needs and problems related to drugs and alcohol, change in a positive direction is an unreasonable expectation.

The foundations, theoretical grounding, dedicated personnel, and requisite prioritization of prevention issues serve as foundations for ensuring that campus efforts are on track to achieve the desired outcomes. Throughout this journey, and with an eye toward continuous improvement, attention to areas of progress is vital. Further, attention to areas of limited impact, stalled efforts, challenges, or even unintended negative consequences is essential; understanding both the positive and negative factors aids in formulating new directions.

Because comprehensive campus prevention initiatives are relatively new—only a few decades old—their roots are not particularly deep or wide. With many campuses providing limited efforts and low prioritization, with substance misuse problems continuing, and with campus leaders believing their actions are sufficient to "get by," many challenges exist to achieving the desired impact. By documenting the importance of prevention efforts, enhancing the value and the return on investment, broadening the base of stakeholders, and engaging students more effectively, results can be significantly increased. In addition, as prevention efforts grow in depth and maturity, as more evaluation and documentation is shared, as additional support is garnered, and as communication and advocacy efforts are strengthened, the opportunity for more permanence of these efforts can be expected.

In this chapter, three contributor segments are offered to provide practical orientations held by campus prevention specialists. In the Case Study, Lindsey Hanlon provides the perspective of a new professional working in the field of substance abuse prevention and mental health promotion. Celebrating progress is essential to prevention efforts; in the Lessons From the Field segment, peer education advocate

Ann Quinn-Zobeck offers helpful suggestions for celebrating achievements. The Innovator highlighted in this chapter is Gerardo Gonzalez, a seasoned professional with research, scholarship, administration, and advocacy as central to his decades of service. He highlights the critical role of students and peer education in orchestrating a comprehensive and effective campus prevention strategy.

MAINTAINING PERSPECTIVE

Key to the effective leadership of campus prevention efforts is maintaining a multidimensional perspective, inclusive of the societal context, campus needs, student engagement, personnel support, and ultimate impact. Campus leaders and prevention specialists do not achieve the desired results by chance, nor are they achieved by minimal effort; results require vision, dedication, planning, engagement, and perseverance—some may even say pure grit. This multidimensional perspective is essential for any prevention specialist, regardless of whether they are new to the role or have been working in it or a related position for decades. For prevention specialists, the following points of observation, coupled with a sense of purpose, can sustain professional engagement throughout the process of leading the campus prevention effort.

First, *drug and alcohol abuse prevention is a large and complex job.* Comprehensive campus programs include policies and procedures, staffing and training, education and awareness, support services, resource development, strategic planning, needs assessment and evaluation, community relations, coalition building, and marketing and communication. No one blueprint for success exists; each campus prepares and adapts focus and strategies based on its needs and priorities, as well as the changing nature of its student body.

Second, *change is slow.* Systems change is slow and culture change is difficult—and the specific topic of drug and alcohol abuse brings its own challenges. Further, addressing substance issues is not a blank slate; change requires challenging and reshaping student, faculty, and staff knowledge, attitudes, and experiences. These efforts rarely yield immediate results. Celebrating any progress, even when modest, is important.

Third, *quality and grounded planning, although essential, does not guarantee that negative consequences will not occur.* Situations such as deaths, injuries, assaults, property damage, academic nonperformance, or other adverse consequences may still happen, although their likelihood may be lessened. Examining traffic safety offers some parallels: It is clear that heightened attention to drunk driving, through education, enforcement, and sanctions, has resulted in lowered fatalities. Further, the use of airbags and seat belts, and the installation of rumble strips, automobile crumple zones, and guardrails, all save lives. However, some car crashes are still not survivable. To expect perfection with prevention efforts is not reasonable; what is reasonable is to expect quality.

Fourth, prevention specialists should *focus on both the broad view and focused initiatives.* To implement a strategy because "it seems like the right thing to do" or "because the boss wants it" is not appropriate grounding. The broad view includes having overall goals and objectives, within which are framed the focused, individualized, and systemic strategies. The focused initiatives, such as education, training, curriculum, policies, and campaigns, each have a more narrow focus in support of the overall effort. Collecting data that center on the overall goals and the more focused strategies can help with documenting results and impact, and provide opportunities to highlight and celebrate progress.

Finally, *consistency must exist between the prevention strategies and the campus and organizational division's mission statements.* With so many mission statements focusing on issues such as "student well-being," "ethical foundations," "future directions," "societal impact," and "quality of life," anchors exist for campus prevention strategies. With guiding principles, assessment processes, evidence-informed approaches, innovation, and oversight, prevention specialists have many opportunities to maintain responsiveness to current issues and needs. Worksheet 14.1: Individualized Goals provides an exercise for prevention specialists to reflect on these five perspectives as they engage in their efforts and make plans for the future. With the enormity of the task at hand, these perspectives are vital. To provide perspective about leadership with prevention efforts, Lindsey Hanlon offers some refreshing views in Case Study 14.1 with her experience with campus prevention initiatives.

CASE STUDY 14.1

Being a New Professional to the Field

Lindsey Hanlon, MS, CPH

Network Prevention Manager, Division of Behavioral Health

Nebraska Department of Health and Human Services

When most people say they "fell into a job," it usually means it was out of necessity or by chance. I would say that I fell into my career through unusual circumstances. I had just finished my graduate degree in nutrition and health promotion and I was determined to get everyone eating healthy and living an active lifestyle. But many health careers require grant experience. I sought out a job in which I could obtain some of this experience, and landed one with Nebraska Department of Health and Human Services, working temporarily on a short-term opioid grant. One aspect of the grant entailed prevention. I became interested in learning more about the world of drug prevention through the lens of behavioral health. I then took over as the prevention manager for the division, and I began overseeing prevention-related grants.

It did not take me long to realize that professionals working in substance misuse prevention are some of the most passionate people in any field. The drive and the integrity that I see from people who have worked in the field for years is what did and continues to inspire me to move the needle forward in prevention. I am fortunate to be in a field with so much history, knowledge, drive, and expertise.

What I wish I had known earlier was that this career was even an option. I believe college settings serve as a perfect introduction to the field of substance abuse prevention and mental health promotion. For me, it would have helped to know what classes I should take, what groups I should get involved with, and what my major or minor should be. That would have laid much of the proper foundations for me. Fortunately, however, I have a great network of support both in my own state and through a network of dedicated individuals always willing to share their knowledge.

STRATEGIES

When identifying and celebrating progress associated with campus prevention efforts, it is important to imbed the following 10 approaches within the general implementation plans:

1. **Continuously reflect on overall programmatic aims.** This means maintaining alignment with the overall program's purposes and guiding principles. When reviewing the program, stepping back and examining the "big picture" as well as more focused elements is essential. When reporting individual or collective strategies, articulate clearly the context within which the strategy and its accomplishments is conducted (i.e., show "where it fits").
2. **Ensure that the overall vision, aims, goals, and objectives are reasonable and appropriate.** Although the vision represents the ultimate endpoint, it must be consistent with institutional and departmental mission statements. Specific progress should be assessed based on objectives that, when established, were viewed as attainable. Remember that the work of prevention specialists and the overall prevention strategy is long-range in nature.
3. **Incorporate measures, metrics, and monitoring.** These criteria provide data for restructuring various programmatic

elements and perhaps eliminating those that are not particularly effective. This attention to accountability and willingness to change helps maintain a positive overall perspective and encourages continued diligence with the ongoing work.

4. **Attend to what is being accomplished.** The ongoing metrics and monitoring offer opportunities to highlight impacts, results, improvements, and insights. Continuously honoring progress sustains the engagement of program personnel and partners. Noteworthy positive outcomes should also be shared with marketing and support-generating initiatives.
5. **Maintain documentation of efforts, results, and recommendations.** Planning documents, checklists, written protocols, data codebooks, summary sheets, staff reports, and summary reviews all benefit future strategies. These documents help prevention specialists replicate, modify, or improve on past efforts.
6. **Focus on longevity and institutionalization.** With sound planning and thorough documentation, concerns with staff turnover and potential loss of institutional knowledge can be minimized.
7. **Manage the boundaries.** Prevention specialists and campus leaders benefit from ensuring that the program's strategies remain aligned with the specified aims and goals. By "building a wall" to protect the program's integrity, particularly with naysayers and detractors, priorities can be maintained. Similarly, efforts to "move the wall outward" can engage new partners, address new audiences, or increase or alter the program's services.
8. **Keep a presence in the minds and hearts of campus leaders and stakeholders.** Prevention specialists benefit from finding ways to share the important and quality work with which they are engaged. Prevention work often goes unnoticed and unappreciated, particularly because effective prevention results in the reduction or absence of adverse consequences (e.g., death, injury, property damage, poor academic performance). Prevention specialists benefit from finding opportunities to share, on a regular basis, updates about their efforts with a wide variety

of campus leaders, stakeholders, partners, and other influential individuals and groups. Items to share include programmatic efforts, highlights of strategic initiatives, and data, which can all keep drug and alcohol issues a top priority.

9. **Become interwoven into the fabric of the institution.** By linking to the campus mission, partnering with campus offices, and integrating into support services, campus prevention efforts can be viewed by campus leaders and stakeholders as invaluable for enhancing the quality of life on campus. Academic efforts may include internships, class assignments, service activities, and mentoring. Outreach may incorporate training by prevention specialists; providing positive mutual aid networks for students; and collaborating on campuswide assessments of health promotion, resiliency, and campus culture.
10. **Implement relevant and appropriate evaluation processes.** Using quantitative and qualitative data is vital to monitor efforts, continually assess needs, and provide evidence of impact. With attention to service delivery, accountability, and continuous improvement, quality data collection can enhance the impact of the prevention program. This is a particularly appropriate role for those on campus with evaluation expertise, as they can provide their knowledge, learn more about the prevention efforts, and ultimately become supporters of the campus prevention efforts.

CELEBRATION

Celebrating successful prevention efforts on campus provides appropriate and well-deserved recognition for individuals and groups who have made a positive difference with the campus prevention initiative. In addition, these celebrations can highlight others who have been instrumental to the success of the campus effort; these include external constituencies, community leaders, and the larger public. Internal efforts, such as nurturing and supporting those engaged with prevention efforts, create pride; external approaches promote public awareness of the importance of sustained quality efforts.

Specific approaches for embracing this celebratory effort include the following:

1. **Actively seek ways to tell the story.** This ongoing process identifies ways to share results, progress, needs, and insights. Along with regular reports, highlights can be condensed into short narratives and shared with advisory groups, campus leaders, department/division heads, community leaders, and other stakeholders. Media coverage by local or national sources can be sought, with the assistance of campus media relations staff. Prevention specialists can prepare articles for professional journals, share results at professional conferences, prepare a regular newsletter or blog, or develop a quality website.
2. **Celebrate those doing the good work.** Prevention specialists can regularly sponsor awards or recognition for those who have contributed in remarkable ways to the overall campus prevention effort. Recognition can focus on individuals, groups, departments, or organizations, and can be as simple as a certificate or something more elaborate (e.g., plaque, medal, trophy, engraved item); recipient names can be advertised as well as codified on a permanent plaque or recognition venue.
3. **Have others serve as advocates and share good works.** Having other individuals provide accolades heightens external credibility for the campus prevention effort. This outside perspective is seen by campus and community leaders, as well as others on and off campus, as being neutral and valid, particularly if the spokesperson is from a group not traditionally aligned with prevention services. For example, faculty members in unaffiliated fields of study, community leaders, alumni, or student organization leaders can have a significant impact with their observations.
4. **Use the results of an external review to celebrate a prevention program's efforts.** Whether evaluating the program as a whole or individual components, a neutral external party's review can

validate the efforts. Positive observations and suggestions for enhancement can provide affirmation and generate support for the campus efforts.

5. **Ask partners and collaborators to promote campus strategies.** Co-sponsoring an event, resource, strategy, or initiative with another organization—either on campus or off campus—can broaden the base of participants because multiple membership groups and networks can be used; further, with co-sponsorships, the perception will be that other groups share the goals of the prevention effort. Collaboration can be as simple as asking another group to assist with one aspect of an event or strategy. In addition, having cooperative efforts can result in greater understanding by the collaborators about the prevention effort; as more collaborators become involved, greater support is likely.
6. **Practice ongoing self-reflection.** Engaging in self-reflection with prevention specialists individually, and as a group, provides positive affirmation for identifying and celebrating progress. This process helps individuals and the group become more appreciative of the work being done. Self-reflection may include testimonials from those affected by the campus prevention efforts, as well as data that demonstrate positive outcomes achieved with specific efforts. Self-reflection may also incorporate thoughts about what the campus and campus culture would have been like had there been no prevention effort, and/or no support for recovery initiatives, and/or inadequate policies, and/or no peer education, and/or no training for staff, and/or no awareness campaigns.

Any of these approaches can promote program visibility, which in turn supports further awareness by campus decision makers and other stakeholders, which then generates further support—all critical for sustainability and long-term impact. In Lessons From the Field 14.1, Ann Quinn-Zobeck offers some practical suggestions from the perspective of an advocate of staff members and peer educators.

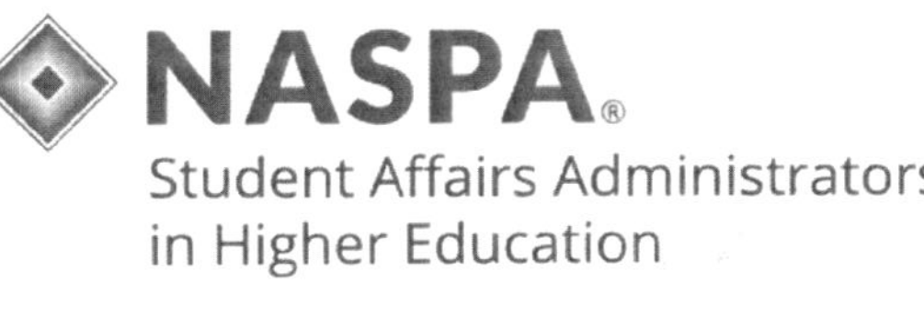

111 K Street, NE, 10th Floor
Washington, DC 20002
Tel: 202.265.7500
Fax: 202.898.5737
www.naspa.org

May 12, 2021

Ann Quinn-Zobeck
BACCHUS / NASPA (ret.)
1858 12th Avenue
Greeley, CO 80631

Dear Ann,

Congratulations on the publication of *Leading Campus Drug and Alcohol Abuse Prevention: Grounded Approaches for Student Impact*. Thank you for contributing to this important text. As a token of our gratitude, we have enclosed a complimentary copy of the book. Additional copies may be purchased at the author discounted price by calling the NASPA Bookstore at 202-265-7500 (press option 4).

Thank you for your continued commitment to NASPA and the student affairs profession. We look forward to sharing this book with NASPA members and encourage you to promote it through your professional networks.

Warm regards,

Melissa L. Dahne
Senior Director of Publications

the leading association for the advancement, health, and sustainability of the student affairs profession

LESSONS FROM THE FIELD 14.1

Prepare to Celebrate Small Wins

Ann Quinn-Zobeck, PhD
Senior Director (retired), BACCHUS
Initiatives and Training
NASPA–Student Affairs Administrators in Higher Education

All types of health promotion efforts in higher education are working to change the campus culture, thereby creating a healthier environment. Culture change, however, takes sustained effort over time. Although we may envision a campus where every student embraces healthy behaviors, focusing on that large goal can become disheartening in the day-to-day work of health promotion. In my own work on college campuses, I learned to recognize and celebrate the progressive steps toward a goal and those who contributed to those small wins.

What do I mean by small wins? Identify the concrete actions needed to create change and find ways to celebrate their completion. Data collection is a good place to start, as it helps identify student attitudes, behavior, and issues. Steps to gathering data may include creating a survey, obtaining internal review board approval of the survey, obtaining permission from faculty to use class time to administer the survey, offering incentives to increase survey return rates, and conducting the survey. As your employees and volunteers meet regularly, take time to announce what data collection benchmarks have been met. Publicly thank the staff, volunteers, and allies who have contributed. Plus, if your data show progress over time, like a shift in attitudes or behavior, that is worth noting.

Look for indicators that show your efforts are having an

impact, even if they seem miniscule (Center for Community Health and Development, n.d.). For example, for a social media campaign, track the number of views, and when you reach a benchmark (say, 500 views or likes), bring cupcakes to the next meeting. Or have a pizza party or play putt-putt golf instead of having a weekly meeting. I once presented each of my peer educators with a small potted plant to emphasize that change takes attention, care, and time before we see the results of our efforts blossom.

Finally, to achieve small wins, it is important to set up your team for success. Keep your staff, volunteers, allies, and yourself motivated by identifying attainable outcomes; this means specifying milestones along the way to the larger goal. Celebrate achievements; this will keep people engaged.

ADDITIONAL OPPORTUNITIES FOR SUPPORT AND GROUNDING

Ongoing attention to and support for the campus prevention effort can be obtained in varied ways. Whether through quality efforts, marketing, outreach, professional development, or networking, these efforts honor the momentum of large and small achievements.

The overarching priority of campus prevention efforts is *maintaining high-quality efforts*. These must remain true to the established purposes, including goals and objectives that are meaningful and current. Regular reporting, updating objectives based on changing student needs, incorporating best practices, continuously collecting data, monitoring for improvement, and engaging campus decision makers regularly are all essential to maintaining relevance and support.

Central to the success of prevention programs is the *marketing of individual and group efforts*. Continuously "telling the story" is essential. Prevention specialists should find opportunities to correct misconceptions common with their audiences, such as outdated information, unsupportive attitudes, and views of lack of impact of personal efforts. Prevention specialists should also cite the challenges they face, and ways other individuals and groups can be supportive. Finding ways to share the campus prevention efforts' strategies, results, and recommendations with various audiences, such as at conferences and articles for professional journals or newsletters, substantiates the role of a prevention effort within an institution of higher education. Engaging others in framing and telling the story helps significantly; this includes students involved with the program's services, professional public relations personnel, and marketing and advertising faculty and students.

Outreach efforts that go beyond the core functions of the prevention specialist, such as is found with a formal position description, further enhance the importance of prevention professionals for the campus. These efforts have an aim of promoting greater understanding and support among other constituencies about the prevention efforts. This commitment can be done by involvement such as serving on other departments' planning or advisory groups, conducting training, giving a public lecture, attending a sponsored event, or being a member of a search committee to fill another department's personnel vacancy. Involvement with academic partners, such as co-teaching or teaching a course within an academic department, conducting a class session, or serving as an academic advisor for students demonstrates that the prevention specialist is engaged with the academic priorities of the institution. Finding ways to infuse professional expertise and understanding into existing or new courses, internships, independent studies, senior seminars, and mentorships advances the integration of prevention science.

Ongoing professional development for prevention specialists is critical for maintaining currency and relevance. Through self-reflection, networking, and reading, professional competencies can be identified and developed. Continuous improvement opportunities abound, with free and low-cost events and webinars sponsored by professional associations, state or federal agencies, and institutions of higher education. Reviewing current research, books, policy briefs, and other documents provides grounding for self-study as well as regular discussions with colleagues. Engaging in regular professional development activities is important for identifying ways to adapt and innovate so approaches of value can be identified.

Networking and collaboration with others on campus and in the community ensures that the prevention effort permeates the campus community and is not an isolated "silo-based" approach. Identifying opportunities for quality relationships with colleagues in units affiliated with drug and alcohol issues is critical; these typically include multiple units within student affairs, such as residence life, student activities, health, and counseling. Also helpful are relationships with colleagues in unaffiliated areas, often including athletics, faculty units, alumni affairs, public relations, and campus police. Engagement in a *statewide consortium* is useful for ongoing support, professional development, and collective action. Finally, identifying *colleagues for grant-funded efforts* can expand the scope of campus efforts, build collaborative relationships, promote greater program awareness, and dramatically expand the impact of the prevention effort.

The premise of these strategies is to institutionalize prevention efforts and ingratiate others on campus to these efforts and their personnel. These are ganglion efforts whereby campus prevention specialists seek, on an ongoing basis, ways of getting intricately involved with other entities and initiatives on campus.

The important work of campus prevention specialists is aided by innovative approaches, such as those embodied with the range of peer education strategies. As described in the Innovator 14.1 segment, Gerardo Gonzalez introduced innovative approaches decades ago with a student-based initiative on one campus; at the time, this approach that focused on peer education was novel. The fact that his initial idea took off, became a national movement, and remains strong is significant; this historical perspective serves to inspire and motivate prevention specialists and campus leaders to dream big and then actualize their dreams for their campuses.

INNOVATOR 14.1

Peer Education: An Idea for the Ages

Gerardo M. González, PhD
Dean Emeritus
Indiana University

In his classic volume titled *Where Colleges Fail*, Nevitt Sanford (1967) called the attitude surrounding drinking on campus "a conspiracy of silence." That began to change in 1975, when the National Institute on Alcohol Abuse and Alcoholism sponsored a meeting of representatives from the major public universities of all 50 states plus 12 private and minority institutions on the campus of the University of Notre Dame. The purpose of the meeting was to review the contents of the *Whole College Catalog About Drinking* (Hewitt, 1977), a publication designed to encourage universities to focus on the issue of alcohol use and abuse on campus and stimulate education and communication efforts to prevent these problems. At the time, I was a graduate assistant in the Office of Student Services at the University of Florida (UF) working under the supervision of Thomas G. Goodale, dean of students.

Dean Goodale represented Florida at the Notre Dame 50+12 meeting. Motivated by what he heard, upon his return to campus, Dean Goodale asked me to lead an effort to develop an alcohol education program at UF. I was excited about the challenge, yet unsure where to begin. Informed by the research literature, I realized that the most successful prevention programs utilized positive peer pressure to get their message across. Just as negative peer pressure was a factor in the onset of alcohol use and abuse, positive peer pressure could raise awareness of the problem and promote moderation.

Armed with that information, I created a local program at UF that ultimately became a national organization known as Boost Alcohol Consciousness Concerning the Health of University Students (BACCHUS). The BACCHUS philosophy was simple: Identify specific behaviors associated with a lower incidence of drinking problems and mobilize students to promote them (Gonzalez, 1978). The idea caught on at campuses nationwide. When I left BACCHUS in 1986, it had chapters in 260 campuses in 47 states and Canada. In 2011, Stephen R. Covey, world-renowned leadership author, wrote, "Gerardo and his friends set in motion an entirely new approach to helping young people avoid risky behaviors, what is now called the 'peer education' or 'peer support' movement . . . and it works, perhaps better than any other approach out there" (p. 188). In 2014, BACCHUS became part of NASPA–Student Affairs Administrators in Higher Education, supporting student leadership and peer education on health and safety issues nationally and internationally.

What Dean Goodale, a small group of committed students, and I started almost 50 years ago as a student-led alcohol abuse prevention effort on one campus has grown to be the largest alcohol and other drug abuse prevention and health promotion student organization in higher education. The basic BACCHUS philosophy used positive peer pressure to promote health and prevent related problems; today, influenced to some extent by that philosophy, every U.S campus provides a variety of peer education programs focusing on alcohol abuse, tobacco, violence prevention, sexual health, safety, physical and mental health, and more. BACCHUS did not eliminate drinking nor all the problems associated with alcohol abuse on campus, but the conspiracy of silence of which Sanford wrote in 1967 has been broken. Could that have happened without BACCHUS? It is hard to say. We know, however, that the peer approach on campus to alcohol problems, specifically, and health promotion, more generally, has made a difference and is growing. Based on solid research, a clear philosophy, and quality student engagement, BACCHUS's foundations provide direction for the future.

CONCLUSION

Prevention specialists and campus leaders aim to make a difference with drug and alcohol misuse and related issues. Acknowledging the mammoth size of this aim, coupled with acknowledging that change is often slow, opportunities must be sought to highlight the successes that do occur. Although continuous improvement is sought and returns on investment are essential, broader perspectives about the nature and scope of the task are critical. Being grounded in reward systems for effort and impact, and recognizing the key roles of individuals and groups on campus and in the community, is important. With the implementation of numerous engagement strategies and celebratory approaches and complemented by other innovative and meaningful efforts, heartfelt efforts are themselves rewarded.

REFERENCES

Center for Community Health and Development. (n.d.). *Chapter 41: Rewarding accomplishments.* University of Kansas. http://ctb.ku.edu/en/table-of-contents/assessment/assessing-community-needs-and-resources/conduct-concerns-surveys/main

Covey, S. (2011). *The 3rd alternative: Solving life's most difficult problems.* Free Press.

Gonzalez, G. M. (1978). What do you mean prevention? *Journal of Alcohol and Drug Education, 23*(3), 14–23.

Hewitt, K. (1977). *The whole college catalog about drinking.* National Institute on Alcohol Abuse and Alcoholism.

Sanford, N. (1967). *Where colleges fail: A study of the student as a person.* Jossey-Bass.

APPENDIX A

Worksheets

WORKSHEET 1.1
CAMPUS ISSUES OF CONCERN

	Current data	Previous data	Audience or population of concern	State/ Regional data	National data
Alcohol use (monthly)					
Alcohol use (daily)					
Heavy (binge) drinking					
Marijuana use (monthly)					
Marijuana use (daily)					
Opiate use					
Other illicit drug use					
Prescription drug misuse					
Public intoxication					
Property damage					
Sexual assault					
Impaired driving					
Emergency room transports					
Health center contacts					
Academic performance					

WORKSHEET 1.2
CAMPUS INCIDENTS

	Total number	Percent alcohol-related	Number alcohol-related
Campus grounds			
Property damage Rowdy behavior Public intoxication Consumption of alcohol Other: ____________			
Residence halls			
Property damage Personal injury Injury to others Behavioral infraction Quality of life Other: ____________			
Health			
Health center contacts Emergency room/Hospital admissions Other: ____________			
Community			
Property damage Noise complaints Trash Parking Other: ____________			
Traffic safety			
Driving while intoxicated Traffic crashes Traffic injuries Bicycle incidents Pedestrian injuries Other: ____________			

Note. Prepared by David Anderson and George Mason University's Center for the Advancement of Public Health.

WORKSHEET 1.3
APPLICATIONS OF THE SOCIAL-ECOLOGICAL MODEL

	Nature of concern	Ways to reduce risk factors	Ways to enhance protective factors
Societal			
Culture			
Historical trauma			
Norms and access			
Socioeconomic status			
Media			
Laws and policies			
Community			
Faith-based institutions			
Schools			
Workplaces			
Neighborhoods			
Relationship			
Peers			
Parents			
Teachers			
Individual			
Knowledge			
Attitudes			
Interpersonal interactions			

WORKSHEET 1.4
REASONS TO BE CONCERNED PLANNING SHEET

Specific Issue	Rating	Ranking
Health and safety		
Death		
Injury		
Harm to others		
Personal health		
Impaired driving		
Safe environment		
Individual factors		
Academic		
Human potential		
Cultural engagement		
Quality learning		
Physical performance		
Management and financial		
Legal liability		
Institutional reputation		
Attrition		
Recruitment		
Alumni support		
Consistency with mission statement		
Faculty engagement		
Staff engagement		
Financial costs		
Property damage		
Other		
Compliance with the law		
Town–gown relationships		
Community support		
Leadership on societal issues		
Preparation of future leaders		

WORKSHEET 2.1
CAMPUS SELF-ASSESSMENT

	Strongly disagree				Strongly agree
Overall					
Adequate funding is being spent on our campus on alcohol abuse prevention.	1	2	3	4	5
Our campus has a comprehensive approach to alcohol abuse prevention.	1	2	3	4	5
Our campus has clearly defined goals and objectives for alcohol abuse prevention.	1	2	3	4	5
Our campus has consensus between students and administrators on the direction of our alcohol abuse and prevention efforts.	1	2	3	4	5
Our campus has formally identified the principles/philosophical underpinnings of its alcohol abuse prevention efforts.	1	2	3	4	5
Our campus utilizes the most effective alcohol abuse prevention strategies (based on professional literature, conference workshops, training, etc.).	1	2	3	4	5
Our campus remains committed to finding and applying effective alcohol abuse prevention strategies.	1	2	3	4	5
Our alcohol abuse prevention efforts have been institutionalized.	1	2	3	4	5

	Not at all	Poor	Fair	Good	Very well
Prevention and education					
Prevention and education efforts overall	1	2	3	4	5
Variety of approaches included in campus substance abuse education and prevention efforts	1	2	3	4	5

Attention paid to unique needs of various groups (e.g., first-year students, student-athletes, people of color, fraternity/sorority, LGBTQIA+)	1	2	3	4	5
Policy and enforcement					
Policy efforts overall	1	2	3	4	5
Enforcement efforts overall	1	2	3	4	5
Reporting and recordkeeping regarding alcohol violations	1	2	3	4	5
Support and intervention					
Support and intervention services overall	1	2	3	4	5
Services for students with a drinking problem	1	2	3	4	5
Services for students in recovery	1	2	3	4	5
Curriculum and training					
Curricular content and training on drug/alcohol issues overall	1	2	3	4	5
Training for paraprofessional staff	1	2	3	4	5
Faculty preparation on policies, problem identification, intervention, referral	1	2	3	4	5
Evaluation					
Needs assessment and evaluation overall	1	2	3	4	5
Campus assessment of program effectiveness	1	2	3	4	5
Student survey on drug/alcohol knowledge, attitudes behavior, perceptions	1	2	3	4	5
Systematic data collection on alcohol involvement with campus issues	1	2	3	4	5
Staffing and resources					
Staffing and resources overall	1	2	3	4	5
Presence of a coordinator/specialist on alcohol/substance abuse	1	2	3	4	5
Campus planning group with strategic plan and measurable outcomes	1	2	3	4	5
Collaboration with various campus groups/organizations	1	2	3	4	5

Note. Prepared by David Anderson and George Mason University's Center for the Advancement of Public Health.

WORKSHEET 2.2
CAMPUS VISION DEVELOPMENT

How would you describe the ideal campus culture, particularly as it relates to drugs and alcohol?		
	Outcomes	Processes
What do you want to prevent?		
What do you want to promote?		

WORKSHEET 2.3
OBSTACLES AND CHALLENGES FOR ACHIEVING VISIONS

Attitudes
Students
Faculty and Staff
Support and Recovery
Resources
Administrative and Managerial
Institutionwide
Other

WORKSHEET 3.1
ACTION FRAMEWORK
Based on the Health Belief Model

	Knowledge	Attitudes	Skills-based knowledge	Skills	Social settings	Socioeconomic factors
Perceived susceptibility						
Perceived severity						
Perceived benefits						
Perceived barriers						
Cues to action						
Self-efficacy						

WORKSHEET 3.2
STAGES OF CHANGE WORKSHEET

Stage	Considerations for change strategies	Planned change strategies
Precontemplation	Increase awareness of need for change Personalize information about risks and benefits	
Contemplation	Motivate Encourage making specific plans	
Preparation	Assist with developing and implementing concrete action plansHelp set gradual goals	
Action	Assist with feedback, problem solving, social support, and reinforcement	
Maintenance	Assist with coping, issuing reminders, finding alternatives, avoiding slips/relapses	

Note. Adapted from "Stages and Processes of Self-Change in Smoking: Toward An Integrative Model of Change," by J. Prochaska and C. DiClemente, 1983, *Journal of Consulting and Clinical Psychology, 5,* 390–395. Copyright © 1983 by the American Psychological Association. Adapted with permission.

WORKSHEET 3.3
PREVENTION TASK FORCE PLANNING GUIDE

Universal	Selective	Indicated
All members of the campus community • Students • Faculty • Staff	First-year students	Self-referral (for self or others)
Members of the surrounding community	Student-athletes • Team leader • First-year member • Member	Grave first offense
Parents	Fraternity/sorority • Leader • First-year member • Member	More than one offense
	Judicial referral	Medical situation
		In recovery
Considerations: Specific substances (e.g., alcohol, marijuana, illicit drugs, prescription drugs); role of intermediaries; direct strategies (e.g., information, signs/symptoms, policies/laws); indirect strategies (e.g., root causes, motivations, alternative activities); timing (i.e., immediate vs. later); roles of self and others		

Note. Adapted from *The Institute of Medicine Framework and Its Implication for the Advancement of Prevention Policy, Programs and Practice* (SMA-4205), by J. F. Springer and J. Phillips, 2007, U.S. Department of Health and Human Services (http://ca-sdfsc.org/docs/resources/SDFSC_IOM_Policy.pdf). In the public domain.

WORKSHEET 3.4
STRATEGIC PREVENTION FRAMEWORK

Assessment	
Capacity	
Planning	
Implementation	
Evaluation	
Sustainability and cultural competence	

Note. Adapted from *Focus on Prevention* (Publication No. [SMA] 10–4120) by Substance Abuse and Mental Health Services Administration), 2017, Center for Substance Abuse Prevention, Substance Abuse and Mental Health Services Administration (https://store. samhsa.gov/product/Focus-on-Prevention/sma10-4120?referer=from_search_result). In the public domain.

WORKSHEET 3.5

COLLEGEAIM STRATEGY PLANNING WORKSHEET

COLLEGEAIM

STRATEGY PLANNING WORKSHEET

Use this worksheet or download a copy to capture your thoughts about your current strategies and new ones you'd like to explore. Keep in mind:

Priorities: Which alcohol-related issues are of most concern to your campus? Make sure your school's needs and goals are well defined, and keep them front and center as you fill in the worksheet.

Effectiveness: Does research show that your current strategies are effective in addressing your priority issues? Might others be *more* effective?

Balance: Realistically assess what you can do with your available resources. Strike a balance, if possible, between individual- and environmental-level strategies, and between strategies that will face few barriers and can be put in place quickly and others that may take longer to implement. Consider the financial cost relative to the program's expected effectiveness and the approximate percentage of the student body that the strategy will reach.

CURRENT STRATEGIES

Strategy Name (and the IND or ENV identifier from *CollegeAIM*, if applicable)	**Individual or Environmental?**		***CollegeAIM* Ratings**				**Notes and Next Steps:** Keep as is? Modify to boost effectiveness? Add complementary strategies? Shift to more effective options?
	✓ IND	**✓ ENV**	**Effectiveness**	**Cost**	**Barriers**	**Reach: Broad or Focused (% of students)**	

POSSIBLE NEW STRATEGIES

Strategy Name (and the IND or ENV identifier from *CollegeAIM*)	**Individual or Environmental?**		***CollegeAIM* Ratings**				**Notes and Next Steps:** Staff training or hiring needed? Other resources? Does the strategy require a plan for conducting an outcome evaluation?
	✓ IND	**✓ ENV**	**Effectiveness**	**Cost**	**Barriers**	**Reach: Broad or Focused (% of students)**	

Note. Reprinted from *Planning Alcohol Interventions Using NIAAA's CollegeAIM Alcohol Intervention Matrix* (Publication No. 19-AA-8017, p. 27), by National Institute on Alcohol Abuse and Alcoholism, 2019, U.S. Department of Health and Human Services, National Institutes of Health (https://www.collegedrinkingprevention.gov/CollegeAIM/Resources/NIAAA_College_Matrix_Booklet.pdf). In the public domain.

WORKSHEET 4.1
DRUG AND ALCOHOL POLICIES AND PROCEDURES CHECKLIST

Foundations for Policy

- ☐ Overall constructs and standards
- ☐ Rationale for specific content elements

Policy Dissemination

- ☐ Reach (who)
- ☐ Frequency
- ☐ Approach (print, website)

Policy Updates

- ☐ Frequency
- ☐ Extent of update (minor update vs. significant overhaul)
- ☐ Who involved
- ☐ Approval processes

Policy Review

- ☐ Frequency
- ☐ Extent of review
- ☐ Monitoring of results
- ☐ Impact of policy implementation (desired and unintended consequences)
- ☐ Processes used (internal, external)
- ☐ Who involved

Audiences Affected

- ☐ Students
- ☐ Faculty
- ☐ Staff
- ☐ Paraprofessional staff
- ☐ Visitors
- ☐ Alumni

Settings

- ☐ Entire campus
- ☐ Residence halls
- ☐ Classrooms
- ☐ Offices
- ☐ Athletic facilities
- ☐ Public grounds

Content Areas

- ☐ Alcohol availability
    - Permitted
    - Conditions of availability (e.g., food, alcohol-free beverages, hours)
    - Age restrictions
    - Monitoring of compliance
    - What may be served (e.g., beer, wine, distilled spirits)?
    - Settings
    - Use of trained servers
- ☐ Specified standards for behaviors of concern
    - Public intoxication
    - Engagement and bystander intervention (e.g., Good Samaritan)
    - Medical amnesty (e.g., alcohol, marijuana, illicit drugs)
    - Misuse of prescription drugs
    - Impaired driving
    - Setting (e.g., residence halls, on campus, campus-sponsored events, student organizations, study abroad)

- Hospital admissions (e.g., notification, referral)
- Health center (e.g., notification, referral)
- Parental notification

☐ Underage drinking

- Reduced access by under 21
- ID cards

☐ Event planning

- Standards for events with alcohol
- Registration
- Guest access
- Event host role (e.g., training, preparation, monitoring)
- Law enforcement role

☐ Consequences

- Individual violations
- Group violations
- Repeat offenses
- Monitoring for substance use disorder

☐ Marketing and advertising

- Content permitted
- Sponsors permitted
- Settings and venues
- Nature of marketing and sponsorship

☐ Enforcement

- Consistency
- Consequences for noncompliance
- Handling repeat offenses (e.g., individual, group)

☐ Education and prevention

- Pre-matriculation requirements
- Early intervention
- Staff training (e.g., professional, paraprofessional)
- Faculty preparedness
- Curriculum infusion
- Incorporation within universal, selective, and indicated prevention strategies

WORKSHEET 4.2
ORGANIZATIONAL SELF-ASSESSMENT

Collaboration and Contacts

1. **Over the specified period of time, please report the number of times you had contact with each group/individual regarding campus drug and alcohol issues. Also report the quality of interaction on a 7-point scale, with 1 = poor quality and 7 = high quality; N/A for no contact.**

	Number of times					Quality
Campus leaders	**None**	**1–2**	**3–5**	**6–10**	**More than 10**	**(1–7) (N/A)**
President						
Chief student affairs officer						
Drug/alcohol coordinator						
Counseling center						
Residence life department						
Health services						
Judicial affairs						
Police/security						
Faculty leadership/ council/senate						
Athletic department						
Student government						
Student organizations						
Other:						
	Number of times					**Quality**
Community leaders	**None**	**1–2**	**3–5**	**6–10**	**More than 10**	**(1–7) (N/A)**
Mayor/city council						
Police/sheriff						
Judicial services/ court						
Bar/tavern owners						

Campus leaders	Number of times					Quality
	None	1–2	3–5	6–10	More than 10	(1–7) (N/A)
President						
Chief student affairs officer						
Drug/alcohol coordinator						
Chamber of commerce/bureau of merchants						
Health officials/ hospitals						
Drug/alcohol services						
Recreation/tourism						
Other:						

2. **Please rate the collaboration between your campus and the surrounding community:**

	Poor	Fair	Neutral	Good	Excellent
Campus rules and policies					
Local ordinances, laws, and policies					
Educational programs					
Identifying funding and resources					
Alcohol-free social activities					
Recreational activities					
Treatment and related support services					
Goal setting					
Defining health messages					
Discussing attitudes					
Outlining solutions					
Discussing knowledge gaps					
Specifying underlying philosophical stance					
Resolving problems and obstacles					
Overall					

3. **Is there any forum that brings together the college, local community, and state leaders to address drug and alcohol issues? ❑ Yes ❑No**

If yes, please describe briefly.

4. **How clearly defined are the following for your campus' drug and alcohol prevention strategies?**

	Not at all				To a great extent	Don't know
General mission	1	2	3	4	5	DK
Overall goals	1	2	3	4	5	DK
Measurable objectives	1	2	3	4	5	DK
Action steps	1	2	3	4	5	DK
Communication strategies	1	2	3	4	5	DK
Social norms marketing effort	1	2	3	4	5	DK
Specific roles for campus groups	1	2	3	4	5	DK
Specific roles for community groups	1	2	3	4	5	DK
Agreement on these roles and responsibilities	1	2	3	4	5	DK

5. **Focusing on the high schools in the vicinity of your campus, on how many occasions during the past 4 months has your campus:**

- Provided drug/alcohol prevention or support services and resources to college-bound students?

- Provided information on campus drug/alcohol policies?

- Provided information about the campus drug/alcohol environment?

6. **Does your campus have an established point of contact with local high schools to address drug and alcohol issues? ❑Yes ❑No**

7. **Over the past 4 months, approximately how many times have you initiated contact with each of the following groupings of people in the state or region regarding identification of solutions or problem-solving of campus and community drug/alcohol issues?**

	Face-to-face	**Email**	**Writing**	**Telephone**	**Other (please specify)**
Consortium member					
Colleague at another college that is not in the consortium					
Local agency or organization					
State agency or organization					

8. **If you had a question you wanted to ask, how comfortable do you feel doing so?**

	Not at all comfortable	**Slightly comfortable**	**Somewhat comfortable**	**Fairly comfortable**	**Very comfortable**
Consortium member					
State college colleague					
State agency/ organization					

9. **In the last 4 months, has your campus attempted to acquire external funding (e.g., federal, state, local, or private grants) for its alcohol/drug abuse efforts?**
❑Yes ❑No

10. **In the last 3 years, has your campus been successful in acquiring external funding (e.g., federal, state, local, or private grants) for its alcohol/drug abuse efforts?**
❑Yes ❑No

Data Collection

11. **When did you last conduct a survey of student drug/alcohol behavior? (month/year)**

12. **When did you last conduct a survey of student drug/alcohol attitudes? (month/year)**

13. **When did you last conduct a survey of student drug/alcohol knowledge? (month/year)**

    ☐ Which survey did you use?
    ☐ Core survey
    ☐ NCHA
    ☐ Other (please specify) ____________________

14. **Which data collection process did you use? (check all that apply)**

    ☐ Classroom distribution
    ☐ Residence hall
    ☐ Web
    ☐ Mailed survey
    ☐ Academic department
    ☐ Intercept interview
    ☐ Other (please specify) ____________

15. **What other data collection approaches were used? (check all that apply)**

    ☐ Review of archival data
    ☐ Incorporate new data
    ☐ Key informant interviews
    ☐ Literature review
    ☐ Focus group
    ☐ Observations
    ☐ Meetings/discussions
    ☐ Other (please specify)

16. **Have you conducted a faculty/staff survey on drug/alcohol issues? ❑Yes ❑No**

17. **To what extent does the drug/alcohol programming on your campus address the unique needs of each of the following demographic groups?**

	Not at all				To a great extent	Not appli-cable	Don't know
First-year students	1	2	3	4	5	NA	DK
Transfer students	1	2	3	4	5	NA	DK
Fraternity/sorority members	1	2	3	4	5	NA	DK
International students	1	2	3	4	5	NA	DK
Persons of Color	1	2	3	4	5	NA	DK

Residence hall students	1	2	3	4	5	NA	DK
Gay/lesbian/ bisexual students	1	2	3	4	5	NA	DK
Student-athletes	1	2	3	4	5	NA	DK
Student-veterans	1	2	3	4	5	NA	DK
Student government members	1	2	3	4	5	NA	DK
Club/organization members	1	2	3	4	5	NA	DK
Men	1	2	3	4	5	NA	DK
Women	1	2	3	4	5	NA	DK
Faculty/staff	1	2	3	4	5	NA	DK

18. List three major steps/processes your campus has used to develop its drug/alcohol strategies.

1.

2.

3.

19. To what extent did you use each of the following resources/services to develop your campus' drug/alcohol strategies?

	Not at all				To a great extent	Not appli-cable	Don't know
State/regional conference	1	2	3	4	5	NA	DK
State/regional retreat	1	2	3	4	5	NA	DK
National meeting on drug/alcohol issues	1	2	3	4	5	NA	DK
Informal networking with colleagues	1	2	3	4	5	NA	DK
Regional consortium meeting	1	2	3	4	5	NA	DK
Regular campus task force meetings	1	2	3	4	5	NA	DK

Campus task force planning retreat	1	2	3	4	5	NA	DK
Review of professional literature	1	2	3	4	5	NA	DK
Private meetings with key campus leaders	1	2	3	4	5	NA	DK
Private meetings with key community leaders	1	2	3	4	5	NA	DK
Mandate from campus president/ chancellor	1	2	3	4	5	NA	DK
Other	1	2	3	4	5	NA	DK

20. To what extent does each of the following prevention approaches guide your campus's efforts to reduce alcohol abuse?

	Not at all				**Very Much**		**Not at all**				**Very Much**
Harm reduction	1	2	3	4	5	Responsible drinking	1	2	3	4	5
Abstinence	1	2	3	4	5	Responsible decision making	1	2	3	4	5
Problem reduction	1	2	3	4	5	Lifelong skills development	1	2	3	4	5
Promoting healthy norms	1	2	3	4	5	Values development	1	2	3	4	5
Healthy life choices	1	2	3	4	5	Enforcement	1	2	3	4	5
Other	1	2	3	4	5	Other	1	2	3	4	5

Note. Prepared by David Anderson and George Mason University's Center for the Advancement of Public Health.

WORKSHEET 5.1
COMMUNICATION RESULTS

	Change	Reinforce	Introduce
Intention			
Attitude			
Knowledge			
Belief • Susceptibility • Severity • Barriers • Self-efficacy			
Skills			
Other			

WORKSHEET 7.1
MOTIVATIONAL INTERVIEWING (MI) CHECKLIST

Date/Time:	Provider:	Observer:

What is the ratio of open-ended to closed-ended questions during the session? In the spaces below, place a check mark for each question asked.				
Open-ended:	How...	What...	Tell me about...	Describe...
Closed-ended:				

What is the ratio of MI-compliant statements made during the session? Place a check mark for each statement made.				
Statements:	Affirming:	Directive:	Giving information:	Confrontation:

Place a check mark for each reflected listening strategy used in session.			
Repeating:	Rephrasing:	Paraphrasing:	Reflection of feeling:

How many times in the session are the client's words summarized? Place a check mark for each summarization.
Summarizing:

How many times in the session did the provider use basic or advanced MI strategies? Place a check mark by each selected strategy.	
Basic strategies	
Use of decisional balance	
Therapist expresses optimism	
Focus on health, not illness	
Client makes argument for change	
Shift focus if resistance is present	
Normalize client ambivalence	
Client identifies goals/values	
Advanced strategies	
Amplified reflection	

Double-sided reflection	
Agreement with twist	
Reframing	

Please rate the provider's use of MI principles below.					
Supporting self-efficacy	1 Ineffective	2	3 Neutral	4	5 Effective
Developing discrepancy	1 Ineffective	2	3 Neutral	4	5 Effective
Rolling with resistance	1 Righting reflex	2	3 Neutral	4	5 Avoids argumenta-tion
Did provider change strategies if score is < 3?	Yes			No	

Based on your observation of the session, please note the stage of change that best describes the patient's readiness for change. PC = Precontemplation, C = Contemplation, P = Preparation, A = Action, M = Maintenance, and R = Relapse					
PC	C	P	A	M	R

Note. Developed by Thomas Hall at the University of Central Florida.

WORKSHEET 7.2
ALCOHOL RISK REDUCTION SCALE

Circle only one number that best describes your confidencelevel.

Think about the NEXT 6 weeks: Imagine you are in a social situation where alcohol is accessible.How confident are you that you will use any of these protective strategies?

Please rate your confidence level for each of the following behaviors.

	Not at all confident					**Very confident**
Pace and space drinks (at least 15 min. between drinks).	0	20	40	60	80	100
Mentally keep track of drinks.	0	20	40	60	80	100
Keep track of drinks by recording use (cell phone, monitoring card, etc.).	0	20	40	60	80	100
Eat before and drinking.	0	20	40	60	80	100
Eat a meal or snacks while drinking.	0	20	40	60	80	100
Alternate alcoholic and nonalcoholic drinks.	0	20	40	60	80	100
Avoid rapid consumption of alcohol (chugging, shots, beer funnels, etc.).	0	20	40	60	80	100
Avoid drinking shots of hard liquor.	0	20	40	60	80	100
Set a predetermined limit of drinks.	0	20	40	60	80	100
Avoid drinking with friends who drink excessively.	0	20	40	60	80	100
Choose not to drink in social situations when alcohol is available.	0	20	40	60	80	100
Drink no more than 2 drinks per hour.	0	20	40	60	80	100

Note. Developed by Thomas Hall at the University of Central Florida.

WORKSHEET 8.1
LEADERSHIP GUIDE FOR STUDENT STAFF AND VOLUNTEERS

The Case for a Community Engagement Curriculum

Hundreds of students are peer mentors, peer educators, resident assistants, orientation leaders, teaching assistants, peer advisors, and student office workers across campus.

Students in academic or nonacademic leadership roles benefit from a curriculum founded in strategic community engagement.

- ☐ Curricular applications
  - Service-learning
  - Internships
  - Practica
  - Cooperative and experiential learning opportunities
  - Undergraduate research opportunities
  - Leadership programs
- ☐ Cocurricular applications
  - Community engagement skill building
  - Peer advocates
  - Peer mentors
  - Peer advisors
  - Selected registered student organizations
  - Employment readiness
- ☐ Extracurricular applications
  - Selected registered student organizations
  - Students committed to community engagement and members of an intentional virtual community

Benefits for Students Who Synthesize Scholarship and Community Engagement

- ☐ Explore communication and leadership styles and personal/cultural identities.
- ☐ Examine personal health behaviors, communication patterns, limitations, and dissonance.
- ☐ Examine current social issues on college campuses.
- ☐ Compare your leadership style to that of others.
- ☐ Explore issues relating to social justice and diversity.
- ☐ Examine the theoretical models of behavior change, social justice, and peer advocacy.
- ☐ Focus on leadership, resource, referral, and facilitation skills.
- ☐ Foster environments that engage students in community.
- ☐ Promote protective factors that motivate and facilitate meaningful relationships and healthy behaviors as well as satisfying, productive, and sustainable lifestyles.

Strategies: ASK (Attitudes, Skills, and Knowledge)

A. SELF-APPRAISAL

1. Acknowledges personal strengths and weaknesses
2. Recognizes intrapersonal and interpersonal skills and abilities
3. Seeks feedback from others
4. Articulates personal and educational goals
5. Understands how personal choices and actions impact the community

B. CULTURAL COMPETENCIES

1. Acknowledges personal identity and culture
2. Recognizes the advantages and challenges within diverse communities
3. Seeks feedback about the impact of stereotypes
4. Articulates a common language for discussing social justice issues
5. Understands the impact of diversity on community

C. COMMUNICATION

1. Acknowledges the importance of listening skills
2. Recognizes diverse audiences
3. Seeks feedback and reflects before responding
4. Articulates abstract and concrete ideas coherently and persuasively
5. Understands the impact of communication on community

D. SOCIAL RESPONSIBILITY

1. Acknowledges a need to work cooperatively with others
2. Recognizes the importance of self-respect and respect for others
3. Seeks feedback about behaviors that impact community health
4. Articulates personal values and explains how they influence decision making across multiple contexts
5. Understands how behaviors promote environmental and community sustainability and risk reduction

E. INTELLECTUAL GROWTH

1. Acknowledges the need for continuous learning
2. Recognizes the importance of critical thinking to form an opinion or make a decision
3. Seeks information from a variety of sources including personal experience and observation
4. Articulates leadership as a theory-to-practice process based on a combination of self-appraisal, cultural competencies, communication, and social responsibility
5. Understands personal power to transform environments and communities

F. LEARNING OUTCOMES

- ☐ Students will discover and understand their personal communication and leadership style. (A1, A2, A3; C1, C2, C3; D1; E3)
- ☐ Students will understand the importance of and be able to set one long-term and two short-term goals. (A4; E1)
- ☐ Students will understand and apply the dimensions of self-care by creating a balanced curricular, cocurricular, and extracurricular schedule. (A1, A3; C3; E2, E4)
- ☐ Students will be able to describe personal and cultural identities. (B1)
- ☐ Students will be able to understand the impact of personal and cultural identity on relationships with others. (A5; B3, B5; C5; E5)
- ☐ Students will be able to prioritize current social issues on their college campus. (A5; B2, B5; C2, C3, C4, C5; D3, D5; E3, E5)
- ☐ Students will be able to compare current social issues on their campus with those at selected peer institutions. (A5; B2, B5; C2, C3, C4, C5; D3, D5; E3, E5)
- ☐ Students will know and understand the dimensions of diversity. (B2, B3, B5; C2; D2)
- ☐ Students will develop a common language for discussing social justice issues. (B4; C4; D1; E1)
- ☐ Students will know and understand multiple theoretical frameworks that describe models of behavioral change, social justice, and advocacy. (B2; C4; E2, E3)
- ☐ Students will know and understand the dimensions of community engagement. (A5; B5; C5; D5; E5)
- ☐ Students will develop a common language to describe models of behavioral change, social justice, and advocacy.
- ☐ (B4; C4)
- ☐ Students will develop an intellectual framework to describe models of environmental and community sustainability.

- ☐ (C4; D5; E2, E3)
- ☐ Students will develop a common language for discussing environmental and community sustainability.
- ☐ (C5; D3; E4, E5)
- ☐ Students will understand the importance of engaging the community to promote meaningful relationships as well as satisfying, productive, and sustainable lifestyles. (A5; B5; C5; D5; E5)

Note. Developed by Thomas Hall at the University of Central Florida.

WORKSHEET 9.1
LOGIC MODEL TEMPLATE

Needs	Inputs		Outputs		Outcomes		
	Resources Available	Resources Needed	Activities	Participants	Short Term	Intermediate	Long Term
Issues to be addressed		What is to be invested	Strategies, efforts, services, products to be implemented or delivered	Whom you reach	Initial results 1–3 months	Midcourse outcomes 6–12 months	Ultimate outcomes 2–5 years
	Tangible: Funding, personnel, materials, technology *Intangible*: Time, partnerships, research, regulations, expertise, leadership				Learning	Behavioral action	Conditions and ultimate impact

WORKSHEET 9.2
PLANNING FOR GOALS AND OBJECTIVES

Goals, objectives, and activities	Schedule	Who	Resources
Goal:			
Objective #1:			
Activities: 1. 2. 3. 4. 5.			
Objective #2:			
Activities: 1. 2. 3. 4. 5.			

WORKSHEET 9.3
PLANNING GUIDE WITH EVALUATION MEASURES

Goals, objectives, and activities	Measures
Goal:	
Objective #1:	Outcome measures: • • •
Activities: 1. 2. 3. 4.	Process measures: 1. 2. 3. 4.
Objective #2:	Outcome measures: • • •
Activities: 1. 2. 3. 4.	Process measures: 1. 2. 3. 4.

WORKSHEET 10.1
FORCE FIELD ANALYSIS

1. **Problem specification**: As clearly as possible, state the nature of the problem.

2. **Desired results**: What is the desired state of affairs, and what is the current state of affairs (status quo)?

Desired State of Affairs Current State of Affairs	**FORCE FIELD ANALYSIS** Restraining Forces ↓ ↓ ↓ ↓ ↓ ↓ ↓ ↓ ↑ ↑ ↑ ↑ ↑ ↑ ↑ ↑ Driving Forces

Note. Force Field Analysis from Kurt Lewin (1890–1947); Institute for Social Research, MIT.

3. **Driving forces**: Consider the present status of the problem as a temporary balance of opposing forces. What are the forces driving toward change or helping to achieve the desired outcomes?

   a.

   b.

   c.

   d.

   e.

   f.

4. **Restraining forces**: What are the forces restraining or hindering change, or blocking movement toward the goal?

   a.

   b.

   c.

   d.

   e.

   f.

5. Prioritization: Rate each of the forces from 1 to 5 (1 = it has almost nothing to do with the force; 5 = it is a major factor for the force).

6. Strategy development:

a. Identify two of the driving forces and outline a strategy for increasing its potency.

Driving Force 1:

Driving Force 2:

b. Identify two of the restraining forces and outline a strategy for reducing its potency.

Restraining Force 1:

Restraining Force 2:

WORKSHEET 10.2
GUIDING PRINCIPLES

Identify factors you believe should be foundational for your efforts and your organization's efforts. These may include items such as (but not limited to) philosophical foundation, interaction style, immediacy of results, importance of various content elements, results desired, programmatic emphases, audience, stakeholders, context, and process of implementation. For each item, indicate its status as a principle for you, the organization, or both.

Self	Organization	Guiding principle

WORKSHEET 10.3
MENU OF STRATEGIES

Policies and Laws	Enforcement
Information Dissemination	Affective Approaches
Campaigns	Curriculum
Skill Building	Peer Approaches and Mentoring
Programming	Training
Community Engagement	Media Involvement

WORKSHEET 10.4
PREVENTION/OUTREACH CHECKLIST AND AFTER ACTION REPORT

<table>
<tr><td>Date:</td><td colspan="2">Event:</td></tr>
<tr><td colspan="3">Check target population: ☐ Universal ☐ Selective ☐ Indicated

Brief event description:</td></tr>
<tr><td>Prevention strategy
(check all that apply)</td><td colspan="2">☐ Information dissemination
(increase awareness and knowledge of risks of substance abuse and available prevention services)
☐ Education
(improve skills, reduce negative behavior, improve responsible behavior)
☐ Alternatives
(a constructive activity that excludes substance abuse and encourages harm reduction)
☐ Problem identification and referral services
(identify emerging adults who have indulged in the use of tobacco or alcohol and those who have indulged in the initial use of illicit drugs—to assess for prevention services or treatment)
☐ Community-based
(enhance the ability of a community to provide prevention and treatment services more effectively)
☐ Environmental
(establish or change local laws, regulations, or rules to strengthen the general community)</td></tr>
<tr><td>Harm reduction
(check all that apply)</td><td>Risk factors
☐ Group affiliation
☐ Substance-using peers
☐ Favorable attitudes about substance use
☐ Risk taking/thrill seeking
☐ Low academic engagement
☐ Inconsistent enforcement of policy/law
☐ Poor school performance
☐ Easy access to mood-altering substances
☐ Early age of substance use onset
☐ Low perception of risk associated with use
☐ Favorable norms about substance use
☐ Anxiety, depression, or other behavioral health concerns</td><td>Protective factors
☐ Promoting well-being
☐ Promoting meditation/mindfulness
☐ Promoting self-help and/or professional counseling
☐ Promoting physical activity
☐ Promoting “safer” behaviors
☐ Promoting academic support services
☐ Promoting self-control/self-regulation
☐ Promoting self-sufficiency
☐ Delaying the age of substance use onset
☐ Promoting substance-free social activities
☐ Promoting access to support resources
☐ Disseminating accurate information about the health and safety of alcohol/drug use</td></tr>
</table>

Duration of activity	
Location of activity	
Number of participants	
See additional page for comments.	

Note. Developed by Thomas Hall at the University of Central Florida.

WORKSHEET 11.1
PLANNING FOR COLLABORATION

Potential collaborator	Benefits for involvement	Concerns about involvement
College president/ chancellor		
Vice president for student affairs		
Provost		
Admissions/enrollment services		
Dean of students		
Student activities		
Fraternity/sorority		
Health center		
Counseling and psychological services		
Athletics department		
Faculty member		
Academic department		
Student organizations		
Student government		
Alumni		
Community member		
Community organization		
Other:		

WORKSHEET 11.2
COALITION LEADERSHIP ACTION STEPS

- ☐ **Personal:** What would you commit yourself to do in the short term and the longer term?
- ☐ **Coalition, group, or organization:** What would you like the coalition, group, or organization to do in the short term as well as the longer term?
- ☐ **For other groups (regardless of whether a member of the coalition):** What would you like them to consider for the short term and/or longer term?

	Short term	Longer term
Personal		
Coalition, group, or organization		
Group:		
Group:		
Group:		
Group:		

WORKSHEET 12.1
COMMUNICATION FOUNDATIONS

This worksheet helps identify the audience(s) to be reached, the overall aim with each audience, and the messages desired regarding what the audience should know, feel, or do.

Audiences	**Aim**			**Message**
	Change	**Reinforce**	**Introduce**	
Universal				
Selective				
Selective				
Selective				
Indicated				
Indicated				
Indicated				

WORKSHEET 12.2
PERSUASION WORKSHEET

Background Documentation – Needs, Issues, and Concerns

-
-
-

Audience Needs and Attributes

-
-
-

Specific Desired Outcomes

-
-
-

Programmatic Issues, Resource Needs, and Costs

-
-
-

Data, Impact, and Cost Equivalents

-
-
-

Testimonials, Examples, and Other Strategies

-
-
-

WORKSHEET 13.1
SYNTHESIS AND REVIEW

As you work toward the conclusion of your project, what insights or recommendations do you have? Consider each of the following issues, and have individuals prepare this document and share their results.

Issue	What went well?	What could be improved?	Other suggestions
Overall aims			
Staffing			
Campus collaboration			
Student involvement			
Faculty involvement			
Evaluation			
Impact			
Resources and budget			
Community role			
Other:			
Other:			

WORKSHEET 14.1
INDIVIDUALIZED GOALS

What are your plans . . .

	Personal	Professional
In 2 weeks?		
At the end of the academic year?		
Within 1 year?		
Over a longer time period?		

APPENDIX B

Resource Bibliography

Research Supporting the Social Norms Approach to Reduce Harmful Drinking and Drug Use in Higher Education

H. Wesley Perkins, PhD
Hobart & William Smith Colleges

Jessica M. Perkins, PhD
Vanderbilt University

Studies Documenting Misperceived Norms About Alcohol Consumption and Drug Use and the Association Between Misperceived Norms and Personal Use

Arbour-Nicitopoulos, K. P., Kwan, M. Y. W., Lowe, D., Taman, S., & Faulkner, G. E. J. (2010). Social norms of alcohol, smoking, and marijuana use within a Canadian university setting. *Journal of American College Health, 59*(3), 191–196. https://doi.org/10.1080/07448481.2010.502194

Boyle, H. K., Merrill, J. E., & Carey, K. B. (2020). Location-specific social norms and personal approval of alcohol use are associated with drinking behaviors in college students. *Substance Use & Misuse, 55*(10), 1650–1659. https://doi.org/10.1080/10826084.2020.1756849

Bustamante, I. V., Carvalho, A. M. P., Oliveira, E. B. D., Oliveira Júnior, H. P. D., Santos Figueroa, S. D., Montoya Vásquez, E. M., Cazenave, A., Chaname, E., Medina Matallana, L. S., & Ramirez Castillo, J. (2009). University students' perceived norms of peers and drug use: A multicentric study in five Latin American countries. *Revista Latino-Americana de Enfermagem, 17*, 838–843.

Corbin, W. R., Iwamoto, D. K., & Fromme, K. (2011). Broad social motives, alcohol use, and related problems: Mechanisms of risk from high school through college. *Addictive Behaviors, 36*(3), 222–230. https://doi.org/10.1016/j.addbeh.2010.11.004

Cox, M. J., DiBello, A. M., Meisel, M. K., Ott, M. Q., Kenney, S. R., Clark, M. A., & Barnett, N. P. (2019). Do misperceptions of peer drinking influence personal drinking behavior? Results from a complete social network of first-year college students. *Psychology of Addictive Behaviors, 33*(3), 297–303. https://doi.org/10.1037/adb0000455

Dempsey, R. C., McAlaney, J., & Bewick, B. M. (2018). A critical appraisal of the social norms approach as an interventional strategy for health-related behavior and attitude change. *Frontiers in Psychology, 9*, Article 2180. https://doi.org/10.3389/fpsyg.2018.02180

Dempsey, R. C., McAlaney, J., Helmer, S. M., Pischke, C. R., Akvardar, Y., Bewick, B. M., Fawkner, H. J., Guillen-Grima, F., Stock, C., Vriesacker, B., Van Hal, G., Salonna, F., Kalina, O., Orosova, O., & Mikolajczyk, R. T. (2016). Normative perceptions of cannabis use among European university students: Associations of perceived peer use and peer attitudes with personal use and attitudes. *Journal of Studies on Alcohol and Drugs, 77*(5), 740–748. https://doi.org/10.15288/jsad.2016.77.740

Dumas, T. M., Davis, J. P., & Neighbors, C. (2019). How much does your peer group really drink? Examining the relative impact of overestimation, actual group drinking and perceived campus norms on university students' heavy alcohol use. *Addictive Behaviors, 90*, 409–414. https://doi.org/10.1016/j.addbeh.2018.11.041

Edwards, K. A., Witkiewitz, K., & Vowles, K. E. (2019). Demographic differences in perceived social norms of drug and alcohol use among Hispanic/Latinx and non-Hispanic White college students. *Addictive Behaviors, 98*, 106060. https://doi.org/10.1016/j.addbeh.2019.106060

Figueroa, S. D. S., Cunningham, J., Strike, C., Brands, B., & Wright, M. D. G. M. (2009). Normas percibidas por los estudiantes universitarios hondureños acerca de sus pares y el uso de tabaco, alcohol, marihuana y cocaína. *Revista Latino-Americana de Enfermagem, 17*, 851–857.

Grossbard, J. R., Geisner, I. M., Mastroleo, N. R., Kilmer, J. R., Turrisi, R., & Larimer, M. E. (2009). Athletic identity, descriptive norms, and drinking among athletes transitioning to college. *Addictive Behaviors, 34*(4), 352–359. https://doi.org/10.1016/j.addbeh.2008.11.011

Gündüz, A., Sakarya, S., Sönmez, E., Çelebi, C., Yüce, H., & Akvardar, Y. (2019). Social norms regarding alcohol use and associated factors among university students in Turkey. *Archives of Clinical Psychiatry (São Paulo), 46*, 44–49.

Guo, Y., Ward, R. M., & Speed, S. (2020). Alcohol-related social norms predict more than alcohol use: Examining the relation between social norms and substance use. *Journal of Substance Use, 25*(3), 258–263. https://doi.org/10.1080/14659891.2019.1675791

Helmer, S. M., Mikolajczyk, R. T., McAlaney, J., Vriesacker, B., Van Hal, G., Akvardar, Y., Guillen-Grima, F., Salonna, F., Stock, C., Dempsey, R. C., Bewick, B. M., & Zeeb, H. (2014). Illicit substance use among university students from seven European countries: A comparison of personal and perceived peer use and attitudes towards illicit substance use. *Preventive Medicine, 67*, 204–209. https://doi.org/10.1016/j.ypmed.2014.07.039

Helmer, S. M., Pischke, C. R., Van Hal, G., Vriesacker, B., Dempsey, R. C., Akvardar, Y., Guillen-Grima, F., Salonna, F., Stock, C., & Zeeb, H. (2016). Personal and perceived peer use and attitudes towards the use of nonmedical prescription stimulants to improve academic performance among university students in seven European countries. *Drug and Alcohol Dependence, 168*, 128–134. https://doi.org/10.1016/j.drugalcdep.2016.08.639

Helmer, S. M., Sebena, R., McAlaney, J., Petkeviciene, J., Salonna, F., & Mikolajczyk, R. T. (2016). Perception of high alcohol use of peers is associated with high personal alcohol use in first-year university students in three Central and Eastern European countries. *Substance Use & Misuse, 51*(9), 1–8. https://doi.org/10.3109/10826084.2016.1162810

Hummer, J. F., LaBrie, J. W., & Lac, A. (2009). The prognostic power of normative influences among NCAA student-athletes. *Addictive Behaviors, 34*(6–7), 573–580. https://doi.org/10.1016/j.addbeh.2009.03.021

Hummer, J. F., LaBrie, J. W., Lac, A., Sessoms, A., & Cail, J. (2012). Estimates and influences of reflective opposite-sex norms on alcohol use among a high-risk sample of college students: Exploring Greek-affiliation and gender effects. *Addictive Behaviors, 37*(5), 596–604. https://doi.org/10.1016/j.addbeh.2011.11.027

Kenney, S. R., Ott, M., Meisel, M. K., & Barnett, N. P. (2017). Alcohol perceptions and behavior in a residential peer social network. *Addictive Behaviors, 64,* 143–147. https://doi.org/10.1016/j.addbeh.2016.08.047

Kilmer, J. R., Geisner, I. M., Gasser, M. L., & Lindgren, K. P. (2015). Normative perceptions of non-medical stimulant use: Associations with actual use and hazardous drinking. *Addictive Behaviors, 42,* 51–56. https://doi.org/10.1016/j.addbeh.2014.11.005

Kilmer, J. R., Walker, D. D., Lee, C. M., Palmer, R. S., Mallett, K. A., Fabiano, P., & Larimer, M. E. (2006). Misperceptions of college student marijuana use: Implications for prevention. *Journal of Studies on Alcohol and Drugs, 67*(2), 277–281.

Larimer, M. E., Parker, M., Lostutter, T., Rhew, I., Eakins, D., Lynch, A., Walter, T., Egashira, L., Kipp, B. J., & Duran, B. (2020). Perceived descriptive norms for alcohol use among tribal college students: Relation to self-reported alcohol use, consequences, and risk for alcohol use disorder. *Addictive Behaviors,* 102, 106158. https://doi.org/10.1016/j.addbeh.2019.106158

Lehne, G., Zeeb, H., Pischke, C. R., Mikolajczyk, R., Bewick, B. M., McAlaney, J., Dempsey, R. C., Val Hal, G., Stock, C., Akvardar, Y., Kalina, O., Orosova, O., Aguinaga-Ontoso, I., Guillen-Grima, F., & Helmer, S. M. (2018). Personal and perceived peer use and attitudes towards use of non-prescribed prescription sedatives and sleeping pills among university students in seven European countries. *Addictive Behaviors, 87,* 17–23. https://doi.org/10.1016/j.addbeh.2018.06.012

Lewis, M. A., & Neighbors, C. (2004). Gender-specific misperceptions of college student drinking norms. *Psychology of Addictive Behaviors, 18*(4), 334–339. https://doi.org/10.1037/0893-164X.18.4.334

Loverock, A., Yakovenko, I., & Wild, T. C. (2021). Cannabis norm perceptions among Canadian university students. *Addictive Behaviors, 112,* 106567. https://doi.org/10.1016/j.addbeh.2020.106567

McAlaney, J., Boot Cécile, R., Dahlin, M., Lintonen, T., Stock, C., Rasmussen, S., & Van Hal, G. (2012). A comparison of substance use behaviours and normative beliefs in North-West European university and college students. *International Journal on Disability and Human Development, 11*(3), 281. https://doi.org/10.1515/ijdhd-2012-0032

McAlaney, J., Helmer, S. M., Stock, C., Vriesacker, B., Hal, G. V., Dempsey, R. C., Akvardar, Y., Salonna, F., Kalina, O., Guillen-Grima, F., Bewick, B. M., & Mikolajczyk, R. (2015). Personal and perceived peer use of and attitudes toward alcohol among university and college students in seven EU countries: Project SNIPE. *Journal of Studies on Alcohol and Drugs, 76*(3), 430–438. https://doi.org/10.15288/jsad.2015.76.430

McAlaney, J., & Jenkins, W. (2017). Perceived social norms of health behaviours and college engagement in British students. *Journal of Further and Higher Education, 41*(2), 172–186. https://doi.org/10.1080/0309877X.2015.1070399

McAlaney, J., & McMahon, J. (2007). Normative beliefs, misperceptions, and heavy episodic drinking in a British student sample. *Journal of Studies on Alcohol and Drugs, 68*(3), 385–392. https://doi.org/10.15288/jsad.2007.68.385

McCabe, S. E. (2008). Misperceptions of non-medical prescription drug use: A web survey of college students. *Addictive Behaviors, 33*(5), 713–724. https://doi.org/10.1016/j.addbeh.2007.12.008

Neighbors, C., Dillard, A. J., Lewis, M. A., Bergstrom, R. L., & Neil, T. A. (2006). Normative misperceptions and temporal precedence of perceived norms and drinking. *Journal of Studies on Alcohol and Drugs, 67*(2), 290–299.

Pedersen, E. R., & LaBrie, J. W. (2008). Normative misperceptions of drinking among college students: A look at the specific contexts of prepartying and drinking games. *Journal of Studies on Alcohol and Drugs, 69*(3), 406–411.

Pedersen, E. R., LaBrie, J. W., & Hummer, J. F. (2009). Perceived behavioral alcohol norms predict drinking for college students while studying abroad. *Journal of Studies on Alcohol and Drugs, 70*(6), 924–928.

Pedersen, E. R., Neighbors, C., & LaBrie, J. W. (2010). College students' perceptions of class year-specific drinking norms. *Addictive Behaviors, 35*(3), 290–293. https://doi.org/10.1016/j.addbeh.2009.10.015

Perkins, H. W. (1995). Scope of the problem: Misperceptions of alcohol and drugs. *Catalyst, 1*(3), 1–2.

Perkins, H. W. (2007). Misperceptions of peer drinking norms in Canada: Another look at the "reign of error" and its consequences among college students. *Addictive Behaviors, 32*(11), 2645–2656. https://doi.org/10.1016/j.addbeh.2007.07.007

Perkins, H. W. (2014). Misperception is reality: The "reign of error" about peer risk behaviour norms among youth and young adults. In M. Xenitidou & B. Edmonds (Eds.), *The complexity of social norms* (pp. 11–36). Springer International Publishing.

Perkins, H. W., Haines, M. P., & Rice, R. (2005). Misperceiving the college drinking norm and related problems: A nationwide study of exposure to prevention information, perceived norms and student alcohol misuse. *Journal of Studies on Alcohol and Drugs, 66*(4), 470–478. https://doi.org/10.15288/jsa.2005.66.470

Perkins, H. W., Meilman, P. W., Leichliter, J. S., Cashin, J. R., & Presley, C. A. (1999). Misperceptions of the norms for the frequency of alcohol and other drug use on college campuses. *Journal of American College Health, 47*(6), 253–258. https://doi.org/10.1080/07448489909595656

Pischke, C. R., Helmer, S. M., McAlaney, J., Bewick, B. M., Vriesacker, B., Van Hal, G., Mikolajczyk, R. T., Akvardar, Y., Guillen-Grima, F., Salonna, F., Orosova, O., Dohrmann, S., Dempsey, R. C., & Zeeb, H. (2015). Normative misperceptions of tobacco use among university students in seven European countries: Baseline findings of the "Social Norms Intervention for the prevention of Polydrug usE" study. *Addictive Behaviors, 51*, 158–164. https://doi.org/10.1016/j.addbeh.2015.07.012

Riou Franca, L., Dautzenberg, B., Falissard, B., & Reynaud, M. (2010). Peer substance use overestimation among French university students: A cross-sectional survey. *BMC Public Health, 10*(1), 169. https://doi.org/10.1186/1471-2458-10-169

Sanders, A., Stogner, J. M., & Miller, B. L. (2013). Perception vs. reality: An investigation of the misperceptions concerning the extent of peer novel drug use. *Journal of Drug Education, 43*(2), 97–120. https://doi.org/10.2190/DE.43.2.a

Sanders, A., Stogner, J., Seibert, J., & Miller, B. L. (2014). Misperceptions of peer pill-popping: The prevalence, correlates, and effects of inaccurate assumptions about peer pharmaceutical misuse. *Substance Use & Misuse, 49*(7), 813–823. https://doi.org/10.3109/10826084.2014.880485

Stappenbeck, C. A., Quinn, P. D., Wetherill, R. R., & Fromme, K. (2010). Perceived norms for drinking in the transition from high school to college and beyond. *Journal of Studies on Alcohol and Drugs, 71*(6), 895–903.

Steyl, T., & Phillips, J. 2011). Actual and perceived substance use of health science students at a university in the Western Cape, South Africa. *African Health Sciences, 11*(3), 329–333.

Factors Contributing to the Growth and Persistence of Misperceived Norms

Boyle, S. C., LaBrie, J. W., Froidevaux, N. M., & Witkovic, Y. D. (2016). Different digital paths to the keg? How exposure to peers' alcohol-related social media content influences drinking among male and female first-year college students. *Addictive Behaviors, 57*, 21–29. https://doi.org/10.1016/j.addbeh.2016.01.011

Boyle, S. C., Smith, D. J., Earle, A. M., & LaBrie, J. W. (2018). What "likes" have got to do with it: Exposure to peers' alcohol-related posts and perceptions of injunctive drinking norms. *Journal of American College Health, 66*(4), 252–258. https://doi.org/10.1080/07448481.2018.1431895

Davis, J. P., Pedersen, E. R., Tucker, J. S., Dunbar, M. S., Seelam, R., Shih, R., & D'Amico, E. J. (2019). Long-term associations between substance use-related media exposure, descriptive norms, and alcohol use from adolescence to young adulthood. *Journal of Youth and Adolescence, 48*(7), 1311–1326. https://doi.org/10.1007/s10964-019-01024-z

Perkins, H. W. (2003). The emergence and evolution of the social norms approach to substance abuse prevention. In H. W. Perkins (Ed.), *The social norms approach to preventing school and college age substance abuse: A handbook for educators, counselors, and clinicians* (pp. 247–258). Jossey-Bass.

Yang, B., & Zhao, X. (2018). TV, social media, and college students' binge drinking intentions: Moderated mediation models. *Journal of Health Communication, 23*(1), 61–71. https://doi.org/10.1080/10810730.2017.1411995

Strategies to Correct Misperceived Norms

Bewick, B. M., Trusler, K., Mulhern, B., Barkham, M., & Hill, A. J. (2008). The feasibility and effectiveness of a web-based personalised feedback and social norms alcohol intervention in U.K. university students: A randomised control trial. *Addictive Behaviors, 33*(9), 1192–1198. https://doi.org/10.1016/j.addbeh.2008.05.002

Borsari, B., & Carey, K. B. (2003). Descriptive and injunctive norms in college drinking: A meta-analytic integration. *Journal of Studies on Alcohol and Drugs, 64*(3), 331–341.

Buckner, J. D., Neighbors, C., Walukevich-Dienst, K., & Young, C. M. (2019). Online personalized normative feedback intervention to reduce event-specific drinking during Mardi Gras. *Experimental and Clinical Psychopharmacology, 27*(5), 466–473. https://doi.org/10.1037/pha0000259

Burchell, K., Rettie, R., & Patel, K. (2013). Marketing social norms: Social marketing and the "social norm approach." *Journal of Consumer Behaviour, 12*(1), 1–9. https://doi.org/10.1002/cb.1395

Cadigan, J. M., Martens, M. P., Dworkin, E. R., & Sher, K. J. (2019). The efficacy of an event-specific, text message, personalized drinking feedback intervention. *Prevention Science, 20*(6), 873–883. https://doi.org/10.1007/s11121-018-0939-9

Carey, K. B., Merrill, J. E., Boyle, H. K., & Barnett, N. P. (2020). Correcting exaggerated drinking norms with a mobile message delivery system: Selective prevention with heavy-drinking first-year college students. *Psychology of Addictive Behaviors, 34*(3), 454–464. https://doi.org/10.1037/adb0000566

DeJong, W., Schneider, S. K., Towvim, L. G., Murphy, M. J., Doerr, E. E., Simonsen, N. R., Mason, K. E., & Scribner, R. A. (2006). A multisite randomized trial of social norms marketing campaigns to reduce college student drinking. *Journal of Studies on Alcohol and Drugs, 67*(6), 868–879. https://doi.org/10.15288/jsa.2006.67.868

Glider, P., Midyett, S. J., Mills-Novoa, B., Johannessen, K., & Collins, C. (2001). Challenging the collegiate rite of passage: A campus-wide social marketing media campaign to reduce binge drinking. *Journal of Drug Education, 31*(2), 207–220. https://doi.org/10.2190/u466-epfg-q76d-yhtq

Haines, M., & Spear, S. F. (1996). Changing the perception of the norm: A strategy to decrease binge drinking among college students. *Journal of American College Health, 45*(3), 134–140. https://doi.org/10.1080/07448481.1996.9936873

Haines, M. P., & Barker, G. P. (2003). The Northern Illinois University experiment: A longitudinal case study of the social norms approach. In H. W. Perkins (Ed.), *The social norms approach to preventing school and college age substance abuse: A handbook for educators, counselors, and clinicians* (pp. 21–34). Jossey-Bass/Wiley.

Hembroff, L. A., Martell, D., Allen, R., Poole, A., Clark, K., & Smith, S. W. (2019). The long-term effectiveness of a social norming campaign to reduce high-risk drinking: The Michigan State University experience, 2000–2014. *Journal of American College Health*, 1–11. https://doi.org/10.1080/07448481.2019.1674856

LaBrie, J. W., Hummer, J. F., Neighbors, C., & Pedersen, E. R. (2008). Live interactive group-specific normative feedback reduces misperceptions and drinking in college students: A randomized cluster trial. *Psychology of Addictive Behaviors, 22*(1), 141–148. https://doi.org/10.1037/0893-164X.22.1.141

LaBrie, J. W., Lewis, M. A., Atkins, D. C., Neighbors, C., Zheng, C., Kenney, S. R., Napper, L. E., Walter, T., Kilmer, J. R., Hummer, J. F., Grossbard, J., Ghaidarov, T. M., Desai, S., Lee, C. M., & Larimer, M. E. (2013). RCT of web-based personalized normative feedback for college drinking prevention: Are typical student norms good enough? *Journal of Consulting and Clinical Psychology, 81*(6), 1074–1086. https://doi.org/10.1037/a0034087

Lewis, M. A., & Neighbors, C. (2006). Social norms approaches using descriptive drinking norms education: A review of the research on personalized normative feedback. *Journal of American College Health, 54*(4), 213–218. https://doi.org/10.3200/JACH.54.4.213-218

Merrill, J. E., Boyle, H. K., Barnett, N. P., & Carey, K. B. (2018). Delivering normative feedback to heavy drinking college students via text messaging: A pilot feasibility study. *Addictive Behaviors, 83,* 175–181. https://doi.org/10.1016/j.addbeh.2017.10.003

Miller, M. B., Leffingwell, T., Claborn, K., Meier, E., Walters, S., & Neighbors, C. (2013). Personalized feedback interventions for college alcohol misuse: An update of Walters & Neighbors (2005). *Psychology of Addictive Behaviors, 27*(4), 909–920. https://doi.org/10.1037/a0031174

Neighbors, C., Larimer, M. E., & Lewis, M. A. (2004). Targeting misperceptions of descriptive drinking norms: Efficacy of a computer-delivered personalized normative feedback intervention. *Journal of Consulting and Clinical Psychology, 72*(3), 434–447. https://doi.org/10.1037/0022-006X.72.3.434

Neighbors, C., Lewis, M. A., Atkins, D. C., Jensen, M. M., Walter, T., Fossos, N., Lee, C. M., & Larimer, M. E. (2010). Efficacy of web-based personalized normative feedback: A two-year randomized controlled trial. *Journal of Consulting and Clinical Psychology, 78*(6), 898–911. https://doi.org/10.1037/a0020766

Neighbors, C., Lewis, M. A., LaBrie, J., DiBello, A. M., Young, C. M., Rinker, D. V., Litt, D., Rodriguez, L. M., Knee, C. R., Hamor, E., Jerabeck, J. M., & Larimer, M. E. (2016). A multisite randomized trial of normative feedback for heavy drinking: Social comparison versus social comparison plus correction of normative misperceptions. *Journal of Consulting and Clinical Psychology, 84*(3), 238–247. https://doi.org/10.1037/ccp0000067

Perkins, H. W. (Ed.). (2003). *The social norms approach to preventing school and college age substance abuse: A handbook for educators, counselors, and clinicians.* Jossey-Bass.

Perkins, H. W. (2009). Learning about student alcohol abuse and helping to prevent it through service learning initiatives: The HWS Alcohol Education Project. In C. A. Rimmerman (Ed.), *Service-learning and the liberal arts: How and why it works* (pp. 151–169). Lexington Books.

Perkins, H. W., & Craig, D. W. (2003). The Hobart and William Smith Colleges experiment: A synergistic social norms approach using print, electronic media, and curriculum infusion to reduce collegiate problem drinking. In H. W. Perkins (Ed.), *The social norms approach to preventing school and college age substance abuse: A handbook for educators, counselors, and clinicians* (pp. 35–64). Jossey-Bass.

Perrault, E. K., Hildenbrand, G. M., Loew, T. F., & Evans, W. G. (2020). Evaluation of a university's smart partying social norms campaign including emoji-style messaging. *Journal of Communication in Healthcare, 13*(1), 35–45. https://doi.org/10.1080/17538068.2020.1753471

Ridout, B., & Campbell, A. (2014). Using Facebook to deliver a social norm intervention to reduce problem drinking at university. *Drug and Alcohol Review, 33*(6), 667–673. https://doi.org/10.1111/dar.12141

Schroeder, C. M., & Prentice, D. A. (1998). Exposing pluralistic ignorance to reduce alcohol use among college students. *Journal of Applied Social Psychology, 28*(23), 2150–2180. https://doi.org/10.1111/j.1559-1816.1998.tb01365.x

Su, J., Hancock, L., Wattenmaker McGann, A., Alshagra, M., Ericson, R., Niazi, Z., Dick, D. M., & Adkins, A. (2018). Evaluating the effect of a campus-wide social norms marketing intervention on alcohol-use perceptions, consumption, and blackouts. *Journal of American College Health, 66*(3), 219–224. https://doi.org/10.1080/07448481.2017.1382500

Thompson, K., Burgess, J., & MacNevin, P. D. (2018). An evaluation of e-CHECKUP TO GO in Canada: The mediating role of changes in social norm misperceptions. *Substance Use & Misuse, 53*(11), 1849–1858. https://doi.org/10.1080/10826084.2018.1441306

Turner, J., Perkins, H. W., & Bauerle, J. (2008). Declining negative consequences related to alcohol misuse among students exposed to a social norms marketing intervention on a college campus. *Journal of American College Health, 57*(1), 85–94. https://doi.org/10.3200/JACH.57.1.85-94

Using the Social Norms Approach in Selective Target Populations

Boyle, S. C., LaBrie, J. W., & Witkovic, Y. D. (2016). Do lesbians overestimate alcohol use norms? Exploring the potential utility of personalized normative feedback interventions to reduce high-risk drinking in Southern California lesbian communities. *Journal of Gay & Lesbian Social Services, 28*(3), 179–194. https://doi.org/10.1080/10538720.2016.1190677

LaBrie, J. W., Hummer, J. F., Grant, S., & Lac, A. (2010). Immediate reductions in misperceived social norms among high-risk college student groups. *Addictive Behaviors, 35*(12), 1094–1101. https://doi.org/10.1016/j.addbeh.2010.08.003

LaBrie, J. W., Hummer, J. F., Huchting, K. K., & Neighbors, C. (2009). A brief live interactive normative group intervention using wireless keypads to reduce drinking and alcohol consequences in college student athletes. *Drug and Alcohol Review, 28*(1), 40–47. https://doi.org/10.1111/j.1465-3362.2008.00012.x

LaBrie, J. W., Lewis, M. A., Atkins, D. C., Neighbors, C., Zheng, C., Kenney, S. R., Napper, L. E., Walter, T., Kilmer, J. R., Hummer, J. F., Grossbard, J., Ghaidarov, T. M., Desai, S., Lee, C. M., & Larimer, M. E. (2013). RCT of web-based personalized normative feedback for college drinking prevention: Are typical student norms good enough? *Journal of Consulting and Clinical Psychology, 81*(6), 1074–1086. https://doi.org/10.1037/a0034087

Larimer, M. E., Parker, M., Lostutter, T., Rhew, I., Eakins, D., Lynch, A., Walter, T., Egashira, L., Kipp, B. J., & Duran, B. (2020). Perceived descriptive norms for alcohol use among tribal college students: Relation to self-reported alcohol use, consequences, and risk for alcohol use disorder. *Addictive Behaviors, 102,* 106158. https://doi.org/10.1016/j.addbeh.2019.106158

Perkins, H. W., & Craig, D. W. (2006). A successful social norms campaign to reduce alcohol misuse among college student-athletes. *Journal of Studies on Alcohol and Drugs, 67*(6), 880–889.

Perkins, H. W., & Craig, D. W. (2012). Student-athletes' misperceptions of male and female peer drinking norms: A multi-site investigation of the "reign of error." *Journal of College Student Development, 53*(3), 367–382. https://doi.org/10.1353/csd.2012.0046

Turner, J., Perkins, H. W., & Bauerle, J. (2008). Declining negative consequences related to alcohol misuse among students exposed to a social norms marketing intervention on a college campus. *Journal of American College Health, 57*(1), 85–94. https://doi.org/10.3200/JACH.57.1.85-94

The Authors

David Anderson, PhD, is professor emeritus of education and human development at George Mason University. With professional work spanning 5 decades, his specialty areas include drug and alcohol abuse prevention, health promotion, strategic planning, communication and education, and needs assessment and evaluation. Anderson conducts training, delivers keynote speeches, and leads webinars; he also prepares needs assessments, prepares evaluation and analysis, and assists with strategic planning. The audience for his work focuses on program planners, policy makers, school and community leaders, college students, and youth.

At George Mason University, Anderson served on the faculty for 28 years, finishing his career there as professor and director of the Center for the Advancement of Public Health. In addition to teaching graduate and undergraduate courses on drug and alcohol issues, community health, and health communications, he served as project director and researcher for over 180 grants and contracts. These projects encompassed research, evaluation, program implementation, curricula, and community service at the national, state, and local levels. He has also produced, moderated, or been a guest on several television programs and has produced several multimedia resources.

Anderson's research and evaluation experience is extensive. Since 1979, he has coauthored the triennial *College Alcohol Survey*, the nation's longitudinal assessment of alcohol, drug, tobacco, violence, and related issues on 4-year campuses. He co-directed the Understanding Teen Drinking Cultures in America research project, which focused on alcohol use among high school youth. He also coauthored the *Wellness Assessment for Higher Education Preparation Programs* and the *Student Affairs Professionals Wellness Assessment.*

Anderson's numerous publications span over 4 decades and are applied in focus. He authored *Leadership in Drug and Alcohol Abuse Prevention: Insights From Long-Term Advocates* (Routledge, 2019) and coauthored *Health and Safety Communication: A Practical Guide Forward* (Routledge, 2017). He edited *Wellness Issues for Higher Education* (Routledge, 2015) and *Further Wellness Issues for Higher Education* (Routledge, 2016). He co-directed the Promising Practices: Campus Alcohol Strategies project from 1994 to 2001, which distributed the following nationwide products: *Sourcebook 2001*, *Action Planner*, and *Task Force Planner*. Anderson produced *COMPASS: A Roadmap to Healthy Living* and *COMPASS Roadmap: Destination Health*, both CD-based and internet programs and resource focusing on a positive approach to wellness choices among young adults. For over 2 decades, he has served as evaluation consultant for the National Collegiate Athletic Association, for which he authored the *IMPACT Evaluation Resource* and produced *Best of CHOICES: Alcohol Education 1998–2008*. Early in his career, Anderson served as senior editor for *A Winning Combination: An Alcohol, Other Drug and Traffic Safety Program for College Campuses* (U.S. Department of Transportation, 1988) and *That Happy Feeling: An Innovative Model for a Campus Alcohol Education Program* (Southern Area Alcohol Education and Training Program, 1979).

Anderson began his career as a student affairs administrator, with positions as director of residence life at Ohio University, director of residential life at Radford University, and residence hall director at The Ohio State University. He received his Bachelor of Science degree from Duke University, with a major in psychology and a minor in business administration. He received his Master of Arts in student personnel administration from The Ohio State University, and a PhD in public policy/public affairs from Virginia Polytechnic Institute and State

University. In Celebration, Florida, Anderson serves on the board of directors of the Celebration Residential Owners Association, having served as president and vice president. He also serves on the American College Health Association's COVID-19 Task Force.

Thomas Hall, PhD, is director of the Orange County Government Drug-Free Coalition. In this role, he oversees Orange County Government Prevention, Treatment, and Recovery initiatives and advises Mayor Jerry L. Demings on relevant policy issues. Before his appointment, Hall directed on-campus prevention/wellness programs for 19 years. His professional experience as a clinician, researcher, and adjunct faculty spans 27 years. His specialty areas include marriage and family therapy, substance use disorder treatment, child and adolescent treatment, and psychosocial oncology.

Hall's research interests include developing substance use and mental health disorder brief intervention and recovery services for college students. In 2013, he was a recipient of a Substance Abuse and Mental Health Services Administration technology-based challenge to prevent high-risk drinking among college students. In 2010, the U.S. Department of Education recognized his work on comprehensive campus alcohol prevention intervention as a Model of Exemplary Prevention Program in Higher Education. Hall received the Outside the Classroom Prevention Excellence Award, Highest Honors for the University of Central Florida in 2008. In 2002, he coauthored the recommendations for higher education in a white paper commissioned by Governor Jeb Bush, "Florida Can—Changing Alcohol Norms." In 2004, Hall was honored by the state of Florida for his contributions to the prevention of binge drinking on college campuses. Hall has served in numerous state and national leadership roles, including for the Drug Enforcement Administration, the American College Health Association, ACPA–College Student Educators International, and the Florida Higher Education Alliance for Substance Abuse Prevention. He has served as a subject matter expert on the development of substance misuse and mental health curriculums being implemented on high school and college campuses across the country.

Hall's publications span over 18 years. He has been invited to author or coauthor segments in the following books: *Leadership in Drug and Alcohol Abuse Prevention: Insights From Long-Term Advocates* (Routledge, 2019); *Wellness Issues for Higher Education: A Guide for Student Affairs and Higher Education Professionals* (Routledge, 2015); and the *International Encyclopedia of Social and Behavioral Sciences* (2nd ed.; Oxford, 2015). Hall has designed and implemented research projects related to changing alcohol expectancies, the development of a brief treatment intervention for college students, homelessness and sobriety, and the use of protective strategies during and after football tailgating, the results of which are published in peer-reviewed journals.

As director of the Orange County, Florida, Government Coalition for a Drug-Free Community, Hall's work includes developing community initiatives on a range of services related to substance use disorder prevention, treatment, and recovery. His priorities of pragmatic and integrated services are informed by a collective impact framework.

The Contributing Authors

Ellen J. Bass, PhD, is interim senior associate dean for research of the College of Computing and Informatics, professor and chair of the Department of Health Systems and Sciences Research, professor in the Department of Information Science, and affiliate professor in the School of Biomedical Engineering, Science and Health Systems at Drexel University. She has over 30 years of human-centered systems engineering research and design experience in air transportation, health care, and other domains. Bass is a fellow of the Human Factors and Ergonomics Society, and a senior member of IEEE and the American Institute of Aeronautics and Astronautics.

Whitney M. Boroski is the manager of student health and well-being at Michigan Technological University. She is a recipient of the National Collegiate Athletic Association (NCAA) CHOICES Grant, is the state coordinator of Michigan for BACCHUS Initiatives of NASPA, and was accepted into the College Health and Wellness Professional Certification program. At Michigan Technological, she is part of a university wide conversation about student well-being, helping orchestrate the development of a well-being curriculum focusing on mental health, exercise, nutrition, and sleep. Boroski is an active member of the Michigan Higher Education Network, where she is currently working on an initiative to educate and encourage healthy behaviors with all students in the campus community.

Susie Bruce, MEd, is director of the University of Virginia's Gordie Center, which works to end hazing and substance misuse among college and high school students nationwide through evidence-informed, student-tested resources. She has expertise in collegiate health promotion, particularly the social norms approach, peer education, and curriculum infusion strategies. Bruce directs the NCAA-funded APPLE Training Institutes, the leading national strategic training program for substance misuse prevention and health promotion for student athletes and athletics departments; is a faculty affiliate of Youth-Nex, the Center to Promote Effective Youth Development; and is an executive board member of the Step UP! Bystander Intervention Program.

Carolyn Capern is co-founder of CTS Agency in Orlando, Florida, which has served as a strategist for multiple nationally and regionally recognized cause-based marketing campaigns. She is an instructor at the Edyth Bush Institute for Philanthropy and Nonprofit Leadership at Rollins College in Winter Park, Florida, and regularly speaks at conferences and events across the Southeast. Capern is a contributing writer for the *Orlando Business Journal* and the International Society of Business Communicators. She serves on the board of directors for Central Care Mission in Orlando.

Thomas S. Castor, PhD, MA, CHES, is an assistant professor in the Department of Public Health and Healthcare Leadership at Radford University Carilion in Roanoke, Virginia. He teaches the following courses: Personal Health, Issues in Community Health, Principles of Health Education and Promotion, Program Planning and Evaluation for Health Education, Health Communication and Social Marketing, and Special Topics (Alcohol & Other Drug [AOD]). His research addresses substance use and addictive behaviors among college students. Castor also conducts health communication interventions to enhance and promote wellness among adolescents and young adults.

Robert J. Chapman, PhD, is the former AOD program coordinator of La Salle University, an educator, and a program consultant. For over 45 years, his work with AOD programs included both the inpatient and outpatient treatment of substance use disorders. Since 1988, his professional interests and responsibilities have focused on high-risk and dangerous collegiate drinking. Chapman is a retired associate clinical professor of behavioral health counseling at the College of Nursing and Health Professions at Drexel University in Philadelphia. In his retirement, he remains active professionally as a consultant and blogger regarding the prevention of high-risk collegiate behaviors and affecting change in maladaptive behavior.

M. Dolores Cimini, PhD, is a New York State licensed psychologist and director of the University at Albany's Center for Behavioral Health Promotion and Applied Research. She has led comprehensive efforts in research-to-practice translation at the University at Albany for the past 28 years, with over $9 million in support from the National Institute on Alcohol Abuse and Alcoholism (NIAAA), National Institute on Drug Abuse, Substance Abuse and Mental Health Services Administration (SAMHSA), U.S. Department of Education, and U.S. Department of Justice. Cimini's areas of expertise include leadership development, peer education, and brief interventions addressing mental health and substance use–related concerns.

Dave Closson, MS, is the owner of DJC Solutions, LLC, a consulting company with a combined focus of serving substance misuse prevention professionals, law enforcement officers, and military veterans. He is the director of the Mid-America Prevention Technology Transfer Center, and previously worked for SAMHSA's Center for the Application of Prevention Technologies and the Illinois Higher Education Center. Closson is the author of *Motivational Interviewing for Campus Police* (DJC Solutions, 2015) and brings a unique experience to substance misuse prevention, having served as a police officer at Eastern Illinois University. He served in the Illinois Army National Guard for 6 years and was deployed under Operation Iraqi Freedom.

Eric S. Davidson, PhD, serves as the interim director for Eastern Illinois University Health and Counseling Services, overseeing the university's health service, counseling center, student insurance, and health promotion programs. Since 2009, he has directed the Illinois Higher Education Center for Alcohol, Other Drug, and Violence Prevention, overseeing statewide training and professional development for higher education practitioners implementing campus substance use programming. Davidson possesses a PhD in health education from Southern Illinois University and a master's degree in clinical psychology from Eastern Illinois University.

Laura A. Dean, PhD, is a professor in the College Student Affairs Administration/Student Affairs Leadership program at the University of Georgia. A member of ACPA–College Student Educators International, NASPA–Student Affairs Administrators in Higher Education, and the American College Counseling Association, she has also been active in the Council for the Advancement of Standards in Higher Education (CAS) for over 20 years, including service as publications editor and as president. Dean is the coauthor of *Assessment in Student Affairs* (2nd ed.; Jossey-Bass, 2016) and coeditor of *Using the CAS Professional Standards: Diverse Examples of Practice* (NASPA, ACPA, CAS, 2017). Her research focuses on assessment of campus-based interventions and the use of professional standards.

William DeJong, PhD, formerly a professor of community health sciences at the Boston University School of Public Health, is an adjunct professor of public health and community medicine at the Tufts University School of Medicine. He directed the U.S. Department of Education's Higher Education Center for Alcohol and Other Drug Prevention from 1995 to 2004. DeJong was awarded the first College Leadership Award by the American Public Health Association's Alcohol, Tobacco and Other Drug Section in 2000, and received the Outstanding Contribution to the Field Award from The Network Addressing Collegiate Alcohol and Other Drug Issues in 2008.

Michael E. Dunn, PhD, is director of the Health, Expectancy & Addiction Laboratory, co-director of the Substance Use Research

Group, and a founding faculty member of the clinical psychology PhD program at the University of Central Florida. He teaches courses in psychotherapy and treatment of substance use disorders, and supervises doctoral students providing treatment for university students and community members. Dunn's work has been supported by grants from NIAAA, SAMHSA, and the U.S. Department of Education, and prevention programs based on his research are used in high schools and colleges nationwide.

Eric Gipson, MA, is a prevention coordinator for the Center for Health Advocacy and Wellness at Florida State University (FSU), concentrating on alcohol and other substances as well as facilitating recovery efforts on campus. His responsibilities include the coordination and facilitation of Smart Choices, an alcohol/marijuana harm reduction program infused with BASICS (Brief Alcohol Screening and Intervention for College Students) and CASICS (Cannabis Screening and Intervention for College Students). Gipson received his BS in healthcare administration from Florida A&M University and his MA in international affairs/Asian studies from FSU.

Tavis J. Glassman, PhD, MPH, CHES, CCPH, is a professor in the School of Population Health at the University of Toledo, where he teaches the following courses: Drug Awareness, Mental Health, Social Marketing, Health Behavior, and Health Communication. Previously, he served as the coordinator of alcohol and other drug prevention at the University of Florida and orchestrated the reduction of high-risk drinking by 19% over a 4-year period, through a combination of social marketing and environmental management strategies. Glassman's extensive research and scholarship address substance misuse/abuse and other prevention issues among college students.

Gerardo M. González, PhD, is the former founder and president of BACCHUS. Starting in 1978, he served in various professorial and administrative roles at the University of Florida in Gainesville. In 2000, he was appointed professor and dean of education at Indiana

University Bloomington—a position he held until his retirement in 2020. González is a recognized authority on higher education and regularly speaks to global audiences about his Cuban immigrant journey and the profound difference education can make to both individuals and society.

Michael P. Haines, MS, is a private consultant and former director of the National Social Norms Resource Center. He and his staff implemented the first successful use of the Social Norms Approach to reduce heavy alcohol use. The effort was chosen as an Exemplary Program by the U.S. Department of Education and as a national model by *The New York Times*, and featured in *The Chronicle of Higher Education* and *USA Today*. Haines is a fellow of the American College Health Association (ACHA) and was a developer of its National College Health Assessment, for which he received the Hitchcock Award. He was honored with the Northern Illinois University Presidential Award for Excellence and the Outstanding Service Award for National Drug Abuse Prevention from the U.S. Department of Education.

Carlton Hall, MHS, is president and CEO of Carlton Hall Consulting, LLC. He has been providing intensive substance abuse prevention and community problem-solving services across the country for more than 25 years, supporting the highest levels of such national prevention systems as the Community Anti-Drug Coalitions of America, SAMHSA, the Drug Enforcement Administration (DEA), and the White House Office of National Drug Control Policy. Hall's responsibilities, unique set of skills, and experience have made him one of the most highly sought after instructors and guides for community problem solving in the United States as well as internationally, with successful achievements in South Africa, Uganda, Ghana, Bermuda, and Kenya, among other countries.

Lindsey Hanlon, MS, CPH, serves as network prevention manager with the Division of Behavioral Health, Nebraska Department of Health and Human Services, and oversees substance use, mental health, and suicide prevention efforts. She received her undergraduate degree from the University of Nebraska-Lincoln (UNL) in child, youth, and family studies with an emphasis in nutrition. Hanlon then returned to UNL, where she received her Master of Science in nutrition and health promotion and a certificate in public health from the University of Nebraska Medical Center.

David J. Hanson, PhD, is professor emeritus of sociology at the State University of New York at Potsdam. His scholarly publications number over 300, and textbooks in 15 fields of study report his research. His research and opinions have also been reported in *The New York Times* and other major newspapers. Hanson has appeared as an alcohol expert on the *NBC Nightly News*, the BBC's *The World Tonight*, MSNBC's *Live*, CBC's *Daybreak*, National Public Radio programs, the *Voice of America*, and the ABC national radio news. He has been quoted in *Family Circle*, *Health* magazine, *Ladies' Home Journal*, *Parade*, and many other popular publications.

Frances M. Harding served for 11 years as the director of the Federal Substance Abuse and Mental Health Services Administration's Center for Substance Abuse Prevention. She is recognized as one of the nation's leading experts in the field of behavioral health prevention. Prior to her federal services, Harding worked for the New York State Office of Alcoholism and Substance Abuse Services for 26 years, completing her tenure with the state as the associate commissioner for prevention and recovery. She has held numerous other state and national positions, including president of the National Prevention Network, and received the Science to Practice Award from the Society for Prevention Research.

Ahmed Hosni, MSW, is assistant director of the Student Life Student Wellness Center at The Ohio State University and director of recovery at the Higher Education Center for Alcohol and Drug Misuse Prevention and Recovery. Having been in long-term recovery since 2007, he knows firsthand the destructive nature of addiction and the restorative power of recovery. Hosni received a BS in community, family, and addiction sciences from Texas Tech University and received his MSW from The Ohio State University. He serves as a board member of the Association of Recovery Schools and the Association of Recovery in Higher Education.

Anthony L. Jenkins, PhD, is president of Coppin State University. He serves on the Association of Public and Land-Grant Universities Council of 1890 Presidents and Chancellors, the 1890 Universities Executive Committee, and the NCAA President's Council. He has been inducted into several of the most prestigious academic honor, business, and leadership societies in the nation: Alpha Kappa Psi, Phi Kappa Phi, Sigma Alpha Pi, Alpha Sigma Lambda, Omicron Delta Kappa, Alpha Phi Sigma, and Order of Omega. Jenkins is a U.S. Army veteran and first-generation college graduate.

Jason R. Kilmer, PhD, is an associate professor in psychiatry and behavioral sciences at the University of Washington (UW) School of Medicine. For years, he has served as an investigator on several studies evaluating prevention and intervention efforts for alcohol, marijuana, and other drug use among college students. In addition to research and teaching, Kilmer has worked extensively with college students and student groups (including student-athletes, fraternity and sorority members, students in residence life, and first-year students) on alcohol and other drug prevention programming, and has presented on this work throughout his career both at UW and on campuses across the nation.

Heather Kovanic, MEd, serves as the director of orientation and transition programs at the University of Delaware and is the 2020 president of NODA: Association for Orientation, Transition, and Retention in Higher Education. Prior to joining the University of Delaware, she worked at Georgetown University in student programming and orientation and at Providence College in undergraduate admissions. Kovanic holds an MEd in higher education and student affairs administration from the University of Vermont, and a BA in classics from the College of the Holy Cross.

Peter Lake, JD, is professor of law, Charles A. Dana Chair, and the director of the Center for Excellence in Higher Education Law and Policy at Stetson University College of Law. He is an internationally recognized expert on higher education law and policy and frequently lectures on issues related to college student safety, including student mental health, alcohol and drug abuse, Title IX and sex discrimination, and First Amendment issues such as managing controversial speakers on campus, academic freedom, and the rights of religiously affiliated colleges. Lake is a graduate of Harvard College and Harvard Law School and also serves as a part-time senior higher education consulting attorney at the law firm of Steptoe & Johnson, PLLC.

James E. Lange, PhD, holds a faculty position as the coordinator of alcohol and other drug initiatives within the Well-Being and Health Promotion Department of San Diego State University's Division of Student Affairs. He also serves as the executive director of the Higher Education Center for Alcohol and Drug Misuse Prevention and Recovery (HECAOD), an academic center of The Ohio State University College of Social Work. The HECAOD serves as a technical advising resource for colleges and universities across the United States on topics concerning the continuum of issues involving student alcohol and drug misuse. From his various research grants, Lange has authored over 60 scientific articles and chapters that have been cited within more than 3,600 publications.

Margo Leitschuh, BS, is the communications coordinator with Missouri Partners in Prevention (PIP), a health and safety–focused coalition of 23 colleges and universities. She graduated from the University of Missouri-Columbia with a Bachelor of Health Science and has been working with PIP since 2017 to implement evidence-based strategies at campuses across the state. In her time with PIP, Leitschuh has presented at the Higher Education Center's National Meeting and the

NASPA Strategies Conferences, authored multiple research briefs on statewide survey data and publications on prevention, and overseen social media management and strategic communications for Missouri Partners in Prevention.

Jeff Linkenbach, EdD, is the director and research scientist at The Montana Institute. He holds a Doctorate of Education with a focus on community education, and a master's degree in counseling. He has over 30 years of experience in the field of public health leadership. He has developed national award-winning research-based programs to change norms through the Science of the Positive and Positive Frameworks. Linkenbach founded the Center for Health and Safety Culture at the Western Transportation Institute, the National Conference on the Social Norms Approach to Prevention, and the Montana Summer Institutes on Positive Community Norms.

Richard Lucey Jr., MA, is a senior prevention program manager in the Drug Enforcement Administration's Community Outreach and Prevention Support Section. He plans and executes educational and public information programs, evaluates program goals and outcomes, and serves as an advisor to the section chief and other DEA officials on drug misuse prevention and education programs. Lucey formerly served as special assistant to the director for the Center for Substance Abuse Prevention, and worked as an education program specialist in the U.S. Department of Education's Office of Safe and Drug-Free Schools.

Joan Masters, MEd, is the senior coordinator of Partners in Prevention (PIP). She serves as primary investigator for PIP's grant projects, including the implementation of the annual Missouri Assessment of Collegiate Health Behaviors survey of college students. Masters is a Missouri Advanced Prevention Specialist and served as a reviewer for the Drug Enforcement Administration's publication *Prevention With Purpose: A Strategic Planning Guide for Preventing Drug Misuse Among College Students* (DEA, 2020). An active member of NASPA, she currently serves on the Peer Education Advisory Board as the Region

IV-West board chair. She received her MEd in counseling psychology from the University of Missouri.

Phil McCabe, CSW, CAS, CDVC, DRCC, is a health educator for the Rutgers University School of Public Health in the Center for Public Health Workforce Development. Additionally, he serves as an adjunct instructor for the Rutgers School of Nursing, Rutgers School of Social Work. He is also the faculty advisor for the Sexuality and Gender Alliance Group at Robert Wood Johnson Medical School. McCabe has over 30 years' experience providing educational training. He is currently the president of The Association of Lesbian, Gay, Bisexual, Transgender Addiction Professionals and Their Allies.

Michael P. McNeil, EdD, CHES, FACHA, is the Columbia Health chief of administration and faculty in Sociomedical Sciences, Mailman School of Public Health, both at Columbia University. His career in higher education has been focused on student center college health and pushing innovation in the field. As a faculty member and researcher, McNeil has a robust scholarship and publication record, with writings on partnerships, marijuana and hookah use, mental health, sleep, time management, and managing infectious disease outbreaks on college campuses.

Karen S. Moses, EdD, is the director of wellness and health promotion at Arizona State University (ASU). For 30 years, she has provided leadership for ASU student wellness initiatives, developing programs, services, policies, and practices that engage students in leading a healthy lifestyle and create a healthy campus environment. Initiatives and grants under her direction have addressed substance abuse prevention and recovery, mental health promotion, suicide prevention, sexual and relationship violence prevention, sexual wellness, healthy eating, physical activity, stress, and coping. Moses is a frequent speaker at conferences, and has served as consultant to assist institutions of higher education establish and enhance their prevention and wellness programs.

Aditya Narayan, BS, is a Fulbright fellow and former education and outreach coordinator of the University of Virginia's Gordie Center, combating hazing and substance misuse through evidence-informed educational outreach. He provides varied experience in biochemical research, social entrepreneurship, curriculum development, and peer-led harm reduction efforts. Narayan sat on the Virginia Higher Education Substance Use Advisory Committee and is a workshop leader for the national Step UP! Bystander Intervention Program.

H. Wesley Perkins, PhD, is professor of sociology at Hobart and William Smith Colleges and director of the Alcohol Education Project, which provides research, educational resources, and strategies to reduce problem behaviors among youth and young adults and has received multiple national awards from the U.S. Department of Education. Perkins developed the theory underlying the social norms approach to preventing risk behavior; has delivered over 500 guest lectures, keynote addresses, research presentations, and workshops for universities, secondary schools, and professional conferences throughout the United States, Canada, and Europe; and has been frequently cited in U.S. and international publications.

Jessica M. Perkins, PhD, is an assistant professor with the Department of Human and Organizational Development at Vanderbilt University. She studies how social norms and social networks drive health-related attitudes and behavior. The overarching goal of her research is to design community-based interventions to increase health-promoting behavior, reduce inequalities, and improve the health and well-being of individuals and communities in vulnerable settings. Perkins's current projects focus on HIV and substance use prevention in Uganda and in the United States. She is supported by funding from the National Institute of Mental Health.

Jim Peters, MEd, is the founder and president of the Responsible Hospitality Institute (RHI), a nonprofit organization founded in 1983 that promotes the planning and management of safe and vibrant places to socialize. Prior to guiding RHI for more than 3 decades, he developed a unique background in education and 26 years of operational management in restaurants and nightclubs. Peters holds a degree in hospitality management and a graduate degree in counseling, and has worked as an alcoholism counselor.

Ann Quinn-Zobeck, PhD, has 30 years' experience working in health promotion and higher education. She most recently served as senior director of BACCHUS Initiatives and Trainings for NASPA. Prior to working at NASPA, she served as director of training and education for The BACCHUS Network and assistant director of student activities at the University of Northern Colorado (UNC). Quinn-Zobeck established the Drug Prevention and Education Program during her time at UNC. She has a master's degree in rehabilitation counseling and a doctorate in college student personnel administration.

Diane Rullo, PhD, is a core faculty member at the Barbara Solomon School of Social Work and Human Services at Walden University. She has been teaching master's-level students for 28 years, with the past 12 years in an online environment. Rullo has been treating people with addiction for 40 years and has a private practice in Orlando, Florida.

Steve Schmidt, MS, is senior vice president of public policy and communications for the National Alcohol Beverage Control Association. He oversees the research and development of policy, best practices, and communication strategies to assist states as they manage alcohol control and regulatory systems. Schmidt has consulted with state and national organizations; authored several articles; and presented at numerous international, national, and state conferences on multiple alcohol-related topics. He has been professionally employed for over 40 years in positions leading efforts to address alcohol-related issues at the local, state, and national levels, and received the Outstanding Contribution to the Field Award from the Network of Colleges and Universities Committed to the Elimination of Drug and Alcohol Abuse in 2006.

Ryan Snow, MEd, is an instructor with Preventionleaders.com. He has served as a police officer for 10 years, with specialties in impaired driving and drug investigations. In his current assignment, he serves on a multijurisdictional task force, helping fight the flow of drugs into the community he serves. Snow is an instructor at the Police Training Institute, where he educates new officers on drugs, consent law, and rights of citizens against unlawful search and seizure. He also serves as a trainer for schools on emerging drug trends and a conference speaker emphasizing the impact of drugs and alcohol on communities.

Greg Trujillo is co-founder of CTS Agency in Orlando, Florida, where has served as a strategist for multiple nationally and regionally recognized cause-based marketing campaigns. He is an instructor at the Edyth Bush Institute for Philanthropy and Nonprofit Leadership at Rollins College in Winter Park, Florida, and regularly speaks at conferences and events across the Southeast. Trujillo is an engineer and former interactive projects manager at GoConvergence Digital, where he collaborated on projects for clients including the USS Intrepid Museum, Cirrus Aircraft, and the Orlando Magic. He is a board member for the Homeless Services Network of Central Florida.

Jennifer B. Wells, PhD, is an assistant professor of higher education in the Department of Educational Leadership at Kennesaw State University. She is a scholar in student development and higher education assessment; is the publications editor for CAS; is the former Kennesaw State University assessment administrator in institutional effectiveness and student affairs; and was actively involved in the institution's recent reaffirmation process. Wells's current focus is on the effectiveness of the CAS standards, the importance of continuous improvement efforts, and the psychosocial development of students with the Broad Autism Phenotype.

Delynne Wilcox, PhD, MPH, CHES, serves as assistant director of the Department of Health Promotion and Wellness at the University of Alabama. She also serves as an adjunct faculty member in the

College of Education and the College of Human Environmental Sciences. With over 25 years' experience in the public health, health promotion, and higher education fields, her University of Alabama work since 2000 has focused on alcohol and other drug prevention as well as health promotion. Wilcox has also served in national leadership roles with NASPA and ACHA. She serves as the primary researcher for the LessThanUThink campaign.

Cynthia Wilson, PhD, is the executive director of the Florida Center for Prevention Research and is a faculty member in the Department of Family and Child Sciences at Florida State University (FSU). She is the principal investigator for the Real Project, a social norming campaign to reduce alcohol-related harm on the FSU campus. Wilson received her BS in family, child, and consumer sciences and her MS and PhD in family relations from FSU, and is a Certified Family Life Educator.

Index

Figures and tables are indicated by f and t following the page number.

A

B

C

D

E

F

G

H

I

J

K

L

M

O

P

Q

R

S

T

U

V

W

Z

Printed in the United States
by Baker & Taylor Publisher Services